endometriosis

AND OTHER PELVIC PAIN

DR SUSAN EVANS
GYNAECOLOGIST

WITH

JANE MARSH RN AND
DR MARGARET TAYLOR

Lothian
BOOKS

Dedication

To my parents, Topsy and David,
who have always encouraged me,
and to my husband, John,
with much love and many thanks

Thomas C. Lothian Pty Ltd
132 Albert Road, South Melbo
www.lothian.com.au

Copyright © Dr Susan F. Evans Pty Ltd 2005
Illustrations © Kathryn Skelsey
First published 2005

National Library of Australia
Cataloguing-in-Publication data:

Evans, Susan F.
    Endometriosis and other pelvic pain.

    ISBN 0 7344 0825 0.

    1. Endometriosis – Popular works. 2. Endometriosis –
    Treatment – Popular works. 3. Pelvic Pain – popular works.
    4. Pelvic pain – Treatment – Popular works. I. Title.

618.14

Cover design by Christa Moffitt, Christabella Designs
Cover image courtesy Getty Images
Text design by Patrick Cannon
Typeset by Cannon Typesetting
Illustrations by Kathryn Skelsey
Printed in Australia by Griffin Press

Contents

Note

Words in the text that appear in bold, e.g. **laparoscopy**
are defined in the glossary.

Acknowledgments

MEDICINE DID NOT teach me how to write, so were it not for the guiding assistance of Julie Stanton, and Lois Grant, I am not sure this book would ever have been finished. It would certainly not have happened without the support of the women who keep my life together: Diana Morgan, Kathleen Connelly, and Deborah Adam.

I am very grateful for Margaret Taylor and Jane Marsh's contributions. Without them it would not be the well-rounded book we hope it to be. Thank you.

My medical colleagues Drs Anne Corbould, Jill Benson, Claire Fairweather, Helena Frawley, Jenny Cook, David Redwine, Penny Briscoe, Neil Hotham, Samantha Pillay, Larry Demco, Christine Kirby, Jane Andrews, Wayne Gillett, Fiona Stewart, Katrina Allen, Nesrin Varol, Susan Treloar, and Mark Arens all generously gave their time providing or reviewing the information.

Danielle Drever, John, Phoebe and Jack Allison, Rowena and Michael Vnuk, Joan Evans, Diana Morgan, Lata and Asha Mayer, David, Topsy and John Evans, Leith Banney, Patricia Johnson, Pat Griffiths, Lynne Mitchell, Peter and Betty Dawson, Barbara Dalwood, Belinda and Kelly Loveless, and Anne-Marie Ramsay read the book and offered kind words of very welcome criticism.

From a personal perspective, I would like to thank Maureen Merrick, Thembi Mazeka, Sharon Whitelaw-Jenkins, Draga Tomich, Rob Laing and Graham Van Renen; the best surgical team I could hope for, and Dr Ossie Petrucco who started me on the road to laparoscopic surgery. I would also like to thank Sheryl Klingner, Thom Rebner and Nick Warden who have supported our endometriosis clinic at Burnside War Memorial Hospital from the beginning.

However, most of all, I would like to thank my patients, who have trusted me with their endometriosis surgery over several years. Thank you.

Check with your doctor

The information in this book is intended only as a guide to help you when you are diagnosed with endometriosis, or suffer other types of pelvic pain. Neither the author nor the publisher can accept responsibility for your health or any decisions you make regarding your condition, or the treatments you choose. I would urge you to discuss your own special situation with your doctor and take their advice into account before you decide on any particular treatment.

Introduction

WOMEN FIND OUT they have endometriosis in many ways. Some realise early that there is something wrong and look for help. Others have endometriosis found unexpectedly during investigation for pelvic pain, an ovarian cyst that hasn't gone away or difficulty becoming pregnant.

As most people in the community know very little about endometriosis, few women recognise what their pain might mean. You may have had your pain for many years believing it to be normal, or due to another condition such as irritable bowel syndrome. Finding out that your pain is actually 'endometriosis' may be a relief that your pain has a name, or a cause for anger and disappointment that the diagnosis took so long.

It would be really nice if endometriosis was easy to diagnose, but it isn't. There is no one problem that all women with endometriosis share and we are not born with a label saying endometriosis! It can only be seen clearly at an operation called a **laparoscopy**, where a telescope is inserted through a small cut near the navel to view the inside of the pelvis. This is the operation most commonly used to diagnose and treat endometriosis.

As an endometriosis surgeon, I am very conscious that not *all* pelvic pain is due to endometriosis. Newer surgical techniques can bring substantial or even complete pain relief to women where endometriosis is the *only* cause for their pain. However, even the best surgery will not be enough for women with a mixture of different pelvic pains. These women may leave their gynaecologist disappointed with what their endometriosis treatment has achieved for them. Endometriosis was only part of the problem. Sorting out the cause of the pain becomes difficult and you may feel that your carers have lost interest in your needs. Your problems have become just too hard for them to manage.

The best endometriosis care in 2005 combines best quality surgery, a thorough search for other causes of pelvic pain, emotional support through the personal problems women with endometriosis may suffer and a recognition that complementary therapies can play a useful role. This is the care only a team can provide — individualised and sensitive to each woman's needs and preferences.

So what can this book do for you?

First, it sets out the facts about endometriosis and other types of pelvic pain as we know them to date. Second, it provides the knowledge you need to be actively involved with your doctor in choosing your own care. The cases described are based on real women I have cared for with their names and some details changed for privacy.

Chapters 1, 2, and 3 provide basic information: What is endometriosis? Could I have endometriosis? How is endometriosis diagnosed? Even women with a long history of endometriosis will find something new and useful here.

Chapter 4 provides a history of endometriosis management over the last 30 years. Thankfully a lot has changed. Young women will find it interesting and appreciate how treatment has improved, but older women may recognise their own experience.

Chapter 5 describes what a laparoscopy is, how to prepare for one, what it can show and what the risks are. Many women have had a laparoscopy, but few understand what it involves.

Chapter 6 outlines the medicines used to treat endometriosis. It also describes how to use common pain medications effectively, and manage your periods.

Chapter 7 looks at the situations you may be in yourself. Whether you are a teenager with period pain, a woman who has 'tried everything', or a woman with endometriosis in the family, there are sections for you.

Chapter 8 answers the questions women often ask at our endometriosis clinic. Will I be able to have children? Will I need a hysterectomy? Will it turn to cancer?

Chapter 9 describes other causes of pelvic pain, what you can do about them and who can help you. You may recognise your own pain from among them. If so it will shorten your path to the right diagnosis and the treatment you need.

A good relationship with the people we choose to care for us is important. Chapter 10 explains how to choose a gynaecologist, what questions to ask and how to prepare for your visit.

In Chapter 11 Jane Marsh, the endometriosis nurse counsellor with whom I work, provides coping strategies and practical advice for women and their partners. Treating the whole woman means looking at all the aspects of her life that contribute to her total pain experience.

In Chapter 12 Dr Margaret Taylor, a well-respected general practitioner and herbal and dietary therapist, describes how these treatments relate to endometriosis. There is practical advice on how to balance your hormones and manage premenstrual syndrome.

Twenty years ago, women with pelvic pain were thought to have emotional problems rather than a medical condition. This reflected our lack of knowledge at that time. Looking back, many of these women had undiagnosed endometriosis. There is more to offer now. Fewer women have undiagnosed pain, and far fewer are told that their pain is normal.

We hope this book helps you.

SUSAN EVANS

Chapter 1

What is endometriosis?

E VEN WOMEN WHO have known of their endometriosis for many years may be unsure what endometriosis actually is. That is understandable. Doctors find it confusing too.

Endometriosis is a condition where bits of tissue that are similar to the lining of the uterus, are found in places outside the uterus where they shouldn't be. This tissue is *not* the same as the lining of the uterus, but it looks similar under a microscope.

Areas of endometriosis are called **lesions**. Lesion is just a medical word for any area of abnormality. A mole on your skin, or a wart on your hand can also be called a lesion.

Endometriosis is a problem because it can cause pain and scarring.

What does endometriosis look like?

Most endometriosis is found in the **pelvis**. Endometriosis lesions form a spotty covering on the side walls of the pelvis, or on the surface of the pelvic organs. These organs include the uterus, ovaries, fallopian tubes, bladder, bowel, **ureter** and appendix. More severe endometriosis grows into the pelvic organs themselves.

Figure 1.1 The pelvic organs seen from the front

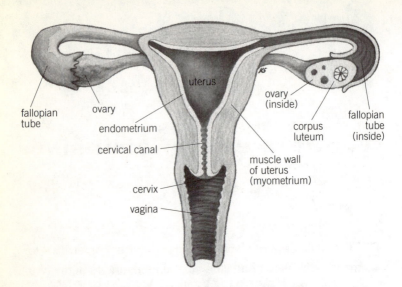

Figure 1.2 The pelvic organs seen through a laparoscope

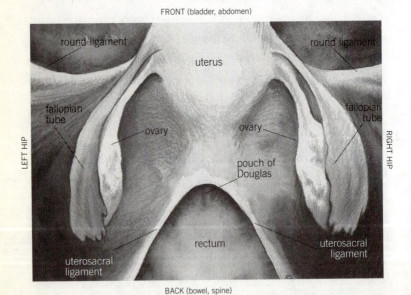

What your pelvis looks like through a laparoscope

At school you learned about what the pelvic organs look like from the front. This is useful for many things, but not showing endometriosis. Endometriosis lies on the surface of organs not inside them, which is why the pictures in this book look different from those you may be used to. They show what your surgeon sees when he or she looks at your pelvis through the laparoscope. If you are shown pictures of your pelvis after your surgery, these are the type of pictures you will see, so you need to understand what they show.

Imagine that you are looking down at your own pelvis through your navel. You will see the pelvic organs from above. In the middle lies the uterus. On either side there is an ovary, and a fallopian tube. Behind the uterus, the uterosacral ligaments extend from the back of the uterus to the back of the pelvis around the pouch of Douglas. The rectum (lower part of the bowel) passes through the centre of the pouch of Douglas and the ureters lie in the pelvic sidewall on both sides. In front of the uterus is the bladder.

All the organs you can see are covered by peritoneum (thin skin) and this is where any endometriosis will lie. Figure 1.2 shows a normal pelvis. Other pictures in the book show a laparoscopy (page 40), an endometrioma (page 45), and an adhesion (page 16).

As both the pelvic organs and the side walls of the pelvis are covered with a thin slippery skin called **peritoneum**, it is in the peritoneum that most endometriosis is found.

Endometriosis lesions come in many colours, shapes and sizes, some easier to recognise than others (see Reference 1). These different colours probably reflect different stages in the development of endometriosis. They include:

- *Red lesions*. These are red because they contain many blood vessels. They look like small red lumps or maybe just a group of blood vessels in one spot. Red lesions may be the first stage of endometriosis.
- *Clear lesions*. These look like tiny bubbles. They are another form of early endometriosis and can be quite difficult to see.
- *Black lesions*. Endometriosis irritates the peritoneum around it causing scarring. Any blood trapped in the scar tissue turns black.
- *White lesions*. Over time, the scarring around the endometriosis blocks any blood vessels. The body absorbs the black colour, leaving a thick white scar.
- *Endometriomas* or *chocolate cysts*. These are larger lumps of endometriosis that grow inside an ovary (see page 45).
- *Peritoneal windows or pockets*. These are oval-shaped areas that look like a dent in the surface. For many years no-one understood what peritoneal windows were. However, small samples (biopsies) of these 'windows' sent to a pathologist and checked through a microscope often show endometriosis.
- *Invisible areas*. Sometimes biopsies taken from peritoneum that looks normal show tiny (microscopic) areas of endometriosis. This is particularly common if the biopsy is taken close to obvious areas of endometriosis.

Young women are more likely to have clear, pink or red lesions. These are the most active forms of endometriosis and the lesions most likely to cause pain. Unfortunately they are also the most difficult lesions to recognise at a **laparoscopy**. Older women usually have white, brown or black lesions. They have probably been present for longer.

Most endometriosis lesions are thin and small – maybe 1 or 2 mm across. Larger and thicker lesions are called *nodules*. These are usually a few millimetres to a few centimetres across.

Chocolate cysts are the largest form of endometriosis. They may be several centimetres across. The word *cyst* just means a space with fluid inside it. It is the type of cells around the edge of a cyst (the lining) that tells what type of cyst it is. The lining of an **endometrioma** is made up of cells that look like the lining of the uterus. The fluid inside the cyst is dark brown and looks a lot like chocolate sauce. This is why they are called chocolate cysts.

If a woman has only a few endometriosis lesions, her condition is described as *mild* endometriosis. Her endometriosis may never be a problem for her. It may have been found by accident during an operation for another reason, such as a sterilisation procedure in women who have completed their families. If she has many lesions, or the lesions are large, her condition is called *severe* endometriosis. *Moderate* endometriosis is therefore somewhere between the two.

Although almost all endometriotic lesions are found in the pelvis, sometimes they are found in unusual places such as the **navel** (also called the umbilicus or belly button), an old caesarean section scar, or the lungs. Very rarely, they have been found in men who have used estrogen hormone medication.

Although endometriosis is especially common in Western countries, it can be found throughout the world and among women of all ethnic backgrounds.

The good news is that although it can spread, *endometriosis is not a cancer.*

Why is it called endometriosis?

The word endometriosis comes from the word **endometrium**. Endometrium is the medical name for the lining of the uterus (womb). 'Endo' means inside and 'metra' means uterus. It is the endometrium that grows inside the uterus each month, and then bleeds away during a period. Although they look similar through a microscope, an area of endometriosis is *not* the same as the lining of the uterus. Endometri*osis* lesions rarely bleed and make different hormones than normal endometr*ium*.

How does endometriosis cause pain?

No-one knows exactly why endometriosis causes pain. It can certainly cause pain if it makes an ovary stick to other organs in the pelvis. This is called an **adhesion**. However, many women with endometriosis have pain but no adhesions.

What *is* known is that endometriosis lesions make many chemical substances that can cause irritation or scarring of the tissue around them. It may be these chemicals that cause the pain. Deeper areas of endometriosis may press on tiny nerves in the pelvis causing pain. This is especially likely if the endometriosis involves the **uterosacral ligaments** (see Chapter 2, page 14).

It is commonly said that endometriosis lesions cause pain because they bleed during a period and the trapped blood has nowhere to go. However, as many painful endometriosis lesions don't bleed, this is unlikely to be true in most cases.

. . . .

Could I have endometriosis?

YES. ANY WOMAN OLD ENOUGH to have periods could have endometriosis, but luckily most don't. Around one in ten women will develop endometriosis at some time during their life, but as much of this is mild endometriosis they may never realise it is there, and it may never be a problem.

What symptoms fit with endometriosis?

Symptoms are health problems you notice when you are unwell. For example, a runny nose, headache and fever are symptoms of a cold, and painful joints are symptoms of arthritis.

The commonest symptoms of endometriosis are:

- Painful periods
- Pain at ovulation
- Pelvic pain between periods
- Painful sex
- Pain opening bowels

- Bleeding between periods
- Difficulty becoming pregnant
- Pain passing urine
- Tiredness
- Unusual symptoms

Luckily very few women have all these symptoms. While most have pain, others have no pain. Some find it difficult to become pregnant, whereas others conceive easily. If you do have endometriosis, your particular symptoms will depend on where in your pelvis the endometriosis is. The symptoms of endometriosis vary so much that few women have the same experience.

If you do have any of these symptoms, it does not mean that you definitely have endometriosis. There are so many other conditions that cause similar problems that it may be due to something else. The only reliable way to diagnose endometriosis is with a laparoscopy, but as no-one wants an operation they don't need it is a good idea to think about what else it might be before booking your surgery. There may be another explanation for your pain, and you may want to try medications, or have other tests first.

For example, most teenagers have period pain but less than one in ten has endometriosis. It is not reasonable to do a laparoscopy on all teenage girls with period pain, yet some need one. Trying other treatments first, and leaving a laparoscopy for those teenagers for whom other treatments don't help saves a lot of surgery on otherwise healthy young women (see Chapter 7, page 87).

Your general practitioner can help you work through this, but ultimately you are the one with the pain and you are the one best able to decide if you need a laparoscopy. So regardless of what your family, friends or doctor say, if your symptoms are a major problem to you, and other treatments have not helped, then look further. You may have endometriosis. Trust your own judgement.

The following sections describe each of the common symptoms of endometriosis and how you might decide if they could mean endometriosis for you.

Painful periods

Endometriosis anywhere in the pelvis can cause period pain (**dysmenorrhoea**) — it's the most common symptom. In fact, if you have period pain bad enough to seek a doctor's advice then you have around a 50 per cent chance of having endometriosis. The chance is even higher if you also have endometriosis in your family.

The other causes of period pain apart from endometriosis include prostaglandin pain (Chapter 9, page 155) due to chemical substances made in the uterus, **adenomyosis** (Chapter 9, page 151) due to changes in the wall of the uterus, and clot colic (Chapter 9, page 158) in women with very heavy, clotty periods. You may have more than one cause for your period pain.

How can I tell if my period pain is due to prostaglandins, endometriosis, or adenomyosis?

Think about when you get the pain and whether medicines help it.

Prostaglandins cause the 'normal' period pain that young women suffer before having their first baby. Although called 'normal', this downplays just how severe the pain may be. Prostaglandin pain usually comes at the beginning of a period. It should only last for one or two days and is much better on the contraceptive pill or with normal period pain medications such as Ibuprofen or Naproxen (Chapter 6, page 70). If your pain goes away with any of these medications then you have prostaglandin period pain and your chance of having endometriosis is low. Period pain medications need to be taken correctly if they are to work well. There are instructions on how to take them in Chapter 6 on page 70.

Endometriosis period pain usually lasts longer than a day. There may be pain leading up to, or right through a period. Period pain in the lower back is especially common in women with endometriosis near the uterosacral ligaments. These ligaments pass from the uterus back to a part of the spine called the sacrum, which lies at the back of the pelvis. While they may help relieve the pain a little, neither the contraceptive pill nor period pain medications usually get rid of endometriosis pain.

Adenomyosis period pain is more common in middle-aged rather than young women, although this is not always true. It causes pain similar to endometriosis, but no endometriosis is found when a laparoscopy is done. The uterus is often a little enlarged. Gynaecologists use the word 'bulky' for a slightly enlarged uterus.

Will my pain get better if I have a baby?

Young women with period pain are often told not to worry because 'You will be fine once you have had a baby'. This may be true of prostaglandin pain, but is *not* true for the pain of endometriosis or adenomyosis. It is also small comfort for women who don't plan to have children. Pregnancy is a poor treatment for endometriosis. If you have already had a baby and your period pain is still severe it is quite likely that you have either endometriosis or adenomyosis.

So one way to tell whether you may have endometriosis is to try the oral contraceptive pill or a period pain medication. If your pain goes away on either medication then endometriosis is still possible, but less likely. If it does not go away, endometriosis is more likely and the decision to have a laparoscopy may be easier for you. It is time to discuss your pain with a gynaecologist.

If you prefer to avoid using the contraceptive pill long term, just two months of treatment is enough to see if it helps your pain.

After two months you can stop the Pill if you prefer. Your pain will return, but you may feel reassured that the chance of endometriosis is low.

Remember that endometriosis can occur at any age after periods begin. Teenagers are definitely *not* too young to have endometriosis.

J thought all women had pain like mine

Pauline is a 35-year-old married accountant who has chosen not to have children. She suffered severe period pain each month for many years despite the contraceptive pill and period pain medication. Pauline was very determined to cope and never missed a day at work, even if that meant using strong pain relief just to get through the day. Pauline thought that all women had pain like hers, so she never sought help. Finally the pain became so severe that she made an appointment to discuss an operation to remove her uterus (hysterectomy). We decided to look for endometriosis first. The laparoscopy showed extensive endometriosis, which was completely removed. Pauline was very pleased. The mild pain she still had with periods could now be managed with normal period pain medication, and she still had her uterus. Her concern was for the many women who, like her, do not seek treatment because they believe that their pain is normal.

Ovulation pain

Ovulation is the time of the month when an egg is released from an ovary. Some pain at ovulation may be normal, but if so it should only last for a day, swap sides approximately every second month, and be much better with period pain medications. This type of pain is called *mittelschmerz* (it means 'middle pain' in German). Contraceptive pills that stop ovulation should stop **ovulation pain**, so be suspicious if you notice ovulation pain while you're on the Pill. There is information on how to work out when you ovulate in Chapter 8 on page 123.

Sometimes endometriosis forms scar tissue that sticks the pelvic organs together. The places where the organs are stuck together are called *adhesions*. Adhesions or endometriosis near an ovary can tie the ovary to the side wall of the pelvis, causing ovulation pain that is *not* normal (see Figure 2.1, below).

If you have pain on one side of your pelvis with periods *and* at ovulation time, you may have endometriosis near that ovary. Ovulation pain on both sides of the pelvis at once may mean adhesions or endometriosis near both ovaries. To make it even more complicated, there are some women who have *crossover*

Figure 2.1 Adhesions

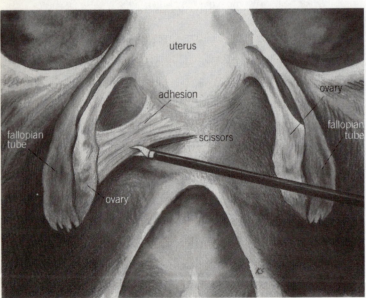

An adhesion between the left ovary and the uterus. Tiny scissors can be used to divide the adhesion and free the ovary.

pain. This is pain felt on one side of the pelvis, when the actual problem is on the other side.

> ### Period pain and ovulation pain
>
> Aisha is a 23-year-old university student with no children, nor any need for contraception. She had severe period pain for every day of her period even with period pain medications. Each month at ovulation she also suffered two or three days of pain on her left side. A laparoscopy showed endometriosis and adhesions tying down the left ovary. The right ovary was normal. The left ovary was freed and the endometriosis removed. After her operation, Aisha's period pain was much better. She still had pain on the first day of her period, but this was now easily treated with period pain medications. The ovulation pain on her left was gone.
>
> Before her surgery, Aisha had both endometriosis and prostaglandin pain. After her surgery only the prostaglandin pain remained.

Pelvic pain between periods

While women who only have pain with periods can do their best to 'live with' the pain and plan their life around those days, it is very hard to live with pain present on most days that can come at any time. What is more, the longer you do 'live with it' the more it affects your work, education, relationships, mood, self-esteem and general health. If you have this type of pain, it may or may not be endometriosis, but you do need to work on a solution.

How can I tell if these pains are endometriosis?

Pain between periods that is due to endometriosis usually feels similar to period pain. It may not be as bad as your period pain, but it feels similar in quality. As a period comes closer, the pain usually becomes more severe and more frequent. The week after your period should be your best time of the month. Pain felt in one particular spot, that follows this pattern, is often endometriosis.

If your pain comes at any time of the month, regardless of when your period is due, then it is probably something else. Remember that you may have a mixture of endometriosis *and* another condition. As pain starting in the bladder, bowel, muscles, ligaments, uterus or pelvic nerves all travels to the brain through similar pathways, it is hard for your brain to separate out all the different pains and decide where each pain came from. Many different pains can feel similar.

Treating endometriosis can only help those symptoms that are due to endometriosis. It is an important first step, but pains from other organs will remain unless they are treated too.

But I have pain all the time!

Pain almost every day over a long period of time is called *chronic pain*. Chronic pain is enough to wear anyone down. It is miserable. It is also something that we as doctors do not know enough about. If you have chronic pain, your situation is complicated but certainly not hopeless. Knowledge about what causes chronic pelvic pain has improved greatly. As time goes by, more and more of what could not be diagnosed in the past has a name. Women knew all along that there was something wrong with them. Sure they were stressed. They had chronic pain!

To me, there is rarely one simple cause (or solution) for this type of pain. Endometriosis is usually only part of the picture. This is why the sections on pages 107 and 143 have been written. If you can recognise yourself in any of the descriptions in Chapter 9, it will be easier to decide where to go for help. A laparoscopy will only be part of the treatment you need. Other types of pain need their own care.

Painful sex

Painful intercourse (**dyspareunia**) is common in women with endometriosis. As well as the physical pain, there is the emotional pain and guilt that women feel when they are unable to enjoy sex with their partner. No one feels like sex if they know it will hurt.

There are many other causes of painful sex apart from endometriosis, so the best person to see first is your general practitioner. Endometriosis rarely causes pain near the opening of the vagina and does *not* cause vaginal itching, a smelly vaginal discharge or vulval skin irritation. These problems are due to other conditions. Skin conditions of the vulva (checked by biopsy and examination), troublesome vaginal muscle contractions (*vaginismus*), vaginal infections ('thrush'), an irritated bladder (see Chapter 9, page 188), or occasionally a uterus that lies at the back of the pelvis (retroverted uterus) can all make sex painful. Your general practitioner can check for some of these causes. A difficult relationship with your partner may also be a factor.

Vaginismus is very treatable, but is not something that an operation will fix. It often happens when sex has been painful for some time. The muscles at the opening of the vagina tighten any time that sex is attempted. You will not be able to 'just relax' (even if you want to) and stop it happening. In most Australian and New Zealand cities, there is a doctor who specialises in sex counselling for couples. They can help your vaginismus. If intercourse has been painful for some time, you and your partner may have many issues to work through to regain a satisfying sexual relationship.

Painful intercourse due to endometriosis is felt deep inside the pelvis. It may be worse in some sexual positions (depending on where the endometriosis is) and can last for one or two days afterwards. Dyspareunia is especially common when the endometriosis lies behind the uterus near the top of the vagina. This area includes the *pouch of Douglas*, the uterosacral ligaments, and the *rectovaginal septum*, which can be seen in Figure 5.1 on page 40.

An operation to remove endometriosis from these places is quite difficult to do because they lie so close to the bowel. However, these are also areas where most medicines or herbal preparations are less effective, and so surgery is often the only effective treatment. If sex is still painful after *all* your endometriosis has been removed, there may be another reason for your pain.

Who was Douglas, and why was the pouch named after him?

James Douglas lived in England from 1675 to 1742. He is described as a 'man-midwife' (gynaecologist) and physician to the queen. His particular interest was the structure of the human body (anatomy). He described the area of the pelvis between the back of the uterus and the lower bowel that we now call the pouch of Douglas. When seen through a laparoscope it is the deepest part of the pelvis. It is also a common place to find endometriosis.

Endometriosis with painful sex — Case 1

Joanne is a married woman of 30 with two young children. Neither her periods nor sex had been a problem for her in the past, but over two years she had noticed pain with intercourse. She described the pain as being in one spot, deep inside and a little to the left. She was exactly right! At her laparoscopy, there was a nodule of endometriosis in the left uterosacral ligament between the uterus and the bowel. The rest of her pelvis was normal. The nodule was removed and her pain was gone.

Endometriosis with painful sex — Case 2

Jacinta is a 25-year-old married university student. Despite periods that were only mildly uncomfortable, and a strong relationship with her husband, intercourse had always been painful. A laparoscopy showed endometriosis in the pouch of Douglas, behind the uterus. The endometriosis was removed but her pain only partially improved. Much of her pain was found to be a vaginal skin condition.

Pain opening bowels or bleeding from the bowel

The bowel lies very close to the uterus, fallopian tubes and ovaries. It is also a common place to find endometriosis. Because of this, it is not surprising that many women with endometriosis have bowel problems, especially at period time. Sorting out how much of the problem is due to the bowel itself and how much is due to endometriosis can be very difficult. There is more information on irritable bowel syndrome in Chapter 9 on page 160.

Endometriosis near the bowel may be difficult to remove surgically. It may also be difficult to see during a laparoscopy because it hides below the surface of the peritoneum. Sometimes it is easier to see (or feel) as a lump (nodule) in the back wall of the vagina. Most women with endometriosis here will have bowel pain, back pain and painful intercourse.

When bleeding from the bowel occurs at period time it is more likely to be due to extra blood vessels in the bowel wall than endometriosis that has grown through the wall of the bowel. It may also be due to other conditions such as haemorrhoids, bowel disease or occasionally a cancer. So if you have bleeding from the bowel you should tell your general practitioner straightaway.

> It is important *not* to assume that the bleeding is due to endometriosis until you are sure that other conditions have been excluded.

My laparoscopy only showed 'mild' endometriosis but lots of scar tissue near the bowel. So why do I have so much pain?

Endometriosis lesions are often found in particular patterns. One of these patterns involves endometriosis in both uterosacral ligaments and the pouch of Douglas (see Figure 1.2 on page 6). There may be only a few brown lesions (which is why it is sometimes mistakenly called 'mild' endometriosis), and the uterosacral ligaments may just look white and scarred. The ovaries are often normal. These women usually have back pain, pain with intercourse and pain when opening their bowels. What is not understood is that the white scarring is usually endometriosis too! *This endometriosis is not 'mild' at all.* Removing this type of endometriosis requires a skilled endometriosis surgeon. It is difficult and can be dangerous. The good news is that completely removing *all* the scar tissue, often with some of the uterosacral ligaments, usually makes a big difference to the pain.

Bleeding between periods (intermenstrual bleeding)

No one knows why bleeding between periods is common in women with endometriosis, but as the endometriosis lesions produce so many hormones and chemicals, it is not surprising that bleeding happens sometimes. If the amount of blood is small, it is called *spotting*.

Before presuming that your bleeding is due to endometriosis, other causes of bleeding need to be excluded. Your general practitioner can help you with this. The contraceptive pill, an unexpected pregnancy or soft fleshy lumps called *polyps* can all cause bleeding between periods. Very occasionally, bleeding between periods is a sign of cancer of the cervix or uterus so you must make sure that your cervical smear tests are up to date and you may also need an ultrasound scan to check the lining of the uterus.

> **Bleeding between periods is not normal, so you should always discuss it with your doctor.**

If the bleeding *is* due to endometriosis, it is more likely in the week before a period than the week after a period. You may have tried several types of contraceptive pill, hoping to find one that didn't cause bleeding between periods, only to find later that endometriosis was the cause of the bleeding, not the Pill. Once the endometriosis is removed, the spotting usually improves.

Difficulty falling pregnant (infertility)

Most of us expect that when we decide to become pregnant, it will happen. Few conditions are more distressing than infertility. As well as the pain of endometriosis, there is the disappointment as each period arrives. There may also be a feeling of guilt at 'letting down' your partner.

While endometriosis *is* more common among women who have difficulty becoming pregnant, this does not mean that all women with endometriosis are infertile. Many women with endometriosis become pregnant easily. What it does mean is that endometriosis is one factor that *may* affect your fertility. It is one factor not in your favour. However, it takes two to become pregnant and there are many factors that affect fertility (both yours and your partner's). If all the other factors are normal, you may never have a problem.

Those women with endometriosis who do have problems becoming pregnant often have either more severe endometriosis or there are other factors involved. More information about endometriosis and fertility is given in Chapter 8 on page 119.

> **If you don't want to become pregnant, then reliable contraception is just as important for you as any other woman.**

Pain passing urine (dysuria)

Most **dysuria** is due to problems with the bladder itself rather than endometriosis. These bladder problems include bladder infections and another condition called *interstitial cystitis* (IC) (see Chapter 9 on page 188). Both can cause pain in the lower **abdomen** or make you want to pass urine more often (**frequency**).

It is true that endometriosis can cause these problems too, but unless you have other reasons to believe you have endometriosis (like painful periods), it is best to talk to your general practitioner or a bladder doctor (urologist) about your bladder. A laparoscopy looking for endometriosis is only necessary if they are unable to help you and endometriosis seems possible.

No one knows why, but many women with endometriosis *also have interstitial cystitis*. This is one reason why some women may be disappointed with their endometriosis treatment. Some of their symptoms improved once the endometriosis was removed, but their bladder symptoms remained. A laparoscopy will not help IC: it needs its own treatment plan (see Chapter 9, page 188).

Occasionally endometriosis grows on the inside of the bladder itself. About one in five of these women will notice blood in their urine at period time.

Tiredness

There is no easy explanation why women with endometriosis often feel tired. It may be that whenever the body is unwell in some way, energy is the first thing to fail. Pain itself is very wearing. So are the worry and stress involved in trying to maintain a normal life and normal relationships despite pain. Chapter 11, written by Jane Marsh, looks at ways to live better with your pain.

Unusual symptoms

The symptoms that I have described so far cover almost all endometriosis. Occasionally endometriosis is found in unusual places and can cause unusual symptoms. For example:

- Pain just below the ribs, worse on breathing in, and only present with periods might be endometriosis of the **diaphragm**. It is rare.
- Pain in one part of a caesarean section scar that is much worse with periods may be due to endometriosis in the scar. It is uncommon.
- Pain down the back of the leg (sciatica) present only during periods, might be endometriosis of the sciatic nerve. It is very rare indeed.
- A lump in the navel that is tender at period time may be endometriosis of the navel. It is uncommon.

Endometriosis in unusual places is painful at the time of a period because no matter where it is, it still responds to the normal hormonal changes of the menstrual cycle. However, these examples are rare.

> If you have any of these symptoms but they come at any time, regardless of whether a period is due or not, then they are much more likely to be due to something else and you should see your general practitioner.

Women with endometriosis have symptoms that other people can't see and don't understand. Even friends and relatives who are kind, caring and patient may become frustrated when your symptoms don't improve. No matter how kind, considerate, and caring your partner is, he has never had period pain. Other women with trouble-free periods may wonder why your periods should be such a problem, and be very unsympathetic. It is therefore not surprising that many women with undiagnosed endometriosis lose faith in their ability to judge their pain.

> ### Why can't I cope with the pain like other women?
>
> The reason may be that you have endometriosis.

Trust your own judgement and ask your doctor about endometriosis if you believe this could be the cause of your pain.

Chapter 3

. . . .

How is endometriosis diagnosed?

LIFE WOULD BE MUCH SIMPLER if endometriosis was easy to diagnose. There are no blood tests that diagnose it reliably and most women with endometriosis will have a normal ultrasound scan. The only reliable way to diagnose or exclude endometriosis is a laparoscopy done by a gynaecologist who is experienced in recognising endometriosis. This is a big step for many women, and one that should not be taken without reason. Then again, most women with severe pelvic pain *do* have good reason. Their pain is severe. I find that a woman who requests a laparoscopy because she is concerned about her pelvic pain is usually right.

What can a laparoscopy show?

A laparoscopy can show whether endometriosis is present, where it is and how severe it is. It also allows removal of the endometriosis at the same time or at least a plan for removal of the endometriosis on another day.

A laparoscopy where no endometriosis is found is not wasted

27

effort. Many women are less concerned about their pain once they know that their pelvic organs are healthy. A normal laparoscopy may have excluded endometriosis as a cause for the pain, but does *not* mean that the pain does not exist. It does, but it's now time to move on and consider other possible causes (see Chapter 9).

You should never be disappointed with a normal laparoscopy. A normal pelvis is *always* the best outcome.

What can an ultrasound show?

Most endometriosis does *not* show on an ultrasound scan. The endometriosis lesions are too thin. An ultrasound scan will show the size of an ovary clearly, but not whether it has spots on its surface. As most endometriosis changes the surface appearance of pelvic organs, rather than their size, most ultrasound scans in women with endometriosis are normal.

One form of endometriosis that *is* large enough to show on an ultrasound scan is an endometrioma, or chocolate cyst (see Figure 5.2, page 45). The 'chocolate sauce' inside the cyst gives it a special appearance on an ultrasound scan. The cyst looks like ground glass, which means that it has a grainy look. This appearance on an ultrasound usually means one of two things:

- That you have an endometrioma, or
- That you have a type of cyst called a *haemorrhagic corpus luteum*.

A corpus luteum is the normal cyst that an ovary makes each month after ovulation, and the word 'haemorrhagic' means that it has blood inside. This type of cyst goes away by itself. So, if you have a cyst on ultrasound scan with a grainy, ground-glass appearance, then time will tell what type of cyst it is likely to be. A haemorrhagic corpus luteum will usually go away by itself within three months, whereas an endometrioma will not. If your cyst is still there at a second scan done two or three months later, then your cyst is probably an endometrioma, and you should discuss it with a gynaecologist. The endometrioma may need to be removed, but depending on your particular situation and wishes, the ovary can usually be saved.

An American study (see Reference 2) showed that if an endometrioma can be seen on an ultrasound scan, it is 99 per cent likely that there will be other areas of endometriosis present too. These other areas may not show on a scan, but they *are* there. So, if you have a laparoscopy to remove an endometrioma from your ovary, you should expect that other areas of endometriosis could be found too.

An ultrasound scan is also useful in women with pelvic problems because it may show other conditions such as **fibroids** in the uterus or ovarian cysts that are unrelated to endometriosis.

What can blood tests show?

There is *no* blood test that will reliably diagnose endometriosis. Occasionally blood is taken to check the amount of a substance called CA-125 in the blood. Many different pelvic conditions, including endometriosis can make the CA-125 level a little high. However, as a normal CA-125 result does not exclude endometriosis, this test is only useful in special situations.

One of these special situations is where an ultrasound has shown an unusual looking ovarian cyst, especially in a woman over 40 years of age. Such a cyst may occasionally be a cancer of the ovary. A cancer of the ovary sometimes makes the CA-125 level very high. Unfortunately, it is not a reliable test for cancer either, because some women with cancer of the ovary have a normal CA-125 level.

A CA-125 is rarely useful in younger women, or women with normal looking ovaries on ultrasound scan.

Why did it take so long for my endometriosis to be diagnosed?

As all the symptoms of endometriosis may be due to other conditions, it is disappointing, but not surprising, that it may take years for a woman's endometriosis to be diagnosed. How many years? In Norway and Australia it takes an average of six years, and in the USA an average of nine years from the beginning of symptoms to diagnosis. This is a long time to have pain. In the USA studies, half the time was lost because women did not report their problems to their doctor, but the other half was medical time lost before a reliable laparoscopy was done (see References 3 and 4).

How is endometriosis of the bowel diagnosed?

The bowel is a long coiled-up tube running from your stomach to your anus. It has an inside and an outside. The outside of the lower bowel and the appendix can be seen at a laparoscopy. The inside of the lower bowel can only be seen by passing a flexible camera through the anus and up into the bowel. This procedure is called a *colonoscopy* and is usually only recommended in women with severe endometriosis that may have spread through the bowel wall, or in those women with other bowel symptoms.

As a laparoscopic surgeon, I am frequently surprised by what I find at a laparoscopy. Women with very few symptoms may have many endometriosis lesions, while others with many symptoms have a normal pelvis. So, how many symptoms you have or how severe your pain is may not be a reliable indicator of how much endometriosis you have.

Without a laparoscopy, you will never know.

Chapter 4
....

How has the management of endometriosis changed?

MANY WOMEN ASK ME about the treatments they have had in the past. Why weren't they offered better options earlier? Why did it take so long to get a diagnosis? Generally I find that they were offered the best that was available at the time. Treating endometriosis effectively remains a challenge, but thankfully improved treatments are now available.

A history of endometriosis treatment

Endometriosis in its most severe form has been known for centuries. From time to time, women had operations through large cuts on their abdomen (a **laparotomy**), and chocolate cysts full of dark brown fluid were found. Endometriosis was believed to be an uncommon condition affecting women in their thirties and forties.

Before the 1970s, diagnosing pelvic pain was very difficult, particularly when no abnormality was found on examination. Neither ultrasound scanning nor laparoscopy were available. If enlarged ovaries were found on vaginal examination, then a large cut was

31

made in the abdomen to investigate the cause of the problem. If a chocolate cyst was found it was removed, together with part or all of an ovary. There was little else that could be done, particularly in women who hoped for a future pregnancy. Endometriosis in other areas of the pelvis was rarely removed because of the difficulty and dangers in doing so, and because many abnormalities we now know to be endometriosis were thought to be normal at that time.

It takes at least six weeks to recover from a laparotomy and fertility may be affected if adhesions form after the surgery. Because of this, gynaecologists were loath to operate on young women with pain, unless a specific lump was found on examination. They wished to avoid doing more harm than good.

As many women with endometriosis did not have a lump that could be felt at vaginal examination, most remained untreated. Understandably, women felt let down and angry when their pain was diagnosed and dismissed as emotional or bowel issues. Once childbearing was complete, many had an operation to remove the uterus (**hysterectomy**), frequently with both ovaries removed at the same time (**bilateral oophorectomy**). There was little else to offer.

Once laparoscopy became available in the 1970s and 1980s, pelvic pain could be investigated without a large cut, without risking fertility, and without a long hospital stay. The skills and instruments needed to remove even small areas of endometriosis through these small holes had not yet been developed, so a laparoscopy at that time gave only a look at the pelvis. If an abnormality were found, a large cut would be made to fix the problem. Even with this new tool to view the inside of the pelvis more easily, it took many years for gynaecologists to recognise what was normal and what was *not* normal. Laparoscopy gave a better, but different, view of the pelvis so there was a lot to learn.

Gynaecologists knew that chocolate cysts in the ovaries, and black lumps around the pelvis were endometriosis, but many other lesions were considered normal. If black or brown areas were seen at laparoscopy, many women were prescribed a six-month course of a medication called **danazol**, in an attempt to remove the endometriosis. Some women did well on danazol, especially those with mild endometriosis, but half of those treated suffered side effects that were too troublesome to continue the treatment.

After danazol came a group of medications that aimed at removing the endometriosis by turning off estrogen production and creating a reversible menopause-like environment. These medications are called Gonadotrophin Releasing Hormone analogues or **GnRH analogues**. They include such medications as goserelin (*Zoladex®*) or nafarelin (*Synarel®*).

I have patients who say they have never felt so good as when they were on GnRH analogues, and a few who have never felt better than when taking danazol, but side effects are often a problem. In addition, none of these medications treat large, scarred or deep areas of endometriosis effectively, and no endometriosis medications improve fertility.

During the 1980s and 1990s, gynaecologists started taking small samples of tissue called *biopsies* whenever they saw something unusual through the laparoscope. These biopsies were sent to a pathologist for diagnosis using a microscope. By the mid-1990s it became clear that many of these abnormalities were actually endometriosis. Endometriosis became a condition with variable appearance. The lesions could be clear, pink, red or white, as well as black or brown. Once these more subtle lesions were included, it became obvious that endometriosis was a lot more common than once thought. It was also recognised that endometriosis was a condition affecting young women as well as older women.

In the 1990s, as laparoscopic skills and instruments improved, techniques were developed to remove endometriosis, and so avoid the need for medication.

The first technique, and one still commonly used today, was electrocautery. **Cautery** uses an instrument to touch the top of the endometriosis lesion, and burn it with electricity. The lesion is 'cauterised' in the same way as a blood vessel that causes nose-bleeds may be cauterised. Cautery works best for small thin areas of endometriosis, particularly those on the ovary or uterus. Unfortunately, it often leaves deeper endometriosis untreated and may cause scar tissue. As endometriosis is often found near delicate organs, and the heat from cautery can spread further than desired, gynaecologists tend to *under*-cauterise rather than *over*-cauterise endometriosis lesions. This decreases the risk of damaging important pelvic structures, but does tend to leave some endometriosis behind. Women often feel better for a short time, but once the remaining endometriosis becomes active again, the pain may return.

Since the late 1990s, the emphasis has changed to **excisional surgery**. This means cutting out the endometriosis wherever possible. Excisional surgery aims to remove the endometriosis completely to decrease the chance of endometriosis recurrence and achieve a longer pain-free time. It takes longer to do and is technically more challenging than cautery, but it does mean that the endometriosis is removed completely. The surgeon can also operate closer to delicate organs such as the ureter (the long tube that carries urine from the kidney to the bladder), or the bowel. Even so, surgery in some areas, particularly those near the bowel or where extensive adhesions have glued the pelvic organs together, remains challenging even for experienced surgeons.

An alternative energy source to electricity is *laser*. It became popular in the early 1990s and can be used to cauterise *or* to excise endometriosis. Laser surgery is not different surgery, rather a different way of doing the same thing. When used to excise endometriosis rather than cauterise (ablate), it is an effective treatment.

Theoretically, if all the endometriosis is removed, there should be less recurrence, better management of pain or fertility, and less need for medication.

All the above treatments are used today, although excisional surgery is currently considered the most effective treatment for endometriosis. Cautery, danazol, GnRH analogues and other medications still have a place in some situations. Excisional surgery has its problems too. It is major surgery through small holes. It has risks, and may cause scarring. In ten years time, the treatments we are able to offer may be different again.

Current endometriosis management

None of us — whether we are surgeons, doctors who prefer to use medications, or complementary therapists — have all the answers. I like to think that we are closer to effective treatment now, but perfect treatments are still some way off.

As a surgeon who specialises in endometriosis, the treatments I recommend tend to be more surgically orientated. That does not mean that other treatments are not useful. They are. I offer medications to women whose endometriosis has not been completely removed, or those who have widespread but tiny thin lesions. Our patients also spend time with a nurse counsellor who supports their emotional needs, as well as considering the benefits other health professionals may be able to provide for each individual woman. Endometriosis is a complex condition and there is no 'right' way to treat everyone.

Regardless of treatment preference, most women with endometriosis will have an operation at some stage. This is because it is the only reliable way to diagnose endometriosis. My own philosophy is that if a laparoscopy is needed to diagnose the condition, why not remove the endometriosis at the same time? If this is possible then the medicines used to treat endometriosis described in Chapter 6 on page 63 can usually be avoided.

However, depending on where you are, and the services available to you, the diagnosis and removal of endometriosis at the same time may not be possible. Sometimes, even if it is possible, it is not a good idea because the best conditions for your surgery may not be present. Surgery to remove endometriosis requires special surgical skills, specialised theatre staff, more operating theatre time, and specialised equipment. It is expensive care for a hospital to provide, even if a suitable surgeon is available. So, if time, personnel or equipment are not available, treatment is better planned as a two-step procedure. The first laparoscopy is done to see whether or not endometriosis is present, and to assess how severe the endometriosis is. The second laparoscopy is booked for a time when appropriate staff, equipment and theatre time are available for the endometriosis to be completely removed. This can work well, even if it is less convenient.

An alternative is one laparoscopy to diagnose the endometriosis, and then a trial of medication (see Chapter 6, page 63).

No matter how good the surgery, it cannot solve the other problems that women with endometriosis may have. Years of pain take their toll on a woman's emotional, employment, educational, relationship and sexual wellbeing. An operation, even if very successful, will not reverse this damage. However, effective surgery may be an opportunity to put some problems away and work on others.

The search for better, more effective and less intrusive treatment continues. So does the search for the cause of endometriosis, and ways to prevent it. Even so, endometriosis remains a challenge for both the women with the condition and the doctors who care for them.

What if J do nothing? Can endometriosis go away by itself?

Yes, especially if it is mild. An Australian study (see Reference 5) followed a group of women with endometriosis who each had two laparoscopies, done six months apart. Half the women had their endometriosis removed at the first laparoscopy. The other half had their endometriosis diagnosed but not removed until their second laparoscopy. None of the women knew which surgery they had had.

Of those women who had their endometriosis diagnosed but *not* removed at the first laparoscopy:

- 45 per cent had more endometriosis six months later
- 33 per cent had the same amount of endometriosis six months later, and
- 22 per cent had less endometriosis six months later.
  After the first laparoscopy, pain improved in:
- 80 per cent of the women who had had their endometriosis removed, but only
- 30 per cent of the women whose endometriosis had been diagnosed but not removed.

Twenty per cent had pain that did not improve even after their endometriosis was removed. These women certainly had endometriosis but there may have been another cause for their pain.

Can surgery fix all my pelvic pain?

Surgery to remove endometriosis will only help pain that is due to endometriosis. Surgery will not help pain due to other causes. So, if endometriosis is your *only* problem, then complete removal of the endometriosis may be able to help all your pain. However, I find that most women with endometriosis have more than one cause for their pain. So even the best surgery does not fix all their pain. It is more realistic to expect your pain to improve, or be easier to manage with medications after surgery, than for it to go completely.

The symptoms that are most likely to be due to endometriosis, and therefore most likely to improve after *complete* removal of endometriosis are:

- Pain during the month that feels like period pain
- Pain on opening your bowels, especially if this happens near your period
- Spotting between periods, if it is due to endometriosis
- Painful intercourse, if it is due to endometriosis

Pain during a period usually improves, but as this pain is usually a mixture of pains, it rarely goes away completely. Other possible causes of your pain are described in Chapter 9, and other treatments for period pain are included on in Chapter 6 on pages 70 and 76.

Chapter 5

· · · · · · · · · · · · · · · · ·

Laparoscopy

THIS CHAPTER EXPLAINS what a laparoscopy is and answers frequently asked questions about the procedure, how to prepare for the operation, and the risks and benefits involved.

What is a laparoscopy?

A laparoscopy may be the first operation you have ever had. Hospitals can be scary places to women who are unfamiliar with them. They don't need to be. The hospital staff are there to look after you, and both your anaesthetist and your gynaecologist will stay with you throughout your operation. Most operations go very smoothly.

A laparoscopy is done under a general anaesthetic, which means you will be asleep the whole time. Once you are asleep, a small cut is made near your navel and a telescope (called a *laparoscope*) is used to look inside and check your pelvis for any endometriosis.

Because the organs in the pelvis lie close together, a gas is used to inflate your abdomen and separate them. Without the gas, the pelvic organs could not be seen clearly. The cut near the navel

Figure 5.1 A laparoscopy

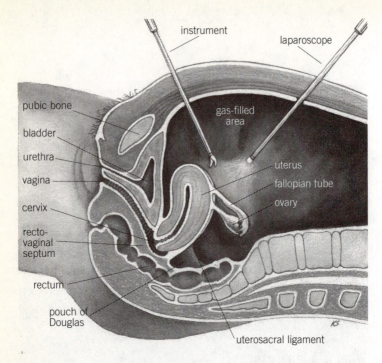

The laparoscope is inserted through a small cut near the navel. It is used to view the pelvic organs. The instruments used to remove endometriosis are inserted through small cuts lower down in the pelvis.

is used to view the pelvis, but if endometriosis is found inside, then more small cuts are needed. Between one and three extra cuts are made, so that the instruments needed to do your surgery can be inserted. What happens next depends on what has been found, and how your gynaecologist treats each problem.

Remember, it is not the small cuts on your abdomen that are the operation; it is what is done inside. Some laparoscopies are minor surgery, whereas other laparoscopies are major surgery through little holes.

After your laparoscopy, you will wake up in the *recovery ward*. This is a special area near the operating theatre where patients are cared for by nursing staff until they are more awake, and feeling comfortable. This usually takes one or two hours depending on what type of surgery you have had and how quickly you wake up. You will be attached to a saline drip (called an intravenous or IV drip) that provides water, salt and any medicine you need into one of the veins in your arm until you are able to eat and drink normally.

Any pieces of endometriosis that are removed during your operation will be sent to a pathologist, and checked with a microscope. This is because some lesions that look like endometriosis turn out to be something else, such as endosalpingiosis (see Chapter 9, page 202) or scar tissue. It is important to know exactly what your problem is before future treatment plans can be made.

How long will my surgery take?

This also depends on what is found. If all looks normal, then your laparoscopy will usually take less than thirty minutes, whereas if you have severe endometriosis, it may take a few hours. Endometriosis surgery is delicate work using small instruments near sensitive structures, so it takes time.

How long will I need off work?

How long you stay in hospital, and have off school, work or normal activities depends on what type of work you do, what surgery was done, and how well you feel. A laparoscopy where nothing abnormal is found can usually be done as day surgery. This means that you are able to go home on the same day as your operation. However, you will still need between three and seven days off to recover.

If endometriosis *is* found at your laparoscopy and removed, the operation will take longer, and there will be more healing required. You will probably stay in hospital overnight, and may need one or two weeks off work.

If this is your first laparoscopy, and you are unsure if you have endometriosis or not, allow a week off after your operation. This will suit most women. However, if you already know that you have endometriosis or if your endometriosis turns out to be severe you may need two weeks off, so don't plan your surgery before an important event. If you need any special bowel preparation before your surgery (see page 51), you may need the day before surgery off too. Some women bounce back quickly, even after major surgery, while others take longer. It is important to accept yourself and your needs whatever group you fit into. Recovering quickly does not make you a better person, just lucky.

Laparoscopies do make your abdomen sore, so you will need pain relief after your operation. Anything stronger than paracetamol or a period pain medication can make you constipated, so a high fibre diet, and a mild laxative are useful. A hot pack on your abdomen is comforting and relaxing. In my experience, women with chronic fatigue, chronic stress, or a lack of support at home, sometimes take longer to recover.

After your operation, you should gradually improve each day, but you will need more rest than normal. A daily walk is good exercise for your recovery, and it is safe to begin walking as soon as you leave hospital. Even a walk around your garden is a start. In general, if an activity hurts, don't do it, and if you are tired, have a rest. If you do too much on one day, you will be more tired the next day. If you are worried that you are not improving as quickly as you expected, ring your doctor. This is particularly important if you notice any of the following signs:

- A high temperature or fever. This can mean an infection.
- Pain in your leg. This can mean a clot in your leg veins.
- Difficulty breathing. This may mean a clot in your lungs or a lung condition such as pneumonia.
- Worsening nausea.
- Worsening pain.

Where does the gas go?

The gas used at a laparoscopy is called carbon dioxide (CO_2). This is the same gas that our bodies make as we turn the food we eat and the oxygen we breathe into energy, so it is a gas that our bodies are used to. CO_2 is breathed out through our lungs.

At the end of your laparoscopy most of the gas will be removed through the navel, but a small amount remains inside. *This gas is* around *the bowel* not *inside it*, so is absorbed by the body rather than passed as wind. This last bit of gas may cause shoulder pain if it lies near the diaphragm, because our brain feels any irritation of the diaphragm in the shoulder. Lying flat or even slightly head down allows the gas to float away from the diaphragm and the pain to improve. It should go away over a few days.

A laparoscopy to look for endometriosis needs to be very thorough. Endometriosis lesions may be subtle and can hide behind other pelvic organs. This means that some women who have had a laparoscopy with no abnormality found in the past, especially if it was more than five or ten years ago, may in fact have endometriosis now. It may have been in a form that was not recognised as endometriosis. This is not an error on the part of the gynaecologist, more a reflection of the lack of knowledge about endometriosis at that time. It is also possible that there truly was no endometriosis at the làst laparoscopy but that it has formed since then.

Which endometriosis lesions cause pain – and what is 'awake laparoscopy'?

Not all lesions seen through a laparoscope are painful.

The question of which lesions hurt, and which do not, has been investigated using *awake laparoscopy*. This means a laparoscopy done with local rather than general anaesthetic. The woman is given just enough sedation to be comfortable, but not asleep. She is awake enough to talk to her doctor during the operation and describe which parts of her pelvis are painful. The gynaecologist uses very delicate instruments to touch each area of the pelvis in turn. As each area is touched, the woman is asked whether she feels pain in that area and whether the pain she feels is the same as her normal pain. This process is called *pain mapping*.

A Canadian study using awake laparoscopy showed that not all endometriosis lesions were painful (see Reference 6). The lesions most likely to be painful were the red lesions or lesions with many blood vessels around them. The next most likely to be painful were the clear or white lesions, and the least likely to be painful were the black lesions. Only about one in four black lesions were painful to touch. They also found that touching normal-looking peritoneum up to 2 cm away from an endometriosis lesion might also cause pain in some women. Peritoneal windows (Chapter 1, page 8) were almost always painful.

Awake laparoscopies are *rare* operations and *never* done without the woman's consent.

How is a 'chocolate cyst' removed at a laparoscopy?

A chocolate cyst (endometrioma) has two parts: the cells around the edge of the cyst (the cyst wall) and the brown fluid inside. Draining the brown fluid from the cyst helps decide what sort of cyst it is, but won't remove the cyst wall. Unless the cyst wall is removed or destroyed, the cyst usually reforms quite quickly.

The cyst wall can be removed by 'stripping' it away from the ovary or 'cauterising' it with electrical or laser instruments. Even when this is done the cyst may still return, but it is much less likely than after drainage alone. The trick is to try and remove the cyst, while leaving as much of the normal ovary behind as possible.

In older women with completed families, removing the ovary may be a better option if the ovary is badly affected by endometriosis. This is rarely necessary in younger women.

Endometriomas are not cancers but they do mean that there is severe endometriosis present. Severe endometriosis like this, if left untreated, is likely to cause scarring and adhesions over time. Scarring and adhesions make surgery more difficult (see Chapter 9 on page 173).

Figure 5.2 An endometrioma

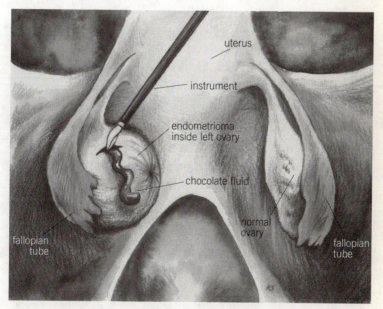

The left ovary is enlarged by an endometrioma (chocolate cyst). Opening the cyst releases a dark brown fluid. Once the cyst fluid and the cyst wall have been removed from inside the ovary, the ovary can return to normal size.

Could I need a larger cut for my surgery?

Sometimes a larger **incision** on the abdomen is necessary so that your endometriosis can be removed completely or for reasons of safety. Almost all endometriosis surgery can be done through small holes, so this is uncommon, but even the best endometriosis surgeons need to make a larger cut sometimes. As larger cuts take longer to heal, it is always a good idea to plan your surgery at least a few weeks before any important events – just in case.

If a larger cut is necessary, then the size and position of the cut will depend on what surgery is needed. Generally it will be either a cut across the lower part of the abdomen, similar to the scar from a caesarean birth, or a vertical cut from near the navel down to the pubic bone.

Do I need an operation?

Endometriosis is a surgical condition. This means that it is a condition where surgery plays a major role. Without a laparoscopy it cannot be reliably diagnosed, and for most women a laparoscopy with complete removal of their endometriosis is the treatment most likely to improve their symptoms for the longest period of time.

However, it is important to understand that the choice of whether or not to have an operation is always *yours*. Endometriosis is *not* a life-threatening condition. You will not die of endometriosis even if it feels like it.

The time to have an operation comes when the benefits *to you* of investigating your problems are greater than the risks *to you* of the operation. This is true of all surgery, but especially true of endometriosis surgery. So, faced with the choice of whether or not to have an operation, different women often make different choices.

However, by the time most women come to me they are ready for an operation. Their quality of life is poor. Other pain treatments have failed and they feel unable to continue as they are. Pain may have interrupted their employment, education or relationships.

The risks of surgery are small in comparison to a life of pain. A laparoscopy with removal of any endometriosis found is often a sensible choice. Even if complications occur, these women rarely regret their operation.

For other women, their pain is minimal. They have no fertility concerns and other treatments control their pain well. These women have less to gain from surgery and the decision whether or not to have a laparoscopy should be considered carefully. If there are complications during their operation these women are more likely to regret their decision.

Occasionally there are women with no symptoms at all but significant concerns who *choose* to have a laparoscopy. This group includes those with a family history of endometriosis who are concerned that they may be affected too, and wish to look after their pelvis for future fertility. A normal laparoscopy is reassuring for them, whereas finding endometriosis allows earlier and, it is hoped, more effective treatment.

Before deciding to have a laparoscopy, you should consider how significant your symptoms or other reasons are. If the following are all true, then a laparoscopy may be a good choice for you:

- Your symptoms are a problem to you, or you have good reason to suspect that you may have endometriosis
- You feel comfortable that you have enough information to decide
- You accept the uncommon but real risk of surgical complications, and
- Your gynaecologist will be able to remove any endometriosis found

> If you have decided to have a laparoscopy, you should discuss with your surgeon what type of surgery you would like if endometriosis were found.

For example, there are two possible options for treating a badly damaged ovary. Either the endometriosis can be removed and as much normal ovarian tissue as possible kept, *or,* the entire ovary can be removed together with its endometriosis. Both types of surgery are reasonable in different circumstances. The first option would suit a young woman, whereas an older woman with a completed family might choose to have the ovary removed and lessen the chance that she will need further surgery in the future (see Chapter 8, page 130).

Do laparoscopies cause scars?

Yes, but they are small and fade over time. How large the scars are, how many there are, and where they are, depends on how much surgery you need and your particular gynaecologist. Surgical techniques vary between different doctors, and the cuts are made in places that suit the surgical technique used.

Almost all laparoscopies start with a cut near the navel. This is usually easy to hide amongst the skin folds. Scars are red soon after the operation, but change to white over one or two years. A white scar will show more on tanned skin.

Keloid scars are a special type of scar. They are very thick, red and rise above the surface of the skin. Keloid scars are related to skin type, not the way a scar was stitched. They are more common in areas around the neck and in dark-skinned women.

How can I prepare for my laparoscopy?

Mental preparation

Having an operation can be daunting as it means giving control of your health to other people (your surgical team) for a period of time. While you are asleep, it is your surgical team who will make decisions for you. If you are someone who controls your life carefully (as many women do), you may find this idea hard to cope with. *However, the chance you won't wake up is virtually zero* and having thought through your options carefully (Chapter 4, page 46), you have a good reason for your surgery.

Anxiety before an operation is normal. If you are nervous, you may be able to visit the hospital before the day of your surgery. This allows you to become familiar with the hospital, and what will be done on the day. You may also wish to discuss a '*pre-med*' with your anaesthetist. This medication will ease your anxiety when you go into theatre. The operation consent form should be signed before a pre-med is given, so plan ahead with your doctor. Pre-meds are not given to everyone as women wake up more quickly without them, and some laparoscopies are done as day surgery.

Remember that you are allowed to look forward to your surgery. Many women do. Sensibly they may be anxious about the risks involved, but the operation is a positive step they have chosen to improve their quality of life.

If possible, be kind to yourself in the days before your operation. With so many responsibilities, work commitments and dependents, many women work extra hard right up to the time of their surgery. They aim to have everyone and everything perfectly organised while they recover. Admirable though this may be, the overwork combined with normal anxiety before an operation means that they arrive in hospital stressed. Once the operation is over they collapse with exhaustion. This is similar to the headache that some overworked men or women get a few days into a holiday. Once the adrenalin stops pumping they fall in a heap. Your time spent in hospital and recovering at home may be the opportunity for your family to learn some useful life skills and take on more responsibility. They may be pleased to feel needed and repay the care you have given them over many years.

Smoking

Smoking is never a good idea and any time is a good time to quit. Before an operation is a particularly good time. As smoking is not permitted in hospitals and the urge to smoke is less after an anaesthetic, it is also an excellent time to make this change permanent. Smoking does not mean you can't have an operation, but it does increase the risk of serious lung infection (pneumonia) in the recovery period.

Telling a smoker from a non-smoker is easy to do as they wake up from an anaesthetic. The smokers are the ones with the terrible cough and sputum. Frequently this is the first time that a smoker is confronted with the consequences of their smoking.

I have a pierced navel. Will I need to remove my ring?

Usually, yes. A ring might get in the way of the telescope, can increase the risk of a skin infection and because it is made of metal may not be safe near electrical instruments. While the risks of leaving it in are small, most surgeons will ask you to remove it. If you cannot remove the ring yourself, ask one of the nursing staff to remove it for you once you are asleep. The ring can be replaced at the end of your operation before you wake up.

Medications

Aspirin, or any medication that contains aspirin, should be stopped at least seven days before your surgery. This is because aspirin increases the risk of bleeding at your operation. Most period pain medications (see Chapter 6, page 70) are related to aspirin but can be continued until three or four days before surgery. Paracetamol and codeine medications are good choices for pain relief at this time because they do not increase the risk of bleeding.

If you are on medications that thin the blood such as *warfarin* or *heparin*, you should discuss this with your doctor and anaesthetist at least two weeks before your operation.

If you are on the *contraceptive pill*, ask your doctor if this should be stopped before your operation. While being on the Pill does increase the risk of leg clots, the risk is still low in young women. Being on the Pill avoids the risk of an unplanned pregnancy, avoids difficulty timing the operation with the menstrual cycle and avoids even worse pain with periods.

Remember to tell your doctor about all the medications you are on, including those you can buy without a prescription, and any complementary therapies.

Bowel preparation

It is important to have an empty bowel during your surgery because:

- An empty bowel lies out of the way during the operation. This makes the operation easier for your gynaecologist to do and makes damage to the bowel less likely
- An empty bowel helps avoid constipation after your operation
- If a hole is made in your bowel, repair of the bowel is simpler and safer if the bowel is empty.

To empty the bowel your gynaecologist may recommend either a small enema or *bowel prep* before your operation, depending on what surgery is planned. The small enema empties the lower bowel, while bowel prep clears your entire bowel. From your surgeon's point of view, bowel prep is preferable, but as bowel prep is more trouble to you, they may reserve this for women where surgery near the bowel is expected. Bowel prep makes your surgery safer and easier.

What is the difference between a small enema and 'bowel prep'?

A small enema involves inserting a small amount of fluid (about 20 ml) just inside the anus, holding it inside for as long as possible (maybe 15 or 30 minutes) and then opening your bowels. It only clears the lower bowel.

Bowel prep involves two days of preparation before the day of your surgery. There are several types of bowel prep. Older bowel prep medications such as Go-Lightly® involved drinking four litres of medication. This was very difficult for women to do. Newer medications such as Picolax® involve two drinks of about 100 ml each. This is much more acceptable. After the medication is taken, diarrhoea starts. How much diarrhoea there is depends a lot on how your bowel works normally. Women who are usually constipated may only open their bowels a few times, whereas women who tend to diarrhoea may have almost continual diarrhoea. Either way, it is advisable to be at home once you start the medication. You may need to open your bowels with little warning. It is important to drink a lot of water during this time.

Pregnancy

It is very *important that you are* not *pregnant at the time of your operation.* A laparoscopy during pregnancy might put your own health or the health of the baby at risk. If there is any chance you may be pregnant, tell your doctor. The date of your surgery may need to be altered, or a pregnancy test done. This is important, even if you would not choose to keep the pregnancy. Pregnancy tests are not reliable until at least the time of a missed period, so there is a window of time when no-one can tell if you are pregnant or not. Diagnosing pregnancy may also be difficult in women with irregular periods.

If you are currently trying to become pregnant, then you are unlikely to be using contraception. Your operation should be booked in the first half of your menstrual cycle after your period, but before ovulation has occurred (see Chapter 8, page 124). This is the time of the month when pregnancy is unlikely. If your periods are irregular or timing is difficult, ask your doctor when will be the best time for your surgery.

Back or joint conditions

Lying in one position on an operating table for prolonged periods of time sometimes aggravates a pre-existing back problem, or occasionally puts pressure on a nerve near the surface of the skin. Luckily, the position used at laparoscopy is one that is comfortable for most women with back conditions. If you do have any back or joint problems, you can ask to be positioned on the operating table while still awake. This allows you to ensure that your position is comfortable before going to sleep.

Other medical conditions and allergies

Any medical conditions such as diabetes or heart disease should be reported to your doctor and anaesthetist. If you have a family history of blood clots, easy bruising or bleeding, be sure to tell your doctor at least two weeks before the operation day. You may need special blood tests to make your operation safer.

Always tell your doctor if you have any *allergies*. A list of the medications that you are allergic to, as well as a list of those that you have taken in the past *without* problems is useful. Ultimately, you will need some medications during your stay in hospital, so knowing which medications do *not* cause you problems will help your doctor decide which medications to use.

What complications could there be?

Endometriosis surgery is difficult surgery. That is why not all gynaecologists do it. Apart from cancer surgery, it is the most difficult surgery we do. With this difficulty come some risks.

Every day throughout Australia hundreds of laparoscopies are done. Only a very small number of these have major complications. However, although they are uncommon, complications from endometriosis surgery are particularly distressing. They occur in otherwise healthy young women.

> **All surgery has risks that must be considered, but
> not having surgery has risks too. If you have
> endometriosis there is *no* option that has all
> benefits but no risks.**

For most women, the risks of a laparoscopy can be divided
into three groups:

- The general risks of an operation. These depend on your
  general health and how long the operation takes
- The risks involved in having a laparoscope and instruments
  inserted into your abdomen, and
- The risks involved with removing your endometriosis.

The general risks of an operation

These include:

- An allergic reaction to any medicines that are used
- A blood clot in the legs which may pass to the lungs
- Temporary aggravation of a previous back injury from lying in
  one position
- Breathing difficulties such as asthma or a lung infection
  (pneumonia) after your operation. This particularly applies to
  smokers.

The anaesthetist who puts you to sleep will stay with you
throughout your operation. He or she monitors your heartbeat,
breathing, temperature and position to make your operation as
safe as possible.

The risks associated with inserting laparoscopic instruments and removing endometriosis

These risks may occur with *any* laparoscopy including a sterilisation operation to prevent pregnancy, removal of the appendix, or
removal of the gall bladder. They can occur even in laparoscopies

where no endometriosis is found. However, the more difficult the surgery is, the higher the risk.

These risks include:

1 Infection in a skin wound

2 A urine infection

3 Constipation or nausea after your operation

4 Shoulder tip pain (see Chapter 5, page 43) for a few days

5 Unintentional pressure on a nerve during an operation (a neuropathy). This pressure sometimes prevents the nerve from working normally for a period of time. Luckily, most neuropathies fully recover without treatment but they may take months to do so.

6 A hernia through one of the small cuts (one in 500 cases). This means a bulge near one of the small cuts. It can be repaired at a separate operation.

7 Adhesions from the surgery (see Chapter 9, page 173). Any surgery can cause adhesions, but they are less common after laparoscopic surgery than after surgery through larger cuts. Endometriosis itself can cause adhesions even without surgery.

8 An unintentional hole (perforation) in a blood vessel or pelvic organ (1 in 250 cases) (see Reference 7).

> **These lists include the most common and the most severe complications. They do not include every possible problem that could occur. If there are particular complications that you are anxious about, you should talk to your gynaecologist about them before your operation.**

What it means to have a perforation of an abdominal organ

This is the complication that worries both women and gynaecologists most. The organs involved might include the bladder, bowel, ureter, or some large blood vessels.

Not all perforations (holes) are a major problem, but some are. Whether or not they are a problem depends on whether the hole can be seen and repaired during the operation, and what type of surgery is needed to fix it.

Sometimes it is *necessary* to make a hole in the bowel or the bladder on purpose so that the endometriosis can be removed completely. Once the endometriosis is removed, the hole is repaired. This is good surgery rather than a complication. Without making the hole, some endometriosis would be left behind and your symptoms might not improve.

Even an *unintentional* hole in an organ may not be a serious problem. If it can be recognised and repaired at the time, and particularly if it can be done through the laparoscope, then although your recovery from surgery may be slower than planned, the long-term results are usually good.

Some of the most difficult cases are those where damage to an important organ, like ureter or bowel, was not recognised at the time of surgery. It may be that the hole was too small to see, or that the hole formed after the operation was finished. The electrical instruments used in most laparoscopic surgery may sometimes cause damage that does not show up until after the procedure is finished. During the operation, the damaged organ looks normal, but over the next few days, the damaged tissue breaks down and a hole forms. It is also possible for an infection in the pelvis to form an abscess that bursts, making a hole.

The effects of a perforated organ depend on which organ it is.

A hole in the bladder

A hole in the bladder can be repaired either through the laparoscope or through a larger cut. A soft rubber tube called a **catheter** is inserted into the bladder for between three and seven days after the operation to keep the bladder empty while it heals. The catheter drains urine into a bag over this time. The bladder heals well, and after the catheter is removed there are usually few problems.

A bladder perforation while dividing adhesions

Eleanor is a 60-year-old retired teacher in excellent health. Her past history included a hysterectomy for an enlarged uterus, and removal of her left ovary due to severe endometriosis many years ago. After some pain on the right side of her pelvis, an ultrasound showed a cyst on her right ovary. At 60 years of age, a cystic ovary could mean a cancer of the ovary. It was important to find out what the cyst was and to remove it.

At laparoscopy her pelvis was full of adhesions. Everything was stuck together. A thick curtain of fatty tissue blocked any view of the right side of her pelvis where the ovary would be. The adhesions were slowly and carefully divided so that the right ovary could be seen. However, during division of these adhesions a hole was made in the bladder. The bladder had been pulled up much higher than normal by the adhesions, and this unusual position had put it more at risk. After dividing all the adhesions, and removing what turned out to be a benign (not cancerous) ovarian cyst, the bladder was repaired through the laparoscope. A catheter was inserted to keep the bladder empty while it healed.

Eleanor stayed seven days in hospital instead of two, but was otherwise well. The catheter was removed after seven days, and she was able to pass urine normally. Although the hole in the bladder was unintended, no long-term damage resulted.

A hole in the bowel

If a hole in the bowel is recognised during an operation, it is repaired at the time. The technique used varies according to whether or not the bowel is empty, which part of the bowel is damaged, and the surgical skills available. The repair might be possible through the laparoscope, but a larger cut may be needed. Repair may be easier in women who have used 'bowel prep' before their surgery (see Chapter 5, page 51).

Sometimes a hole in the bowel forms after the operation is finished. Other holes may be too small to see at the time of the operation. The woman involved may look well after her surgery but become very ill later on, often after she has gone home. Her pain may increase, there may be vomiting and she may have a fever. This is an emergency situation requiring urgent medical attention. Repair of the hole usually requires a large cut on the abdomen, and may require a short-term **colostomy**. A colostomy means that the bowel empties into a bag outside the body on the abdominal wall. After three to six months, when the bowel has recovered, the colostomy is repaired at another operation. Once the bowel is rejoined, faeces can be passed normally again. This complication is a major problem for the woman involved, and her family. It is a complication that we, as surgeons, constantly try to avoid.

A bowel perforation with colostomy

Vivian is a 25-year-old married woman with one child. Her periods were painful and a laparoscopy found endometriosis that was removed. The pain improved, but two years later she returned unable to become pregnant and with painful periods once more. Laparoscopy showed more endometriosis, very close to the rectum (lower bowel), which was removed. Vivian was well the next day, but two weeks later suddenly became very unwell. Vivian had a hole in her bowel with infection throughout her abdomen (peritonitis). She went straight to surgery where a large cut on her abdomen was made. A small hole in the bowel next to where her surgery had been was found and repaired. However, a colostomy was needed in order to rest her bowel and allow the hole to heal. After four months the colostomy was closed at a separate operation and bowel actions emptied normally again. Vivian required major surgery, time in intensive care, and three months off work. No-one wishes to cause such a serious injury to another person. It has been a major problem for Vivian and her family.

A hole in a large blood vessel

There are several large blood vessels in and around the pelvis. They include the aorta, the inferior vena cava and the iliac blood vessels. Damage to one of these blood vessels, although very uncommon, is an emergency situation that usually requires a large cut in the abdomen to repair.

Damage to the ureter

The ureter is an important tube that passes from the kidney to the bladder on each side of the pelvis. The ureter lies in the side wall of the pelvis underneath the ovary. This is the most common place to find endometriosis, so removing endometriosis usually means operating very close to it. Any scar tissue present makes the ureter difficult to see and therefore difficult to avoid.

To make things even more difficult, some women are born with two ureters on one or both sides of their pelvis. Gynaecologists avoid damage to the ureter by finding it, and then staying as far away from it as possible. If there is a second, unknown ureter hidden amongst the endometriosis or scar tissue, then the second one may be damaged despite due care.

A damaged ureter may be very difficult to recognise during an operation. The woman involved may look and feel well after her surgery, but later develop pain in the loin area near the kidney on that side. An operation through a large cut is usually required to repair the ureter.

I have a large scar on my abdomen. Does that matter?

Yes. Women with an 'up-and-down' cut on their abdomen have a higher risk of bowel perforation at a laparoscopy. This is because a piece of bowel may have become stuck to the back of the scar during the healing phase of the previous operation. If so, then it is possible to make a hole in the bowel while the telescope is being inserted, before your doctor has a chance to see what is inside. A vertical scar does not mean that you cannot have a laparoscopy, but you should realise that there is an increased risk.

Does my general health affect the chance of a complication?

Yes, definitely. The two examples below illustrate the different risks among different women.

A healthy, normal weight, non-smoking 20-year-old woman, who has a laparoscopy where no abnormality is found, has the risks associated with having an anaesthetic as well as the risks involved in inserting instruments into the abdomen, but that is all. The risk for her of having an anaesthetic is very low. She is as likely to die driving her car to the hospital as die of the anaesthetic. The risk of a perforated organ as the instruments are inserted is small, but difficult to quantify. It may be approximately 1 in 500 laparoscopies. If endometriosis is found, then removing it will increase the risk, but also the possible benefits of her surgery.

A 45-year-old woman who has smoked for 20 years, is overweight, and has severe endometriosis, has higher anaesthetic, laparoscopy and endometriosis surgery risks to consider. The extra fatty tissue inside her abdomen restricts the view through the laparoscope and pushes the bowel closer to the instruments.

There is less room to work in her pelvis, and more chance of damage to the bowel. Her long-term smoking habit will make breathing difficulties such as asthma or pneumonia more likely after her surgery. Removing her endometriosis makes the operation longer and makes the chance of a hole in a pelvic organ greater. Smoking, middle age, overweight and a longer operation time all increase the chance of a blood clot in her legs. Even so, this woman has risks associated with surgery through a larger cut too, so if she truly does need an operation, a laparoscopy is still a good choice.

So why would any woman choose to have a laparoscopy?

They do so because their pain is severe, they are trying to become pregnant, or they suspect they have endometriosis. Surgery offers the only reliable diagnosis, and the most successful treatment for women with endometriosis.

> **Your surgeon's experience with endometriosis is very important, but all surgeons have complications at some time. In addition, those surgeons with the most experience are sent the most difficult cases requiring the most difficult surgery with the highest risk. There is *no* surgeon who can promise that all will go well, but experience and good laparoscopic surgery skills do count.**

It is very reasonable for you to ask your particular surgeon what complications they have encountered before. Most will be quite open with this information, and welcome the opportunity to be frank about possible problems.

Chapter 6

Which medicines are used to manage endometriosis?

THIS CHAPTER DESCRIBES both the medications used to treat endometriosis and other medications that you may use at different times. They are divided into:

- Medicines that treat endometriosis
- Medicines that treat pain
- Medicines that manage periods or block ovulation
- A progesterone-like medication inserted in the uterus (Mirena)
- Other medications.

> Whichever medicine you take, it is important to discuss possible side effects, other medications you already use, and any medical conditions you have with your doctor first. Only paracetamol and codeine are suitable for women who may be pregnant.

Medicines to treat endometriosis

These include danazol, **gestrinone**, and the GnRH analogues (Zoladex® and Synarel®).

Doctors disagree on how useful these medications are at treating endometriosis. Those gynaecologists who are able to remove endometriosis usually prefer surgery first and leave medications for situations when surgery is not enough. Those gynaecologists who are less comfortable with endometriosis surgery usually diagnose endometriosis at a laparoscopy, and then recommend a course of medication. They keep further surgery for those women in whom medications have failed.

> **All doctors agree that there are *no* medicines (or herbal preparations) that are always effective, always safe, have no side effects, have no long-term risks, are cheap to provide and easily available. If such a treatment existed, no-one would recommend anything else.**

The *advantage* of using a medication is that it avoids *some* of the risks of an operation. It won't allow you to avoid an operation altogether because a laparoscopy is still needed to diagnose endometriosis in the first place. However, a laparoscopy that looks for endometriosis but does not remove it is shorter, safer and easier than a laparoscopy that looks for and removes endometriosis. My concern is that it is also less effective at managing pain.

The *disadvantages* of using a medication include its side effects, the need to avoid pregnancy while taking the medication, the cost involved, and the fact that endometriosis symptoms often return once the medication is stopped. Medications rarely remove endometriosis. They suppress it.

All the commonly used anti-endometriosis medications work by changing your hormone levels to make life uncomfortable for the endometriosis. Unfortunately they sometimes make life uncomfortable for you too! Most are given as a six-month course, during which time periods usually stop.

As there are no periods, these medications are very good at treating period pain. They are less successful (but often still good) at treating pelvic pain during the month, painful intercourse, or bowel pain, probably because women with these symptoms usually have some scar tissue present.

> **None of these medications will remove scar tissue, divide adhesions, remove chocolate cysts from an ovary or improve fertility. They work best on thin, small lesions.**

Even in women with a very good response to medications (and there are many of them), pain often returns once the course of treatment is finished. Any endometriosis that remains becomes active again, and the pain returns, often within about six months of stopping the medication. Even so, medications can offer a welcome break from pain. They are also useful where some endometriosis (but not scar tissue) remains after surgery, or where surgery to remove endometriosis is unavailable.

All these medications have side effects and none will suit everyone. *If your endometriosis has been removed completely at laparoscopy, there is usually no need to use these medications.*

Danazol and Gestrinone

Danazol and gestrinone are similar medications. They both make *estrogen levels lower* and *androgen (testosterone) levels higher*. Estrogen is the 'female' hormone made by the ovary in women before menopause. Androgens are often called 'male' hormones, but women have them too, just as men have estrogen.

The side effects of danazol and gestrinone include:

- Side effects due to higher androgen levels. These include weight gain, slightly bulkier muscles, oily skin, increased body hair and cramps
- Side effects due to low estrogen levels. These include lower libido (interest in sex), smaller breasts, and sometimes hot flushes.

Occasionally, there is a deepening of the voice. This is not a common side effect but unlike the other side effects that go away once the danazol or gestrinone is stopped, a deeper voice may be irreversible. So, if you are a keen singer the small risk of a deeper voice is not worth taking and these medications are not for you.

Danazol is a banned substance for competitive athletes because it increases muscle size and strength. It may also affect blood sugar levels so should be used with care by women with diabetes.

In particular, it is very important *not* to become pregnant on danazol or gestrinone. If taken from more than eight weeks after falling pregnant, it may cause abnormalities of the baby's genital organs.

Danazol is taken in capsule form, at a dose of 600 to 800 mg daily. Gestrinone capsules are taken at doses of 2.5 to 5 mg twice a week. Both medications are usually prescribed for six months. They are not used long term because their effect on blood fats might increase the risk of heart and blood vessel disease later in life. These risks are small when used for six months.

It is estimated that pain returns in 50 per cent of women within 12 months of stopping treatment. If the endometriosis is severe, then symptoms are even more likely to return during this time (see Reference 8). This is the major problem with their use.

After a course of danazol or gestrinone, some women choose to start the contraceptive pill and take it continuously (see Chapter

6, page 77). This sometimes maintains any benefits that have been achieved.

In Australia, danazol and gestrinone are only available on the Pharmaceutical Benefits Scheme (PBS) to women where endometriosis has been seen at a laparoscopy. If endometriosis has not been seen, then their cost is not subsidised by the government. This makes their use more expensive to you.

Gonadotrophin-releasing hormone analogues (GnRH analogues or GnRHa)

These include goserelin injections (Zoladex®) and nafarelin nasal spray (Synarel®).

Natural GnRH is a hormone made by the brain. It tells the ovary to prepare an egg for ovulation and make the hormone estrogen. GnRH analogue medications look like natural GnRH to our bodies, but act differently. They stop natural GnRH from working and block the message from the brain to the ovary. An egg is not released and very little estrogen is made. Estrogen levels become very low indeed: much lower than with danazol or gestrinone. Androgen (testosterone) levels are approximately normal.

The acid in our stomach would destroy GnRH analogues taken as tablets, so they are given either as a nasal spray twice a day (Synarel®) or a long-acting injection once a month (Zoladex®). Treatment is started during a period and must *not* be used if you may be pregnant. There is a possible risk of miscarriage or birth abnormality if used during pregnancy.

The side effects of GnRH analogues are similar to a normal menopause, so while taking these medications, you and your mother may have more things in common than usual! The low estrogen levels mean no periods, hot flushes, tiredness, night sweats, vaginal dryness, headaches, muscle pains, low libido and a tendency to thinning of the bones.

To manage these symptoms while on the treatment, many women take hormone replacement therapy. This contains estrogen and progestogen, the two female hormones. When used with a GnRH analogue, this is called *add-back therapy* and does not prevent its effect on endometriosis. While on this treatment it is a good idea to increase the calcium in your diet, or take a calcium tablet each day. This gives even more protection to your bones. It has been common for add-back therapy to be given only after a month of GnRH analogue treatment alone. However, it has recently been shown that starting add-back therapy from the beginning of GnRH analogue treatment is just as effective (see Reference 9).

Although there have been some concerns about the safety of long-term HRT in women after menopause, there are no concerns over the safety of HRT in women before menopause who are on a GnRH analogue. All doctors agree that it is a good idea. The HRT is only giving back a small amount of the hormone that the GnRH analogue has taken away. It is not providing extra hormone above the woman's normal levels. Once the GnRH analogue and add-back therapy cease, estrogen levels return to normal and periods return.

As with danazol and gestrinone, GnRH analogues suppress rather than remove endometriosis, so even if all has gone well, your pain may return over time. It is also common to start the contraceptive pill, used continuously, after the course of GnRH analogue is completed to try and maintain any benefits that have been achieved.

Danazol, gestrinone or a GnRH analogue. Which one is best for me?

Your choice depends on which side effects you are least concerned about and what other problems you may have. For example, danazol and gestrinone make skin oiler and periods lighter. They are a good choice if you have heavy periods, but a poor choice if you have acne. GnRH analogues stop the menstrual cycle but also lower bone density. They are a good choice if you suffer premenstrual tension or severe headaches with periods (*menstrual migraines*), but a poor choice if you have thin bones. In general, GnRH analogues are better tolerated than danazol or gestrinone especially if 'add-back therapy' is used.

Some women feel really well with low estrogen levels. Those who have suffered hormone-related symptoms such as migraines during periods, or hormonal moodiness, sometimes really enjoy their time on Zoladex® or Synarel®. Their hormonal cycle has been turned off, at least for six months, and they feel the best of their adult life. These women later find menopause a blessed relief.

GnRH analogues are expensive medications. In Australia they are subsidised by our government on the PBS, but only where endometriosis has been seen at a laparoscopy and only for one six-month course over a lifetime.

GnRH analogue treatment and pain

Janine is a 37-year-old office worker. Over the last year she had noticed a severe pain just under her right rib cage with each period. It had taken a while for her to realise that this pain only happened on the first day of her period. Janine also had stress at work. Her boss was difficult and she was working long hours. A laparoscopy showed small areas of endometriosis in her pelvis, which were removed. No endometriosis was seen on the diaphragm, but as the liver hides part of the diaphragm, endometriosis at that site could not be completely excluded. Janine started Zoladex® injections monthly for six months. During this time she had no periods and no right-sided pain. At the end of six months treatment, Janine started the contraceptive pill taken continuously hoping to maintain the benefit achieved with the GnRH analogue medication. Periods were planned every three to four months. Janine also changed her job, became less stressed, and worked on her general health. There have been no further episodes of pain.

Endometriosis of the diaphragm is rare. To remove it may require major chest surgery. We may never know if it was present or not. However, the fact that the pain only happened with periods and that using the GnRH analogue to stop periods also stopped the pain certainly suggests that the pain might be due to endo-metriosis. While her pain can be avoided with the contraceptive pill used continuously, there is no need for further treatment.

What about long-term GnRH analogues and HRT without a laparoscopy?

In some countries, some doctors use GnRH analogues with add-back HRT long term for women with pelvic pain, without first doing a laparoscopy. They are never sure whether or not their patients actually have endometriosis, but it is presumed that they do. This form of treatment is used where a laparoscopy is considered too expensive to offer, or the skills to treat endometriosis surgically are not available. It is not a treatment plan that I use, but may be reasonable in some cases.

My concerns are that:

- Some women without endometriosis will be treated unnecessarily
- Other causes of pelvic pain may be missed

- The treatment will not improve fertility
- This treatment is unlikely to remove large or deep areas of endometriosis
- Some women may have side effects from the medication
- In rare cases, a cancer of the ovary could be missed.

Pain management medicines

If you have long-term (chronic) pain, you will be pleased to hear that 'pain management' is a growing and specialised area of medicine. There are now doctors who specialise in this area. Most large hospitals have pain clinics for men and women who suffer long-term pain, whether it be from their pelvis, back or another body part (see Chapter 9, page 181).

Commonly used pain medications include **anti-prostaglandin medications**, paracetamol, stronger pain tablets (**opioids**), and amitriptyline. Less commonly used medications are described in Chapter 9 on page 179. More recently, an intra-uterine device that releases a progesterone-like medication to the uterus to make periods lighter has been used to treat period pain. It is explained further in this chapter on page 82.

Anti-prostaglandin (period pain) medications (NSAIDs)

These medicines are also known as non-steroidal anti-inflammatory drugs, anti-inflammatory medications or NSAIDs. They include common period pain medications such as ibuprofen (Nurofen®), naproxen (Naprogesic®), diclofenac (Voltaren®) and mefenemic acid (Ponstan®).

NSAIDs stop the uterus or an endometriosis lesion from making *prostaglandins*. Prostaglandins are very powerful chemicals and a common cause of pain. It is prostaglandins that put a woman into labour when she has a baby, so it is not surprising that they can cause very severe pain. *NSAIDs will improve pain that is due (or partly due) to prostaglandins.*

While pain tablets like codeine work because they prevent the brain noticing the pain, an NSAID works by treating the cause of the pain. By themselves they can treat mild or moderate pain, but when combined with other pain tablets such as codeine or paracetamol they are useful for more severe pain.

Anti-prostaglandin medications are particularly useful as one part of the pain relief given after a laparoscopy. When tissues are irritated during surgery they make a lot of prostaglandins, which contribute to the pain. Even when stronger pain medications are needed, adding an NSAID gives a better quality of pain relief, as well as minimising the need for stronger pain medications *(opioids)*. It is the opioids that are most likely to cause nausea, vomiting and constipation.

Most NSAIDs are taken as tablets, but the strongest forms of NSAIDs come as suppositories on prescription. Suppositories are a medication mixed in a soft pellet often made from cocoa butter or paraffin. They are pushed through the anus so that the medication can be absorbed into the body through the bowel wall. They work well for period pain, and last for 12 hours, but I rarely have much luck suggesting them to teenagers!

NSAIDs should *not* be taken in pregnancy. They are also not suitable for women who are elderly, take blood pressure medications, have kidney disease, have stomach ulcers or stomach irritation, or whose asthma is triggered by aspirin-like medications.

How anti-prostaglandin medications work

Prostaglandins are made in the uterus from a substance called arachidonic acid. Arachidonic acid is present in the uterus all the time without causing pain, but at period time an enzyme called *cyclo-oxygenase (COX)* changes it into prostaglandins, and the pain starts.

NSAID medicines block the COX enzyme, and stop the uterus making prostaglandins from arachidonic acid. This is how they treat the pain and why it is important to take these medications either at the first sign of pain or even before the pain starts. Once the prostaglandins have been made, an NSAID will not remove them. This is why they are much less effective when taken once the pain is severe. The individual NSAIDs vary, so you may find that one type of NSAID is more effective than the others.

Figure 6.1 How anti-inflammatory medications work

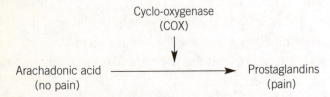

Anti-prostaglandin medications can prevent the COX enzyme making prostaglandins, but cannot remove them once they are made.

Paracetamol

Paracetamol is useful for mild to moderate pain, and is especially effective if taken together with an NSAID or codeine. It is important never to take more than 8 of the 500 mg paracetamol tablets in one day, or liver damage may occur. If you use other tablets that have paracetamol in them, this paracetamol must be included in your total daily dose.

Opioid medications (also called narcotics)

Opioid medications were originally made from opium poppies. Some still are but others are made in laboratories. Tasmania grows large numbers of opium poppies to make into the medications we use in Australia. Opioid medications include codeine, oxycodone, methadone, dextropropoxyphene, pethidine, morphine, tramadol, and fentanyl. Pethidine, fentanyl and morphine are generally only used in hospitals. The common opioids used by women in the community include codeine, dextropropoxyphene and oxycodone. Dextropropoxyphene is mixed with paracetamol to make Capadex® and Digesic®.

All opioid medications can cause constipation and nausea but some women are more sensitive to these effects than others.

Codeine is a 'pro-drug'. This means it must be converted into another drug by our body to have the best effect. Codeine itself has some effect on pain but it is much more effective when converted by the body into morphine. To change codeine into morphine requires an enzyme called *CYP2D6*. As some people don't have this enzyme, some people don't find codeine very useful for their pain. They get a benefit from the codeine itself, but not the morphine benefit that others receive. Codeine is usually prescribed in doses of 8 to 60 mg every 3 to 4 hours. It is often combined in a tablet with either paracetamol or aspirin.

Oxycodone is a strong opioid medication that can be taken in tablet form. It has a similar effect to morphine. Oxycodone can be taken as slow release tablets that work for a longer period of time. This means that they do not need to be taken as often.

Figure 6.2 How codeine is converted to morphine

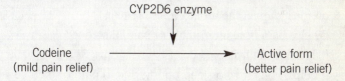

CYP2D6 enzyme

Codeine
(mild pain relief)

Active form
(better pain relief)

Women whose bodies do not make the CYP2D6 enzyme will find codeine less helpful for their pain than other women.

Tramadol

Tramadol is a medication for pain with a mixture of actions. It has a weak opioid effect (like codeine), but more importantly it affects a chemical in the brain called serotonin. Tramadol may be useful for moderate pain but is not strong enough for severe pain. It is quite a complicated medication and can cause side effects that include nausea, dizziness, vomiting, confusion and occasionally epileptic fits. It should be avoided by women with epilepsy and used with care in women who take any of the following medications or herbal preparations:

- Tricyclic medications (this includes amitriptyline)
- St John's wort
- Ondansetron (an anti-nausea medication)
- A group of medications called selective serotonin reuptake inhibitors (SSRIs). These are used to treat depression and anxiety.

Amitriptyline

Amitriptyline is not a medication to treat endometriosis, nor is it a normal painkiller, but it *is* very useful for women with pelvic pain. Amitriptyline helps women with pelvic pain in many ways:

- It treats 'neurogenic pain' (see Chapter 9, page 177), where the pain pathway to the brain becomes overactive with too many pain signals being sent at once. This type of pain is common in women with endometriosis, particularly those who have pain on most days of the month (chronic pain)
- It helps pain from an irritable or painful bladder
- It can slow an irritable bowel
- It helps women who sleep poorly, due to pain or the need to empty their bladder frequently.

With so many possible benefits, it is not surprising that many women with chronic pelvic pain improve on amitriptyline. It rarely cures pain completely, but is a valuable part of the whole treatment plan.

The common side effects of amitriptyline include dry eyes, dry mouth, mild constipation, and drowsiness. However these side effects go away as your body becomes used to the medication. Starting with a small dose taken *at night* avoids most side effects and allows most women to use amitriptyline if they choose to. Even if you have tried amitriptyline before and felt unwell, you may still be able to use it if you start with a low dose, and increase the dose slowly.

There are many different treatment plans, but 5 mg at night is a good dose to start on (half a 10 mg tablet). This dose may not be enough to improve the pain but it usually not enough to cause many side effects either. If you feel well and alert the next day, then the dose can be increased by 5 mg every few days until either your pain has improved or you reach 25 mg. If you feel at all sleepy, or too dry, then stay on the same dose each night until your body adapts to the tablets. This might take a few days or a week. There is no rush: it is more important to feel well and avoid problems.

Very few women need more than 25 mg, so if you have reached this dose without any benefit, then amitriptyline may not be effective for you. If your pain improves at a dose lower than 25 mg, then stay on that dose. Many women find that 10 mg at night is all they need. Chewing gum, or making sure you take extra drinks help a dry mouth.

Amitriptyline is taken at night because it can cause drowsiness. This could be dangerous if you are driving a car or operating machines. If taken at night drowsiness is less of a problem and may be a benefit. Just in case, it is important to start it the evening before a quiet day when you do not need to drive a car or operate machines, until you can tell how you will feel. Amitriptyline does not mix well with alcohol. Any alcohol you do drink will affect you more than usual, so be careful!

Amitriptyline is not a medication to take every now and then. If you do start it, make the commitment to take it every night. Then consider whether it has helped. Amitriptyline is unlikely to completely resolve your pain, but ask yourself: Are you better? Do you sleep better? Is your pain easier to manage? If so, then the amitriptyline should be continued for 3–6 months, or even longer. When you decide to stop it, decrease the dose slowly by 5 mg every few days or so, just as you did at the start. *Do not stop it suddenly.*

Amitriptyline is one of a group of drugs called *tricyclics*. In the past, tricyclics were used in high doses (maybe 150 mg) to treat depression. If your doctor recommends amitriptyline, or a similar medication, it is not because they think your pain is psychological, or that you are depressed. They have recommended it for good medical reasons. Amitriptyline is no longer used to treat depression, because there are better drugs available. It is used in small doses to manage pain, an irritable bladder, an irritable bowel, or interrupted sleep.

Unlike a completely unrelated group of drugs called benzodiazepines, *problems with addiction to tricyclics are uncommon*. Benzodiazepines include drugs such as diazepam (Valium®) or oxazepam (Serepax®). These have very little place in the management of chronic pain, apart from muscle spasm.

> **There are some medical conditions, and some medications, that do not mix well with amitriptyline. This is why it is important that you talk to your doctor before starting it, and don't take it if you may be pregnant.**

Medicines used to manage periods or block ovulation

These include the contraceptive pill, progestogens and the levonorgestrel-releasing intra-uterine device.

The contraceptive pill
The contraceptive pill should really be called a 'hormone management pill'. It has many uses apart from contraception, and is used

by many women who are not sexually active and have no need for contraception. In women with endometriosis, it is particularly useful because:

- *The Pill is a good treatment for prostaglandin pain.* Prostaglandin pain is a major part of most period pain, but particularly in women who have not had children. It is also a part (but not all) of endometriosis pain. The Pill prevents ovulation. Blocking ovulation means fewer prostaglandins and less pain.
- *The Pill can be used 'continuously' to decrease the number of periods per year.* Fewer periods means less period pain. The Pill can also allow periods to be timed to avoid important events like exams or holidays.
- *The Pill may prevent endometriosis in some women.* An Australian study found that women who had used the Pill for more than five years had a 30 per cent lower risk of endometriosis (see Reference 10).

Newspapers and popular magazines frequently report negative things about the Pill but there are some positives too. Women on the Pill have less period pain, lighter periods, less ovulation pain, less premenstrual tension, more regular periods, fewer pimples and a lower risk of developing cancer of the ovary or uterus. It also provides good contraception.

Although you need to carefully consider with your doctor the side effects of the Pill as they apply to you, women with endometriosis may have a lot to gain from being on it.

How to use the Pill continuously (skipping periods)

Most women who use the Pill continuously still have periods, but their periods are two, three or four months apart rather than one month apart. They time their periods to fit their lifestyle.

If you wish to do this, you will need to use a 'monophasic'

contraceptive pill. Monophasic pills have two different coloured tablets in each packet. There is one colour for the hormone tablets, and one for the inactive or 'sugar' tablets. 'Triphasic' pills have four different coloured tablets in the packet. They are not suitable for continuous use as troublesome bleeding usually occurs.

You should take a hormone tablet every day, with no sugar tablets until you plan a period. When you want to have a period, stop the hormone tablets for seven days, have a period and then restart the hormone tablets again.

If you want to have the longest possible time between periods, take a hormone tablet reliably every day, and wait until bleeding starts by itself. Some women can take the Pill for six months without bleeding, whereas others bleed after only six weeks. Almost all women will start bleeding eventually.

Once you start bleeding, you should stop the Pill for seven days and have a period. You don't have to do this straightaway if you are busy, but until you do have a period the bleeding will probably continue. The bleeding that happens on the hormone tablets is bleeding from the lining of the uterus. It does not take the place of a normal period.

After seven days off the hormone tablets, you should start them again and continue them until either you start to bleed or you choose to have a period. Provided that the hormone tablets are taken for at least 21 days between periods, and there is no more than seven days break between hormone tablets, you are no more likely to become pregnant than women using the Pill with monthly periods.

If you have a special event in mind and want to avoid having a period, it is safest to plan a period a couple of weeks before the event, so that it is unlikely you will be bleeding on the day. With seven days off the Pill, and then another week or so to settle, you will hopefully be pain and bleeding free at the chosen time. Students sometimes choose to have periods only during their holiday breaks.

Other women might choose to have the worst days of their period on a weekend. Remember that if you miss any pills this tells the uterus to start a period, and you may bleed or have pain.

Is it dangerous to use the Pill continuously?

Despite the fact that many women skip periods with the Pill, there has been very little research into this question. If you take the Pill continuously for a whole year without any breaks, then you will have taken an extra three months of tablets during the year. This means that if there are any extra risks, they could be due to a higher hormone dose.

However, almost all the information we have on the Pill and its risks is based on old studies that used pills with 35 to 50 micrograms of estrogen in each tablet. As the newer pills have only 20–30 micrograms of estrogen in each tablet, even if extra pills are taken, the total dose for the year is still no higher than the dose on which our current understanding of risk is based.

It is likely that we will soon have 15 microgram pills that are designed to cause a period every three months. These will provide an even lower total hormone dose than currently possible.

Using the Pill continuously provides *more* reliable contraception than the same pill used with a monthly period.

Endometriosis, prostaglandin pain and premenstrual syndrome

Jackie is a nurse aged twenty-one who suffered pelvic pain on most days of her cycle, but particularly with periods. Premenstrual syndrome (PMS) before her period was straining the otherwise good relationship she had with her family and boyfriend. A laparoscopy showed widespread endometriosis that was completely removed. At review a few months later the pain through the month had gone. This pain had been due to her endometriosis.

The first day of her period was still painful and she still had PMS. Jackie had worked hard at her general fitness and stress management. She felt better able to cope with her premenstrual symptoms and was generally healthier but still moody. Adding the contraceptive pill helped her PMS further, improved the prostaglandin period pain, provided contraception, and allowed her to skip periods. Over time it might provide some protection against further endometriosis. Jackie knows that at her age new areas of endometriosis may develop. However, she feels comfortable knowing that if her pains recur then treatment is available.

Progestogens

Women with endometriosis use progestogen medications partly because they can delay periods and block ovulation, but also because they may make the endometriosis lesions less active.

Progestogens are not the same as progesterone. Progesterone is the hormone made by the ovary in the second half of the menstrual cycle after ovulation. A tablet of progesterone would be destroyed by the acid in the stomach, so synthetic versions of progesterone (progestogens) have been developed which survive in the stomach, and act like progesterone in the body.

The commonly used progestogens include norethisterone (Primolut®), medroxyprogesterone acetate (Provera®), levon-orgestrel (Microval®), dydrogesterone (Duphaston®) and depot medroxyprogesterone acetate (Depo-Provera®).

Many women take progestogens without any difficulty, but others find progestogen side effects unacceptable. Once again, we are all different.

The commonest side effect is 'break-through bleeding', which means vaginal bleeding at irregular and unpredictable times. This may be quite prolonged and persistent. Other side effects include moodiness, bloating, and headaches. Women who are 'progestogen sensitive' describe this feeling as being 'constantly premenstrual'. It was in order to provide the benefits of progestogens without many of the side effects that the levonorgestrel-releasing intra-uterine device was developed (see the following section on page 82).

When taken every day (continuously) progestogens prevent periods, at least in most women, and avoiding periods means less period pain.

If you feel well on the contraceptive pill, you are unlikely to have many side effects with a progestogen medication.

A progestogen used to prevent period pain

Jane is a 43-year-old mother of three children. Five years ago, a laparoscopy performed to investigate her painful periods found endometriosis. Apart from severe pain during her period she was well. Jane started a progestogen medication taken every day and continued it for five years. Over this time she had no periods and no pain. Some women feel moody on progestogens, but Jane felt healthy and was happy that she could avoid the pain.

After five years, Jane noticed vaginal bleeding at odd times that became very persistent. An ultrasound showed a normal uterus with a very thin lining. The normal balance between estrogen (which makes the lining thicker), and progesterone (which makes the lining thinner) had been disturbed. On her tablets Jane had more progestogen than estrogen, and the lining of the uterus had become so thin that it bled easily, much like the thin skin on an old person's hands if they are knocked. There was nothing dangerous about a thin lining but the bleeding was annoying and unlikely to stop until the lining of the uterus became thicker and less delicate.

Jane stopped her progestogen tablets. Her estrogen levels increased, the bleeding stopped and her periods returned. Unfortunately with the return of her periods came the period pain she had avoided for five years.

A progestogen-releasing medication intra-uterine device (Mirena®)

Progestogen medications work well at avoiding periods and decreasing pain, so why are progestogen tablets and injections unpopular? They are unpopular because many women just don't like the way that progestogens make them feel.

Most of these side effects can be avoided by putting a smaller dose of progestogen in the uterus itself, rather than taking a larger dose as a tablet or an injection in the hope that at least some of it reaches the uterus. To get the progestogen into the uterus, it is attached to an intra-uterine device (IUCD) and called a Mirena® IUCD. The progestogen used is levonorgestrel, which is the same medication used in many contraceptive pills.

Yes, you *can* use a Mirena® for contraception, just like any IUCD, but many women use it to lighten their periods. Some women now use a Mirena® to treat their period pain, particularly the pain they have on the first one or two days of a period.

An Italian study looked at whether or not inserting a Mirena® during a laparoscopy to remove endometriosis would give women longer lasting and better relief for their period pain. A year after their laparoscopy, 45 per cent of the women who just had a laparoscopy had bad period pain, whereas only 10 per cent of the women who had a laparoscopy *and* a Mirena® had bad period pain (see References 12 and 13).

Figure 6.3 A Mirena® IUCD diagram

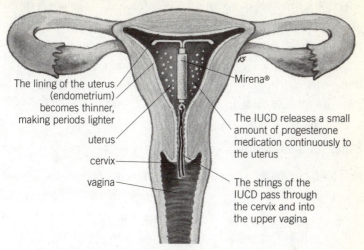

The lining of the uterus (endometrium) becomes thinner, making periods lighter

Mirena®

The IUCD releases a small amount of progesterone medication continuously to the uterus

uterus

cervix

vagina

The strings of the IUCD pass through the cervix and into the upper vagina

A levonorgestrel-releasing intra-uterine device (Mirena®).

If you plan to have a Mirena® inserted, it is important to realise that irregular and annoying bleeding is quite common for the first two or three months after it is inserted. Not everyone gets this, but many women do. Once it settles, there is a good chance that you will have very little bleeding and, it is hoped, less pain. Around 30 per cent of women have no periods at all with a Mirena® IUCD in place.

It is also common to have crampy pains after it is inserted. These pains usually settle within a few days to a few weeks and can be treated with period pain medications (see Chapter 6, page 70).

When the IUCD is inserted, there is a small chance that a pelvic infection may occur. Over time, such an infection may cause pain (see Chapter 9, page 203) or possibly block the fallopian tubes causing difficulty becoming pregnant. If you are considering having an IUCD, talk to your doctor about your individual risk of infection and how an infection can be avoided. This will help you decide whether having an IUCD is a good choice for you.

If you like the Mirena®, it can stay in place and it remains effective for five years. It can then be removed or replaced. If you don't like it for any reason, your doctor can remove it by pulling the strings that pass out through the cervix into your vagina.

In Japan, an IUCD that releases a small amount of danazol to the uterus, rather than a progestogen has been used. This device is not currently available in Australia.

Other medications

Research continues on medications to treat endometriosis. Several types of medications have been suggested, and if your endometriosis has been difficult to manage it is possible that one of these medications might be recommended to you. None of these new medications have been used by enough women for us to know how useful they are, nor what their side effects are. Their use is experimental and generally reserved for those women where more usual treatments have failed. They include:

- Aromatase inhibitors, such as anastrozole and letrozole (see below)
- Anti-estrogen medications, such as tamoxifen or raloxifene
- Anti-tumour necrosis factor (anti-TNF) medications like infliximab
- Medications to discourage new blood vessel formation, such as endostatin and TNP-470
- Medications that affect chemicals called matrix metallo-proteinases
- Medications that affect immunity, such as pentoxifylline.

How do aromatase inhibitors work?
Endometriosis lesions need estrogen to survive. Some of the estrogen they need comes from the ovaries but some is made in the endometriosis lesion itself.

The endometriosis lesion does this using an enzyme called *aromatase* that can convert other hormones into estrogen. An endometriosis lesion likes lots of estrogen and by making its own supply it is able to adapt its environment and promote its own growth. Having the enzyme aromatase also means that an endometriosis lesion can make its own supply of estrogen even after both ovaries have been removed.

As the name suggests, aromatase inhibitors block aromatase and stop the endometriosis lesions from making their own estrogen. In a woman who is through menopause and no longer makes estrogen in her ovaries, this takes away the last supply of estrogen available to an endometriosis lesion.

The major side effects of aromatase inhibitors are bone thinning, tiredness and menopausal symptoms, but there are others. These medications are usually only recommended for women after menopause, but have recently been used in some women before menopause too.

Before considering this medication it is important that you understand the possible side effects and discuss them carefully with your doctor. Aromatase inhibitors are not subsidised on the PBS for endometriosis in Australia, so are expensive to use. They should *never* be taken during pregnancy.

Post-menopausal endometriosis treated with an aromatase inhibitor

The first gynaecologist to report using an aromatase inhibitor to treat endometriosis was a Japanese gynaecologist called Dr Takayama in 1998 (see Reference 11). Dr Takayama treated a 57-year-old woman whose endometriosis had returned even after a hysterectomy, removal of both ovaries, and two extra operations for endometriosis blocking her ureter. Even after this surgery the woman returned with a painful 3 cm endometriosis lesion in the vagina. Because it was in the vagina, the lesion could be easily seen at vaginal examination. Dr Takayama could measure the size of the lesion before and after different treatments to see which treatment was most effective.

Four months of a progestogen medication did not help. The lesion stayed the same size and her pain continued. However, within two months of starting anastrozole (an aromatase inhibitor), the pain had gone. After nine months of treatment the 3 cm lesion had shrunk to 3 mm. To try and minimise bone thinning while on the medication, she was given calcium tablets and a medication called alendronate, which encourages bone formation. Even so, she lost 6 per cent of her bone density over the treatment period. There were no other side effects reported in her case.

Newer aromatase inhibitors in the future may be able to avoid bone thinning.

Chapter 7

Is this your situation?

FACTS ABOUT ENDOMETRIOSIS are one thing, but the most important question is *'What choices do I have now to manage my pain?'* Every woman's situation is different, but this is the question I have tried to answer in this chapter. You may find that one of these sections describes your situation.

The group left out are all the women whose endometriosis has been treated successfully by whatever method they chose. Not surprisingly, most of these women would prefer to forget about endometriosis and get on with their lives.

I am a teenager with severe period pain

Most teenagers have period pain of some sort. For most, this pain is due to chemical substances called prostaglandins that are made by the uterus at period time. Prostaglandin pain is usually quite easy to diagnose. It comes on the first day of bleeding, may be severe, but generally goes away with the Pill, or normal period pain medications if they are taken correctly. A teenager with prostaglandin pain may look quite sick on the first day of her period, yet be fully recovered only a few hours later. This is the pain that is rather unkindly called 'Normal period pain'. It is called 'normal' because the pelvis looks normal at a laparoscopy, *not because it doesn't hurt*. It does.

If you are a teenager, then you will have at least *some* prostaglandin pain, but if your pain doesn't fit the normal picture you may have endometriosis too. You may have worked out already that your pain is different to the other girls. Your friends may argue (very reasonably) that there is nothing 'normal' about their pain, but it is probably not as bad as your pain.

None of us know what another woman's pain is like, but if your pain is *un*-manageable despite the Pill, or period pain medications, then consider endometriosis. It becomes even more likely if you have pain leading up to a period, pain like period pain at other times of the month, severe back pain, pain felt in one spot rather than generally across your abdomen, or pain opening your bowels. Your particular symptoms will depend on where the endometriosis is, so you may not have all these symptoms.

Severe period pain in young women is a bigger problem now than it was in the past. Our grandmothers often had their first baby before they were 20 years old. After that came years spent pregnant or breast-feeding until menopause arrived. Even if their periods were painful, at least they didn't have many of them. Our grandmothers probably averaged about 30 or 40 periods in a lifetime. Prostaglandin pain usually improves after having a baby, so one cause of their pain got better, even if their endometriosis remained.

Girls start their periods earlier now. They delay their first pregnancy and have fewer (if any) children. By 14 years of age, many have had periods for three or four years. They are still girls, but physically they are women. They may have 300 or 400 periods before menopause.

In the past, endometriosis was thought to be rare in teenagers. This is not true. An American study of teenagers with severe period pain, who were no better after trying medications, found that 70 per cent of them had endometriosis (Reference 14). If you have periods, you are *not* too young to have endometriosis.

> **Remember that if you are a young woman who has not had a baby, then at least some of your pain will be prostaglandin pain. So, the questions to consider are: *'Do you have prostaglandin pain with an otherwise healthy pelvis?'* or *'Do you have prostaglandin pain AND endometriosis?'***

If you can manage your pain well with the Pill, a period pain medication or both, then your chance of having endometriosis is low. So, if there are no other reasons to suspect endometriosis, then a laparoscopy is probably not necessary. However, if medications don't help and your pain persists then it is time to talk to your general practitioner or a gynaecologist.

If you do have a laparoscopy and endometriosis is removed, this does not mean you will have no pain. You are still a young woman who has not had a child, so you will still have prostaglandin pain. Removing endometriosis can only help symptoms that are due to endometriosis. What is hoped is that you will have *less* pain and that the pain you have will be easier to manage.

What can I do if my endometriosis has been removed but the first one or two days of my period are still very painful?

This period pain is coming from your uterus. In the old days, you would be advised to have your children quickly then have a hysterectomy. Nowadays, you can almost always manage the pain well with one or more of the following options.

- The contraceptive pill used continuously to cut down the number of periods so you suffer pain less often (Chapter 6, page 77)

- Anti-inflammatory suppositories (Chapter 6, page 171) which seem to work better than anti-inflammatory tablets
- Continuous progestogen medicine to stop periods, either as tablets, a three-monthly injection, or possibly a three-year hormone implant (Chapter 6, page 80).
- A levonorgestrel intrauterine device to provide the benefits of a progestogen without most of the side effects (Chapter 6, page 82). This is a newer treatment, but very promising, and definitely worth considering.
- Complementary therapies to decrease the estrogen effect on your uterus (Chapter 12, page 245)
- Acupuncture
- Working to improve your health and fitness generally – this is always worthwhile. Healthy, happy people have less pain.

A teenager with period pain

Rosetta is a 16-year-old woman who came to see me with several problems. Rosetta had severe period pain for a week before and throughout her period. A similar milder pain bothered her at other times of the month without warning. She noticed spots of blood in her pants at odd times, but especially in the week before a period. Her worst day by far was the first day of her period. The pain was unbearable and she had missed a lot of school.

I explained that there was a good chance that removing her endometriosis would help the pain before her period, the pains during the month and the unexpected spots of blood. These symptoms were probably due to endometriosis. However, the severe pain on the first day of her period was a mixture of endometriosis and prostaglandin pain, so removing her endometriosis would not stop this. She would need other treatment for this pain. It was important that she understood that removing her endometriosis, although worthwhile, would not fix all her pain. Rosetta chose a laparoscopy to remove her endometriosis with a Mirena® inserted at the same time.

Other causes of pain in teenagers

While 70 per cent of the teenagers with severe pelvic pain in the American study had endometriosis, 30 per cent did not. Not all pain is endometriosis, and pain can be a mixture of endometriosis and something else. Chapter 9 describes several other possible causes of pain. These apply to teenagers just as much as older women.

To make everything even worse, many teenagers are stressed or suffer depression. Young women, especially those with chronic pain, often have low self-esteem. They may be studying hard in their last year of school, or feeling anxious about their relationships, their family or their employment prospects. Others struggle with drug or alcohol dependence. The severe distress of sexual assault may also show as pelvic pain. *Just like endometriosis, stress and depression are often missed in teenagers.*

Exercise, maintaining a healthy weight, management of depression, a healthy diet and good self-esteem are so important, especially during the teenage years. While they may not treat the pain, they do prevent many of the other problems that women with pain suffer.

Why has it taken so long to recognise that teenagers get endometriosis?

For many years gynaecologists have been reluctant to do laparoscopies on teenagers. Teenagers were thought too young to have endometriosis. Unfortunately, this is not true. The youngest girl ever reported with endometriosis was ten and a half years old. No woman with periods is too young for endometriosis.

Even when a laparoscopy *is* done, endometriosis in teenagers is often missed. Clear, pink or red areas are much more common in teenagers than the easily seen brown or black lesions. Sometimes, the only abnormality found is an area with extra blood vessels or a pocket in the peritoneum (see Chapter 1, page 8). Endometriosis in teenagers is under-diagnosed.

I know I have endometriosis, but it wasn't removed

This is a very common situation, because many gynaecologists are not comfortable removing endometriosis at a laparoscopy. They have been trained to look for (diagnose) endometriosis, but not to remove it. This is particularly true if your endometriosis is severe.

At a first laparoscopy neither you, nor your gynaecologist, know what (if anything) will be found. If endometriosis *is* found, then your gynaecologist has to consider where your endometriosis is, the skills and resources available to them at the time, and the possible risks involved in removing the endometriosis. If removing endometriosis is not an operation they feel comfortable doing, or the staff, equipment or available time do not permit, then the endometriosis is usually left untreated.

> *This decision should be respected*, because it is not in your interest to have surgery if the conditions are not right. The risk of complications is higher, and it can make later surgery more difficult.

Your laparoscopy has still been useful. You now have a diagnosis for your pain! This is the first step to effective treatment, but on its own will not help your pain. Which treatment you choose now depends on how troublesome your pain is, your own treatment preference and where the endometriosis was found. Unfortunately, it will also depend on the health services available to you.

Endometriosis removed as a two-stage procedure

Danielle is a 17-year-old woman from the country. Her periods were very painful and two days off school every month made it difficult for her to keep up with her schoolwork. A laparoscopy at her local hospital showed endometriosis. Her local gynaecologist recognised that her endometriosis should be removed, but knew that their local hospital was not equipped for such surgery. The extra time needed to recover from a more extensive laparoscopy would also mean even more time off school for Danielle.

Photographs from her laparoscopy were sent to our clinic for review. We agreed that Danielle needed her endometriosis removed and arranged a second laparoscopy in the city during her next school holidays. Danielle used the contraceptive pill continuously to avoid periods while waiting for her surgery.

What can I do about my endometriosis now?

Now you know that you have endometriosis, you can chose to have it removed, or choose to leave it and manage the pain in other ways. You may need to do both, because even removing endometriosis does not always mean that your pains go completely. Equally, endometriosis is not a life-threatening condition (even if it feels like it), so you could choose to do nothing.

Remember that any management choice should be just that. A choice. *Your choice.* Something you have decided on, together with your doctor, because *you* want help with *your* pain. Reasonable options to consider include:

- *A laparoscopy to completely remove the endometriosis, if that is possible.* This is a good option for women who know they have endometriosis. If the endometriosis is not completely removed (see Chapter 7, page 99), then you are more likely to find yourself in this situation again in the future.

- *Endometriosis medications.* There are special medications only offered to women who know that they have endometriosis. You were not eligible for them before your laparoscopy, but you are now. These medications are described more fully in Chapter 6, on page 63. They work best on thin, active areas of endometriosis (the clear, pink or red lesions). They will not remove scar tissue, adhesions, nodules of endometriosis or chocolate cysts. A three to six month course of medication usually gives good pain relief for six to twelve months, but unfortunately pain often returns a few months after stopping the treatment. These medications do *not* improve fertility, and must not be taken while pregnant, so if becoming pregnant soon is your priority don't take them.

- *The contraceptive pill or a progestogen medication used continuously.* Neither medication will remove endometriosis, but they can cut down the number of periods you have each year. As fewer periods mean less period pain, they make it easier to live with your endometriosis. Both options work best for pain with periods or at ovulation. They are less helpful for pain at other times of the month. To have the least number of periods possible on the contraceptive pill, see Chapter 6, page 77.

- *A levonorgestrel intra-uterine device (Mirena®) — see Chapter 6, page 82.* This is a newer option, but one that I believe will become more popular. It works best for pain that comes from the uterus, so might be useful as *part* of your plan.

- *Improved pain management.* Once again, this will not remove your endometriosis, but are you getting the most out of your pain medications? Is there something you haven't tried? Is there a better way of taking it? Your general practitioner can review your medications and offer ideas on what to take, and when. Common pain medications are discussed in Chapter 6, on page 70.

- *Complementary therapies.* This type of therapy is outside my area of expertise, but explained in a thoughtful way by Dr Margaret Taylor in Chapter 12. As knowledge of endometriosis varies widely between different herbal therapists, your general practitioner or endometriosis clinic may be able to recommend someone with whom they deal frequently. Endometriosis management requires cooperation, so pick someone who is comfortable working with your medical team.

- *Acupuncture.* I can only say that some of my patients have found it helpful. I look forward to the results of trials currently under way into acupuncture and period pain.

- *No treatment.* Maybe just knowing what has caused your pain is enough for you. It is important that you feel able to say no to treatment you don't want, whether it is medical, surgical or complementary.

In reality, you will probably need to look at more than one of these options to get the best result for your pain. You will also need to look at the stresses in your life. Period pain on a good day is period pain, but period pain on a bad day is unbearable. You need more good days!

The removal of endometriosis is not a procedure that all gynaecologists offer, so if you decide to have surgery, then now is the time to seek out the best surgical skills available to you. Endometriosis does not change quickly, so you have time. If you do plan to see another gynaecologist, they will need details from your previous laparoscopy. This information might include a copy of the operation sheet showing where your endometriosis is, photos taken at the laparoscopy (if available), or a copy of the letter sent to your general practitioner. If you have any of this information, keep it safely always. If you do not have this information, you can write to your surgeon or hospital requesting copies of the operation sheet. They will need your written, signed permission for this and it takes time, but this information is important. Your new doctor cannot plan your next laparoscopy well without it.

Whether or not a second laparoscopy is successful at improving your pain depends on how completely the endometriosis can be removed, and whether or not there are other causes for the pain.

> **Removing your endometriosis will only treat those symptoms that are due to the endometriosis. Symptoms from other causes will still be there after your surgery.**

Other ideas to improve your pain

- *Are there other health problems I can improve?* Most women with endometriosis have other problems too. These may be physical health problems or life stresses. Fixing any one problem will make it easier to live with the others. Is there something you *can* fix? For example, you may have periods that are heavy as well as painful. Any treatment that lightens your periods means fewer problems to deal with at period time.

- *Look after your mental health.* Any woman with pain benefits from time spent with a counsellor or psychologist. This is why I enjoy working with Jane Marsh so much. She is able to work through many issues that I, as a surgeon, feel ill equipped to handle. Frequently it is the women who were most reticent to see a counsellor who benefit the most.

- *Dietary changes.* Many women with endometriosis complain of bloating and bowel pain. If you already have pelvic pain from endometriosis, then the last thing you need is an irritable bowel to multiply the pain. Margaret Taylor writes on dietary management of pelvic pain in Chapter 12, on page 245 and bloating is discussed in Chapter 9 on page 169. A dietician may be able to check for food intolerances that could be causing your bowel symptoms.

- *Exercise.* Exercise makes us feel better because it releases natural pain killing chemicals called endorphins into our body *and* because it makes us stronger. Remember that the first couple of weeks of exercise just reminds the nerves and muscles how to work well together again. Improved health and strength comes with consistent exercise after this time. Is there exercise you *can* do, despite your pain?

My laparoscopy helped, but now the pain is back

To have had pain go and then come back is pretty depressing. The good news is that your pain improved before. It can improve again and this time, we hope, for longer.

To work out the best treatment for you, it is important to think about why the pain has come back. Generally, it will be for one of three reasons:

1 *Your endometriosis was not completely removed at your laparoscopy, and the remnants have become active again.* Removing endometriosis may be very difficult, so this is common. Cautery certainly reduces endometriosis, but may not remove it completely (see Chapter 7, page 99). Even the best endometriosis surgeons leave endometriosis behind sometimes. They may do this on purpose, particularly if these areas are near delicate structures that could be damaged.

2 *New areas of endometriosis have developed since your laparoscopy.* Endometriosis usually develops over a period of years during your teens and twenties. If you were only partly through this phase of your life at your last laparoscopy, then even after the best surgery new areas might develop. At the first laparoscopy, some of the endometriosis you were destined

to develop had not yet formed. If you have another laparo-scopy now, new areas of endometriosis may be found in areas that looked normal last time. Unfortunately, only another laparoscopy will show whether there are new areas of endo-metriosis or not.

3   *Your pain is due to something else, not endometriosis.* Even if the pain feels similar to your old pain, it is always worth considering if it is a new pain (see Chapter 9).

The first two possibilities both mean that you might have endometriosis in your pelvis again, so the treatment options are the same as those in the earlier section on page 94.

The only difference is that if all your endometriosis *was* truly removed last time and you have now developed new areas of endometriosis, then a three to six months course of a GnRH analogue medication (see Chapter 6, page 66) may be worth trying. The new lesions have only been present a short time, so they are probably small, thin and few in number. These are the lesions most likely to respond to medications. If all goes well with the GnRH analogue, you may be able to avoid surgery. If not, then surgery remains an option.

Alternatively, another laparoscopy may be a good choice *if* the pain you have now is like your old pain, *and* your last laparoscopy really did help you, at least for a while. If your last laparoscopy did not help your pain at all, then consider other causes for your pain.

I think my endo has come back. Again!

Siobhan is a 25-year-old married woman with no children. Her first laparoscopy was done 4 years ago. Endometriosis was found and cauterised, but the pain she suffered for three in every four weeks only improved a little. Within a few months her pain was as bad as ever.

Two years ago she had her second laparoscopy. This time all her endometriosis was completely removed. Her pain was much improved for over a year. There was still pain on the first one or two days of her period, but this was pain from her uterus, rather than pain from endometriosis.

Two years later she returned. She had pain again and felt sure that more endometriosis must be present. A third laparoscopy showed no endometriosis at all. Her pain was now a mixture of bladder pain (see Chapter 9, page 188), neurogenic pain (see Chapter 9, page 177) and anxiety over her ability to have children rather than endometriosis. Siobhan felt relieved that her endometriosis had not returned, and moved on to manage the other causes of her pain.

If you do plan more surgery, it is a good idea to ask your gynaecologist what type of surgery would be done if endometriosis were found. It may be that an area of endometriosis was left behind at your last laparoscopy for a good reason. It may be close to important and easily damaged organs. Your next laparoscopy may be a much larger operation than your first. You need to know what would be involved and what risks there are.

How can I tell if my endometriosis was completely removed?

Complete removal of endometriosis from the pelvis means that at the end of the operation no endometriosis can be found. Endometriosis is removed in one of two ways.

The first technique is called *cautery* or *ablation*. It involves burning the top of any visible endometriosis lesions using electricity, laser or other instruments. It can remove small areas of endometriosis from the surface of the uterus or ovaries well, but is less successful in other areas. There are two reasons for this. First, as endometriosis usually lies close to important organs such as the ureter or bowel, gynaecologists tend to *under*-cauterise, rather than *over*-cauterise any lesions to avoid damaging these organs. This tends to take the top off a lesion but leave deeper areas behind, a bit like an iceberg where only part of the iceberg lies visible above the surface. Second, cautery only treats the spots of endometriosis that can be seen. Microscopic endometriosis in the areas between the endometriosis lesions are not cauterised because they look normal.

The second technique is called *excision* or *excisional surgery*. It can also be done with electricity, laser or other instruments, but rather than burning the top of the lesion, the whole lesion is cut out. With this comes the area of skin (peritoneum) around the endo-metriosis. Any microscopic areas are removed at the same time.

So, if your endometriosis was cauterised or ablated, it may or may not have been completely removed. If it was excised *and* your gynaecologist treated all the affected areas, then complete removal is more likely. *So unless your endometriosis is minor, or lies on the ovaries or uterus, complete removal really means excisional surgery rather than cautery.*

If you are not sure what type of surgery you have had, ask your doctor for details.

What other conditions could be causing my pain?

Other causes of pain in women who have had endometriosis are common. It is very difficult for most women to pick the cause of their pelvic pain because most sensations from the pelvis travel to the brain through similar pathways. This makes it difficult for your brain to decide which part of your pelvis the pain came from.

So, even if your current pain feels similar to the old pain, it may be due to a different condition. You may have two or more causes for your pain. Combinations such as endometriosis and bladder pain (interstitial cystitis), endometriosis and bowel pain, or endometriosis and neurogenic pain are very common. Chapter 9 includes details of how to pick what your pain might be.

The best treatment will depend on the cause of the pain.

Does endometriosis surgery work?

Yes, but not for all women, and not for all pain. An Australian study (Reference 16) asked 176 women to rate their pain as a score between 0 (no pain) and 10 (the worst pain imaginable) both before and after surgery for endometriosis. Period pain scores reduced from an average of 9 before surgery to 3 after surgery. It did not take away all their period pain, but they were certainly better. In women with daily pelvic pain, the pain score fell from 8 to 3, and for women with pain opening their bowels from 7 to 2. The best result was a fall in pain score from 7 to 0 in women with painful intercourse. *These women had expert excisional surgery.* Over a two to five year period, one in three women had further surgery looking for endometriosis, but new endometriosis was only found in two-thirds of these women. The other one-third had pain like endometriosis, but no endometriosis was found.

My endometriosis was removed, but I still have pain

Few things are as disappointing or demoralising as continued pain after an operation you thought would solve your problems. *Why has it happened? Why aren't I better?* In most cases it is a mixture of the complicated nature of pelvic pain, the limitations of surgery and unrealistic expectations (yours or your doctor's) of what surgery can achieve.

This is where the modern management of pelvic pain still needs improvement. As endometriosis surgeons, we have believed that if we could just develop our surgical skills enough, that we could cure our patients' pelvic pain. Sometimes we can, but sometimes we can't. As a surgeon, I believe it is important that I give women a realistic expectation of what can be achieved with surgery. Doctors *want* to help women in pain. They also want to believe that they *can* help women in pain. Women *want* to believe that their pain can be cured. It is easy for unrealistic expectations to develop on both sides. Sometimes the pain *is* gone after surgery, but often an operation is one (important) part of a complete treatment plan. Getting the best results usually means a mix of treatments as well as some lifestyle changes.

Surgery for any condition usually involves *repairing* the body, or *removing* an organ. Even the best repair is just that, *a repair*. Surgery to remove endometriosis can repair the pelvis and, we hope, treat those pains that are due to endometriosis, but it cannot make a new pelvis, nor treat pain from other causes. Even though you had endometriosis this does not mean that this was the only cause for your pain. Not all endometriosis is painful and most women have more than one cause for their pain. This is where it is important to keep in mind the other causes of pelvic pain described in Chapter 9.

What else could the pain be?

Think about your pain. You may notice that your pain is different now. It may come at different times of the month or feel different in some way. Some symptoms may have improved, while others have not. Before your surgery, you may have had two causes of pain, both sending pain impulses to your brain through the same nerve pathways. After your surgery, one cause was removed, but the other cause is still there and is still sending pain signals through the same pathways. Not surprisingly, your brain may feel as though little has changed.

How the brain feels pain and the pain pathways are explained further in Chapter 9, on page 146.

In general, painful periods with good health for the rest of the month might be prostaglandin pain (page 155), adenomyosis (page 151), clot colic or pelvic congestion syndrome (page 198).

Pain present on most days over a long period of time is called *chronic pain*. Chronic pain *and* bladder symptoms might mean interstitial cystitis. Chronic pain that is worse with certain movements or a change in activity may be muscular or joint pain. Pain with a 'burning' or 'sharp' quality may be neurogenic pain and pain with diarrhoea, constipation or bloating may be bowel pain. Adenomyosis can cause either daily pain or period pain.

As well as describing all of these conditions more fully, Chapter 9 also suggests people who can help you with these pains.

Remember that these suggestions presume that there is now no endometriosis left in your pelvis. If your endometriosis was not completely removed, then managing your pain becomes more complicated. To move forward, you need to know what is left and what type of surgery was done. If some endometriosis has been left behind, this does not mean that you have been managed badly by your gynaecologist. It may well have been the best decision at the time considering the skills available and the risks involved.

My doctor said my endometriosis is 'mild', but it still hurts (a lot!)

Catarina is a 38-year-old married woman who would like to have a baby. She has always had painful periods and after two years of trying to get pregnant had a laparoscopy with her gynaecologist. The operation report described only a few spots of endometriosis, but scarring involving both uterosacral ligaments and several adhesions. The brown lesions had been cauterised and some of the adhesions divided, but her pain continued. To me, this usually means that there is more endometriosis present than first realised.

Catarina had no other cause for adhesions apart from endometriosis and yet the amount of endometriosis described did not sound enough to cause so many adhesions. At her second laparoscopy there were a few spots of brown endometriosis, several adhesions around both ovaries, and thick white scarring of both uterosacral ligaments. All the scar tissue, the endometriosis and the adhesions were cut out completely and all showed endometriosis when checked by a pathologist. Whether or not she becomes pregnant will depend on many things (see Chapter 8, page 119), but we hope she will at least have less pain.

How to avoid feelings of abandonment

After all the time spent with your doctors during the diagnosis and treatment of your endometriosis, it is easy to feel abandoned once treatment finishes. Couples who use IVF to become pregnant have similar problems. There is a flurry of activity, but once they become pregnant they are on their own. There is little contact with those people who were once a regular part of their life.

An endometriosis specialist may not offer general gynaecological reviews, and may not feel able to help manage other causes of pain once your endometriosis has been treated. Your general practitioner remains the key to coordinating your care. This is one reason why it is so important to have a general practitioner with whom you have a long-term professional relationship. Some ways to avoid feeling abandoned include:

- An after-treatment appointment with your counsellor, if one was involved with your care. Just because the pain is better, relationships do not always improve, nor jobs become more satisfying.

- A regular monthly visit to your general practitioner until you are truly well. Questions and concerns can be stored up over this time and the stress of 'Do I, or don't I need to see the doctor' is avoided.
- Plan a review visit with your endometriosis surgeon 6 months after your surgery. It will take this long to work out which symptoms are better and which are not, especially if you are spacing periods out with the contraceptive pill. Keep a list of questions ready to ask at your visit. If no endometriosis was found, or your surgeon has nothing more to offer, ask whom you should see for further advice.

Endometriosis is in our family

Some women know all about endometriosis. Their mother, sister, or aunt has suffered and not surprisingly they are worried. Endometriosis *is* more common in families, but just because you have a relative with endometriosis, it does not mean that you will get it too. Even if you do, there is more to offer now.

No-one fully understands how endometriosis is inherited, but some things are becoming clearer.

It seems likely that whether or not a woman inherits a tendency to endometriosis probably involves many different genes. Some things about us (like our eye colour) probably involve only one pair of genes: one gene from each parent. If one of these genes is for brown eyes, then you *will* have brown eyes. There are few other factors involved.

Endometriosis is different. There are probably many genes involved. None of these genes on its own decides whether or not you will get endometriosis, but the more of these 'endometriosis risk' genes you have, the more likely it is that you will. Each gene increases the risk a little. This inheritance is similar to the way asthma or diabetes is inherited in families.

Women with severe endometriosis probably have many 'endometriosis risk' genes. Because they have so many, there is a good chance that their relatives will share at least some of these genes too. This may explain why the chance of having endometriosis is higher if you have a relative with severe endometriosis, than if you have a relative with mild endometriosis. Women with mild endometriosis may only have a few 'endometriosis risk' genes.

Genetics is an exciting area of medicine that is changing rapidly. Within the next few years, it may be able to explain which genes are involved and better predict which women are at highest risk of developing endometriosis.

Whatever our genes, other environmental factors are important too. Some women with endometriosis have no relatives with endometriosis, and other women with a strong family history of endometriosis never have problems.

What is the risk of endometriosis in twins?

An Australian study of twins (see Reference 16) showed that where one *identical twin* had endometriosis, the other twin had endometriosis too 30 per cent of the time. Identical twins share the same genes because they came from the same egg. These results show that our genes play a major part in whether or not we develop endometriosis, but that other factors are important too. If our genes were the only factor, then if one twin had endometriosis, the other twin should have it too in 100 per cent of cases, not just 30 per cent.

Just what these other factors are is not well understood.

If a *non-identical* twin has endometriosis, then the other twin is affected only 10 per cent of the time. This is because non-identical twins only share some genes. Their risk of endometriosis is similar to the risk other children in their family have.

Sisters with endometriosis

Alex was 14 when she came with her mother requesting a laparoscopy. Fourteen is young to have endometriosis, but her pain was severe. Alex herself felt sure of the diagnosis. Her much older sister Valerie suffered severe period pain from the age of 15, but was only diagnosed with endometriosis at 21 when she finally had her first laparoscopy. Before then she was considered 'too young for endometriosis'. Endometriosis has been a continuing problem for Valerie. Alex recognised the symptoms, and wanted to act quickly.

At laparoscopy Alex's endometriosis was widespread and completely removed. She became my youngest patient with endometriosis. Time will tell whether excising her endometriosis completely and promptly, will lessen the major problems her sister has had.

Nothing seems to work for me

Chronic pain despite everything is miserable. This is where endometriosis gets really hard. There is a small group of women for whom no treatment has provided lasting benefit. Over many years their episodes of acute period pain have become daily, chronic pain. Fewer women need suffer this now, but some still do.

If you have severe chronic pain, there is really no choice but to continue looking for ways to improve or cope with the pain. The option of 'just ignoring it' is unrealistic unless your pain is minor. However, there may come a time when you have run out of ideas.

If this is your story, I do not pretend to have all the answers, but the following section has some ideas for a fresh start.

First of all, has all your endometriosis *truly* been completely removed? If you don't know, ask your gynaecologist.

Ideas if you still have endometriosis present

- *Obtain as many details of your previous surgery and endometriosis treatments as you can and seek out the best endometriosis surgeon available to you.* Any surgery now is likely to be difficult.
- *If further surgery is not a realistic option, then consider one of the newer anti-endometriosis medications discussed in Chapter 6, on page 84.* Over time, more information on which of these are effective and safe will become available. There are very few women in whom surgery to remove endometriosis is truly not an option, but the surgery required may be major and does have the risk of significant complications.
- *Review again the options on pages 93–97 or Chapter 9.*

Ideas if all your endometriosis is gone

- *What actually is causing the pain?* Your pain may have started as endometriosis pain, but changed over the years into pain from something else. You are no longer 'an endometriosis patient'. You are a woman with chronic pelvic pain. Read all the types of pain in Chapter 9 and see which fit with your situation. In particular, consider a treatment for neurogenic pain such as low dose amitriptyline (see Chapter 6, page 74), or a treatment for uterine pain such as a Mirena® IUCD (see Chapter 6, page 82). You could try both.
- *Could a pain management specialist or pain clinic help?* Pain management is a specialty in itself. A pain specialist manages chronic pain from many causes, of which endometriosis is just one. He or she has knowledge and medications that are outside your gynaecologist's experience. You will need to take details of your previous surgery with you, particularly those describing your most recent laparoscopy. There are more details on the types of medications used by pain specialists in Chapter 9 on page 179.

- *Are there emotional issues holding back your progress?* No operation or tablet will heal the hurt of infertility, low self-esteem or sexual assault. Tackle the issues complicating your pain. Review your general health, and life stresses. A psychologist, endometriosis counsellor or occupational therapist can help.

- *Is it time to consider a major operation?* Some women only improve after surgery to remove the uterus, any scar tissue, any remaining endometriosis, and sometimes both ovaries. This is a big decision and not reasonable for young women, women who would like to have children, or women who need their uterus to feel good about their body. If you have completed your family, and particularly if you also have heavy periods, an operation such as this may be a good choice. *Remember that a hysterectomy alone, without removal of any remaining endometriosis is not enough.* Before considering an operation such as this you need to feel confident that any abnormal areas in the pelvis will be removed. You must also feel sure that your pain *does* actually have a gynaecological cause. To have a major operation and find that the pain is still present would be disappointing to say the least!

> **A complete cure for chronic pain may not be possible, but worthwhile improvement in the pain almost always is.**

You may find that many of your life goals can still be achieved, even if some of your pain remains. Some occupational therapists specialise in helping people live with chronic pain. They can work with you on what you *can* achieve; to help you maintain or resume the parts of your life that have always been important to you.

It is not surprising that many women with chronic pain become focused on their pain. Many lose sight of the 'non-pain goals' in their life. Before the pain, they had many interests and pleasures. Now there is only the quest for a cure. Maintaining one's personality and appreciation of life is a challenge when confronted with daily pain. Some women succeed. They are inspiring and unsung heroes.

Anger and disappointment after years of pain

Annie is a 45-year-old woman who has always had painful periods. No treatment for her endometriosis had helped. She married at 35, and tried to become pregnant without success. After three failed cycles of fertility treatment, and at 40 years of age, she and her husband decided to accept that a pregnancy was unlikely and stopped trying. Despite knowing that logically she should move on in her life, the bitter disappointment of living without children had never left her. Her experience of medical care had been disappointing, and left her angry. It had delivered her neither pain relief nor children. When we first met, she was angry and suffered daily pain, much worse with periods.

After a discussion of the treatments she had had in the past, Annie felt better. She now understood that although inadequate for her needs, she had at least been offered the best that was available at the time. We discussed what pain management options she had left. These included:

- *A laparoscopy to look for and remove any remaining endometriosis.* At 45 years of age and after previous surgery there was probably no endometriosis left. Her current pain was much more likely to be a combination of adenomyosis, adhesions or neurogenic pain. A laparoscopy alone would only remove any remaining endometriosis, and divide any adhesions. It was unlikely to manage all her pain.

- *A laparoscopic hysterectomy with removal of any remaining endometriosis, any scar tissue, possibly her ovaries, and then the option of HRT if she chose to use it.* Medically, this was the option most likely to help her pain. However, emotionally this would mean confronting her childless state, and putting aside any chance of pregnancy, no matter how small. Annie was a long way from this decision.

- *Medications to improve pain* such as amitriptyline, period pain medications taken regularly, a continuous oral contraceptive pill or a progestogen medication.

- *Referral to a pain management specialist.*

It is important to me as a gynaecologist that women want their surgery. *If they don't want it, I don't want to do it.* Annie was not ready for any of these options. She needed time to think. After speaking with Jane Marsh, Annie decided to work through her emotional needs with a psychologist before considering any surgery. Annie is welcome to return if she chooses to.

Removal of the uterus, ovaries, endometriosis and scar tissue for chronic pelvic pain

Antonia is a 35-year-old woman with a long history of severe endometriosis managed very competently elsewhere. She and her husband, Bill, had healthy six-year-old triplets, conceived using IVF, and no plan for more children. While on a family trip around Australia, Antonia's pain became worse. She always had some pain, but this pain was so severe they were unable to continue their trip. All the surgery possible through a laparoscope had been done. Antonia had thick scar tissue between her bowel, uterus, and ovaries. Despite her young age she felt ready for major surgery. Antonia decided to have a hysterectomy with removal of all her scar tissue, a segment of bowel affected by endometriosis and both ovaries. It was a difficult operation done with the help of a bowel surgeon. All the scar tissue was removed, but the surgery required a large cut on her abdomen. After the operation, Antonia recovered well and left hospital 8 days later. Both estrogen and testosterone replacement medication were started as she was only 35 years old, and her ovaries had been removed. Estrogen replacement avoids hot flushes and other menopausal symptoms. Testosterone replacement avoids the tiredness and low libido common in young women whose ovaries have been removed.

Three weeks after surgery, Antonia developed crampy abdominal pains, vomiting and a swollen abdomen. She was admitted to hospital with a blockage in the bowel (called a 'bowel obstruction'). This settled after a few days of fasting and fluid through a drip. A temporary bowel blockage like this sometimes occurs after surgery near the bowel but usually settles without surgery. We hope it will not recur. Antonia continued on her family trip 6 weeks later with much less pain than before and the promise of no more periods.

Chapter 8

Frequently asked questions

What causes endometriosis?

N O-ONE KNOWS what causes endometriosis, but several possibilities have been suggested.

Most doctors, if asked, will put forward *'Sampson's theory'* which dates from 1921. Sampson noticed that women who had operations during their period often had period (menstrual) blood in their pelvis at the time of their operation. This blood flowed through the fallopian tubes into the pelvis, rather than out through the vagina. This process is called *'retrograde menstruation'* and is normal for most women.

Sampson's explanation was that live fragments of endometrium (lining of the uterus) mixed with the period blood, settled around the pelvic organs, implanted on the surface of these organs and grew into endometriosis. Several factors fitted this theory. It was noted that endometriosis does not occur in girls before menstruation begins, and that endometriosis is more common in those rare women with a blockage in their cervix that prevents their menstrual blood flowing into the vagina normally.

However, there are many factors that do *not* fit with Sampson's theory:

- An endometriosis lesion is *not* the same as endometrium (the lining of the uterus). It is only similar to it in some ways.
- Endometriosis may be found in places outside the pelvis, such as the lung. It is found in rare cases in men who have used estrogen medications to treat cancer of the prostate. Endo-metriosis in these areas cannot be due to retrograde menstruation.
- Genetic tests on areas of endometriosis show that they have a different origin from endometrial tissue from the same woman. If the endometriosis came from cells spread from the uterus, they should be genetically the same.
- Endometriosis usually develops during a woman's teens or twenties, after only a few years of periods. New endometriosis developing after this is uncommon. If Sampson's theory were true, then as time goes by and more periods occur the likeli-hood of new endometriosis should continue to increase.

Sampson lived in 1921, before much of the modern medical knowledge we now take for granted.

So, what other possible causes are there?

Even before the genetics of endometriosis were better understood, came an alternative theory. The *Metaplasia theory* suggests that some cells in the peritoneum lining the pelvis are predestined to change (metaplase) into endometriosis once conditions are right.

Which factors bring about the right conditions? Once again, no-one knows, but one factor appears to be the rise in estrogen level that occurs with puberty. There are probably others that affect in whom and when endometriosis lesions form, but as yet they are poorly understood.

One of these factors probably involves the immune system, but exactly how this happens remains unclear. Women with endometriosis are a little more likely to have illnesses to do with the immune system than other women, but most don't. Research has found other immune differences between women with and without endometriosis too, but so far it has not been easy to put all the known facts together. Research into this area continues.

Another factor may be our environment. Some toxins, such as dioxin (found in air pollution) have been linked to endometriosis.

So which one is the real cause?

It is possible that all these theories have some truth in them.

Endometriosis may be a collection of disorders, each with a different mix of causes. There may be one type of endometriosis due to retrograde menstruation and another due to metaplasia, both influenced by changes in the immune system, the environment and our hormones. Personally I believe that, for most women, their endometriosis is due to metaplasia rather than retrograde menstruation, but many doctors disagree with me on this.

One thing is certain. You cannot 'catch' endometriosis. It is not contagious like an infection, and cannot be passed from one person to another.

What about endometriosis in the rectovaginal septum?

Doctors disagree on how rectovaginal endometriosis forms (see Figure 5.1, page 40). No period blood reaches here, so it is not due to retrograde menstruation (Sampson's theory). Some doctors believe that it is due to metaplasia: that it forms from cells that have been there since birth and then turned into endometriosis when the time was right. Others believe that endometriosis here is really a type of adenomyosis (see Chapter 9, page 151), and thus a different disease altogether.

Can endometriosis be prevented?

Whether or not you believe that endometriosis can be prevented, depends on what you believe causes endometriosis in the first place (see our earlier discussion in this chapter).

If you believe that endometriosis is caused by retrograde menstruation then any treatment that cuts down the number of periods or the amount of blood passing into the pelvis should decrease the chance of endometriosis. Less blood means less opportunity for endometrial cells from inside the uterus to settle in the pelvis.

However, if endometriosis is caused by metaplasia, then the number of periods and amount of blood passed into the pelvis may not matter. Those areas of peritoneum that are destined to become endometriosis in some women will do so, once a suitable environment is present for endometriosis to grow. The only prevention possible is a change in the environmental or immune factors that stimulate the growth of endometriosis. Some of these factors might be changes in hormone levels or avoiding exposure to toxins in our environment. Much more needs to be known about what actually does promote its growth.

The metaplasia theory includes both good and not-so-good news. The not-so-good news is that prevention of endometriosis may not be possible (for now, at least). Endometriosis that is destined to develop will do so if the conditions for its growth are right. The good news is that once an affected area of peritoneum affected by endometriosis has been excised, the peritoneum that grows over the area will be healthy new peritoneum that is unlikely to develop new endometriosis. This is what I see in my patients. In places where endometriosis has been completely excised (not just cauterised) it rarely recurs. Any new endometriosis is usually found in areas of peritoneum that were not removed before, because they looked normal.

Factors encouraging the growth of endometriosis in some women, but not others, are poorly understood. Women with habits that lower estrogen levels, such as exercise, have a lower chance of developing endometriosis (see Reference 10). Regular exercise during the teenage years has other health benefits as well, and is highly recommended.

The Pill may also help. It prevents the high levels of estrogen present during ovulation. So, even though the Pill is an estrogen medication, women who take it often have a lower overall estrogen level than women who do not. An Australian study concluded that women who use the Pill for more than five years have a 30 per cent less chance of developing endometriosis than those not taking the Pill (see Reference 10).

Will my endometriosis come back?

It might, but if it is completely removed, there is a good chance that it will not return.

Many women have been told that 'You can't cure endometriosis — it always comes back'. I do not believe this statement, but I do accept that, even after the best surgery, new areas may form. Understandably, women who have suffered severe pain in the past, then found relief from the pain may worry that their pain will return.

An Australian study (see Reference 15) followed the progress of 250 women for between two and five years after laparoscopic excision of their endometriosis. Of these, 36 per cent had another operation over this time. Another operation was especially likely if their endometriosis was severe at their first laparoscopy. However, only two-thirds of the women who did have more surgery actually had endometriosis found at their next operation. This means that about *one in four* women had new areas of endometriosis develop over this time.

Personally, I believe that the likelihood that new areas of endometriosis will develop after it has been removed is higher in younger women.

I believe that most endometriosis develops during a woman's teens and twenties. If her endometriosis is removed *after* all the endometriosis she was destined to make has formed, then it is unlikely that new areas will grow. She may develop pain from a different cause (see Chapter 9), but new areas of endometriosis itself are uncommon.

However, if her laparoscopy was done *before* all her endometriosis had formed, then the chance of finding new areas at a second laparoscopy is higher. Her first operation could only remove the endometriosis that was visible at the time. When new endometriosis forms, it is usually found in the areas that looked normal last time, rather than in the areas treated at her first operation.

> **So, the younger you are when your endometriosis is first diagnosed and removed, the higher the chance that new areas of endometriosis will develop in the future. The older you are when your endometriosis is removed, the lower the chance that *new* areas of endometriosis will form.**

All of this presumes that the endometriosis has been removed completely. Endometriosis that has been cauterised or laser ablated (rather than laser excised) may improve for a short time, but is more likely to recur. Some women have many laparoscopies, each with cautery, a short improvement and then a recurrence of their pain. This is why many people believe that endometriosis always comes back. Cautery remains a useful treatment for lesions on the surface of the ovaries or uterus, or very thin lesions elsewhere.

When a woman who has had endometriosis in the past gets pain, it is often presumed to be due to endometriosis. This may or may not be true. The pelvis feels many pains in a similar way, so it is easy to be confused about what is actually causing the pain, especially when it is a mixture of different pains. A woman such as this is described in Chapter 9, on page 187, and information about other causes of pain are also described in Chapter 9.

Recurrence of endometriosis in a young woman

Simone came to see me first when she was 22. Her periods were irregular and painful. A laparoscopy showed endometriosis, which was completely removed, and her pain improved. Taking the contraceptive pill made her periods regular and avoided the prostaglandin pain that is usual in most women without children.

Three years later, Simone returned for review. Her pain was coming back despite the contraceptive pill. A laparoscopy showed new areas of endometriosis but only in areas that were normal the first time. The areas removed previously looked healthy. The new endometriosis was once again removed completely and her pain became manageable again. It is hoped that she has now produced all the endometriosis she is destined to develop, and there will be no further recurrence.

Will I be able to have children?

Many women with endometriosis fall pregnant easily. However, others find it difficult to become pregnant. Why?

Becoming pregnant is a complex process. Endometriosis is one factor not in your favour when trying to become pregnant. However, there are so many other factors involved that, if everything else is normal, you may never have a problem becoming pregnant. These other factors include the quality of the man's sperm, the woman's age, whether or not she ovulates each month, and whether or not her fallopian tubes are open.

Most couples who find it difficult to become pregnant have either severe endometriosis present, or other problems apart from the endometriosis.

Possible problems might include a low sperm count, or irregular periods with infrequent ovulation. When two or more 'minor' problems add together, becoming pregnant becomes much harder to achieve. For example, a common situation is a woman with mild endometriosis, and a man with a slightly lower than normal sperm count. Neither problem is severe on its own, but together the chance of becoming pregnant becomes less.

However, even couples with a mixture of fertility problems do become pregnant sometimes. I almost never say that pregnancy is impossible, just unlikely without help.

Once a woman does become pregnant, endometriosis will not hurt her baby. All pregnancies have a chance that the baby may not develop normally, but endometriosis does not increase this chance.

How does endometriosis affect fertility?

This depends on how severe the endometriosis is.

For many years, doctors have disagreed whether mild endometriosis with no scarring of the pelvis has any effect on fertility at all. Although some doctors still believe that mild endometriosis has no effect, most believe that it does affect fertility, but are unsure why. Several possibilities have been suggested. These include a changed environment for the egg or sperm, an effect on ovulation, a toxic effect on the newly formed embryo, or an effect on the hormones made by the ovary.

When there is severe endometriosis present, it is easy to understand how fertility could be affected. It can cause scarring that can block the fallopian tubes, prevent normal ovulation, or prevent the fallopian tubes picking up the egg once it is released. It can also make intercourse too painful to consider. Luckily, most women with endometriosis do not have scarring like this.

Can treatments for endometriosis improve my fertility?

Most doctors believe that an operation to remove any endometriosis, whether it is mild or severe, does improve fertility. The chance of becoming pregnant increases by about 40 per cent after surgical removal of endometriosis, and the first six months after the operation seem to be a particularly fertile time.

So, if your endometriosis is removed, you may be able to avoid the need for more complicated fertility treatments such as IVF. Even if IVF is still required, it is more likely to be successful if your endometriosis is removed first.

Medical therapies such as danazol, GnRH analogues or progestogens (see Chapter 6) *do not* improve fertility. They also take up valuable time, because pregnancy must be avoided during treatment.

What is JVF?

In-vitro fertilisation (IVF) means fertilisation of the egg by sperm in a laboratory, rather than in the body. Eggs are collected from the woman, and a semen sample is collected from the man. The eggs and sperm are mixed together in a dish, allowing the sperm to fertilise the eggs. Between one and three fertilised eggs are then inserted into the woman's uterus.

Becoming pregnant normally is a complex process. Sperm must be deposited in the vagina, penetrate the mucus in the cervix, travel up through the fallopian tubes, and penetrate the outer covering of an egg. There must be an egg ready for the sperm to fertilise. The fertilised egg must then travel back down the fallopian tube to the uterus and implant there.

IVF can help if there are problems with any of these steps.

Low sperm count and endometriosis

Angela is 32 years old. She and her husband Tom began investigation of their fertility after a year of trying to conceive was unsuccessful. Tom was found to have a very low sperm count. Angela ovulated regularly. No laparoscopy was done as Angela had only mild period pain, and it was thought that Tom's low sperm count was their only problem. However, after three unsuccessful cycles of IVF, Angela's fertility doctor wondered if there might be some endometriosis present and referred her to me for a laparoscopy. Although Angela had very little pain, a laparoscopy showed several areas of endometriosis that were then completely removed. Her fallopian tubes were normal and open. Angela and Tom will still need IVF due to his low sperm count. However, their chance of a successful pregnancy with each IVF cycle is increased now that her endometriosis has been removed.

When to ask for investigation of infertility

When you want to become pregnant, every month that goes by feels like one month too many. You may have friends who all seem to get pregnant easily, or all seem to be having babies. It is very stressful waiting to see if you will become pregnant, and worrying that there may be a problem.

Even if all your friends do seem to become pregnant easily, many couples don't. The chance of becoming pregnant after one month of intercourse without contraception is actually only 20 per cent. This means that only one in five couples will become pregnant after one month without contraception. After 12 months of trying, four in five couples will have become pregnant. That means that after a year, one in five couples will be disappointed.

If you have not become pregnant after 12 months of trying to do so, you may wish to discuss your fertility with your doctor. Although some couples would become pregnant without help if they waited another year, 12 months is considered a good time to start any investigations.

However, if you or your partner already know of a reason why becoming pregnant might be difficult, you may wish to talk to your general practitioner or gynaecologist earlier. Irregular periods, a known low sperm count, or where the woman is over 35 years of age are good examples of this.

When is the best time of the month to get pregnant?

Pregnancy is most likely if you have sex at ovulation. This is the time when the ovary releases an egg and you notice a large amount of clear, stretchy, jelly-like mucus. Intercourse every couple of days around ovulation time is enough because your partner needs to replenish his semen count between times.

How can I tell if I am ovulating?

A month where an egg is released from the ovary is called an *ovulatory cycle*. Some women know they are having ovulatory cycles. They have all the telltale signs. Others are less sure, or don't know what to look for.

Think about your periods. Ovulatory cycles are usually regular. This means that the number of days between the first day of one period and the first day of the next period is about the same each month. Ovulatory cycles are usually between 21 and 35 days long.

> **If you have *regular* periods, the day when ovulation should occur can be worked out by the formula:**
> Day of ovulation = Cycle length − 14
> If your period comes every 28 days, then you probably ovulate on day 14 (28 − 14 = 14).
> If your period comes every 35 days, then you probably ovulate on day 21 (35 − 14 = 21).

Check your vaginal mucus. Ovulatory cycles have clear, plentiful and stretchy vaginal mucus for two or three days leading up to ovulation. This change is due to rising estrogen levels. After ovulation the mucus becomes less, whiter, and thicker.

Measure your temperature every morning. A temperature chart filled in each morning shows a 0.2–0.5 degree increase in body temperature after ovulation. Although this is an effective way to tell if ovulation has taken place, I don't recommend temperature charts because this daily reminder of infertility is emotionally stressful and time consuming. A progesterone blood test taken seven days before a period is more reliable and simpler.

Have your progesterone level checked. Progesterone is a hormone made by the ovary in the second half of a normal ovulatory cycle, *if* an egg has been released from the ovary that month. In cycles where no egg is released, there is no progesterone hormone made by the ovary. A blood test for progesterone, taken seven days before a period starts, will tell if ovulation has occurred that month or not. If ovulation did occur, the progesterone level will be high. If ovulation did not occur, the progesterone level will be low. The blood test result only applies to the month in which it is taken. It does not tell whether you will ovulate next month or not.

I have irregular periods. Can I become pregnant?
Some women don't ovulate as regularly as others. They still ovulate but it doesn't happen on the same day each month. This makes

predicting ovulation a bit trickier, but pregnancy is certainly possible. There may be some months where no egg is released at all. These are called *anovulatory cycles*. All women have anovulatory cycles sometimes, but some women have them more often than others. Remember that even women with very few periods ovulate sometimes, so pregnancy is not impossible, even if there have been no periods for some time.

Professor Robert Jansen's book *Getting Pregnant* has detailed information on all aspects of fertility (see Reference 17).

I have endometriosis and don't want to become pregnant. Do I need contraception?

Yes, definitely. If you do *not* want to become pregnant you must use reliable contraception. Never presume that your endometriosis will prevent a pregnancy, even in a very scarred pelvis.

If less reliable methods of contraception have worked well for you in the past, they may not be as reliable once your endometriosis has been removed. Your fertility may increase and you may need to review your contraception.

An unplanned pregnancy after removal of endometriosis

Cassandra is a 30-year-old single farmer. Her periods were regular, and very painful. Although very keen to avoid a pregnancy, she and her partner used condoms, without spermicide, for contraception. Cassandra had used this contraception successfully for years, and was unwilling to consider a more reliable method. A laparoscopy to investigate her period pain found moderate endometriosis, which was completely removed and her pain improved.

Six months later, Cassandra came back for review. She was two months into an unplanned pregnancy, and one month after a split with her boyfriend. Fertility improves after removal of endometriosis even in those who don't want it. After a lot of thought, Cassandra continued with the pregnancy alone.

If you are young, and not even thinking of children for now, you should presume that you could get pregnant easily. If you do have problems one day, we are lucky enough in Australia and New Zealand to have good fertility services available. All women are advised to have babies earlier rather than later if they are socially able to do so, because fertility does decrease with age. This applies to all women, not just those with endometriosis. Leaving pregnancies until you are in your late thirties will work for some women, but will leave others disappointed. As a general guide, it is time to start thinking about pregnancies once you turn thirty.

Will I need a hysterectomy?

Most women with endometriosis do *not* need a hysterectomy.

A hysterectomy is an operation to remove the uterus. It is not a treatment for endometriosis because these lesions usually lie outside the uterus. Removing the uterus but leaving endometriosis behind is unlikely to make your endometriosis go away, and may not help your pain.

However, there are other causes of pelvic pain that a hysterectomy *does* treat well. These causes include adenomyosis (see Chapter 9, page 151), prostaglandins (see Chapter 9, page 155), and pelvic congestion (see Chapter 9, page 198). They all cause pain that feels similar to the pain of endometriosis, but is in fact coming from the uterus. Many women have both endometriosis *and* pain from their uterus. Removing the endometriosis is still the best treatment for endometriosis, but adding a hysterectomy is one way of treating pain from the uterus as well.

A hysterectomy becomes even more reasonable in women who have no plan for future pregnancy, but have other conditions such as heavy periods or troublesome fibroids (see page 128). There are also a few women with very severe endometriosis in whom surgery is easier when the uterus is removed at the same time as their endometriosis.

Even so, you should never feel that you have to have a hysterectomy. With modern surgical techniques, it is almost always possible to remove the endometriosis without removing the uterus. In general, a hysterectomy in women under the age of 35 is rarely necessary. Women who wish to conserve their uterus, for whatever reason, should be able to do so. Their pain management may be more difficult in some cases, but neither adenomyosis, nor prostaglandin pain, are life-threatening conditions. Unless you have a cancer you never have to have a hysterectomy. Even heavy bleeding with periods can usually be managed in other ways. A hysterectomy should always be a choice, made by you, after consideration of the options available.

Women who have never had serious pelvic problems find it hard to believe that a woman would ever want to lose her uterus. Many women who have suffered for years can't wait to do so. We are all different, and our views on hysterectomy depend on our age, fertility, cultural background, and life experience.

Some women choose a hysterectomy, even if this is not absolutely necessary. Their lives have been dictated by pain and bleeding. Social activities depend on the time of the month. Holidays are difficult or impossible. They wish to move on in their lives, and leave periods behind. This is entirely reasonable. Very few women in this situation regret their decision. The vast majority of such women comment afterwards: 'I should have done it years ago.' Hysterectomy remains a popular operation for women with period pain, heavy periods and completed families.

> **Remember that a hysterectomy alone does not remove endometriosis. If the uterus is removed, but the endometriosis is left behind, your pain may continue.**

What is the difference between a hysterectomy and a 'full' hysterectomy?

Actually there is no difference. A hysterectomy is an operation to remove the uterus. The ovaries are conserved.

The word 'full' is often used by non-medical people to describe an operation where both the uterus *and* the ovaries are removed. This is not correct. A full hysterectomy (from a medical viewpoint) means a hysterectomy where both the cervix (lower part of the uterus) and the body (upper part of the uterus) are removed. This is distinct from a 'partial' or 'subtotal' hysterectomy where the body of the uterus is removed, but the cervix is left behind.

If the ovaries are removed, the operation is called a 'bilateral oophorectomy'. Bilateral means both sides. If the fallopian tubes are removed at the same time, it is called a **bilateral salpingo-oophorectomy**. So, an operation where the uterus, both fallopian tubes and both ovaries are removed is described as a 'hysterectomy with bilateral salpingo-oophorectomy'. If you are having a hysterectomy, you should be clear what will be removed and what will be kept.

What are fibroids?

Fibroids are tumours that grow in the muscle wall of the uterus. Only about 1 in 1000 fibroids are cancerous, so almost all are benign (not cancerous). The medical name for a fibroid is *leiomyoma*, and they are sometimes called *myomas*. Fibroids are common. Up to 30 per cent of women will have fibroids by the time they are 40, but many of these are small and not significant.

Fibroids vary a great deal in size. They range from less than 1 cm to several cm across. Fibroids only need removal if they cause symptoms such as heavy periods, or pressure on nearby organs like the bladder or bowel.

The site of the fibroid is very important. A woman with a small fibroid on the inside of her uterus may have very heavy periods, despite its small size. A woman with a large fibroid on the outside of the uterus may have normal periods, but notice pressure on her bladder or bowel.

Hysterectomy after years of pain

Briony is a 45-year-old housewife. Her only painless period was her first one, more than 30 years ago. Over the years, her pain had been treated in many ways, but never with lasting relief. Her first child was conceived easily, but she required IVF assistance for the second. After years of severely painful periods, often requiring pethidine injections, she was completely worn out by pain. We talked about the options:

- Do nothing and hope that menopause brought relief soon.
- Have a laparoscopy to remove any remaining endometriosis. This would improve the part of her pain due to endometriosis but not pain from the uterus itself.
- Six months of danazol or a GnRH analogue medication. This was unlikely to provide long-term relief, but would improve her pain for six to twelve months.
- A laparoscopic hysterectomy, with removal of any endometriosis present, but conservation of her ovaries.
- Investigation of complementary therapies.

Briony chose a hysterectomy. She was sick of the pain, and sick of the effect her pain had on her family. Some old endometriosis was found over one ureter. Her previous surgeon had left this area of endometriosis alone, due to its difficult location. Her pelvis was otherwise normal. The endometriosis was removed, and sent to pathology. The pathologist found adenomyosis too (see Chapter 9, page 151). Her pain had evolved over the years from prostaglandin and endometriosis pain as a young woman, through to old endometriosis and adenomyosis pain. Either way, it was all gone, and she was relieved. Briony described the operation pain as no worse than a period, but unlike a period, this pain would not come again.

Should my ovaries be removed?

In most cases, no.

Ovaries are important organs. They make hormones for wellbeing, and eggs for pregnancy. If your ovaries are healthy and you are not close to menopause then they should be kept, unless there are good reasons to remove them.

In the past, it was common for gynaecologists to recommend removal of both ovaries in woman with even mild endometriosis, to bring on an early menopause. It was hoped that this would cure her endometriosis. The endometriosis itself was left behind, but it was thought that the low estrogen levels of menopause would remove the endometriosis without surgery. This type of treatment is now much less common.

Removing the ovaries worked for some women, but sometimes caused more problems than it solved. The areas of endometriosis left behind sometimes continued to cause pain, and the symptoms of early menopause (low estrogen hormones) were often severe. When estrogen hormone medications were taken to help the menopause symptoms, the endometriosis left behind often became active again, and the pain returned.

It is now almost always possible to remove endometriosis from an ovary without removing it. The ovary is 'repaired'. Repairing the ovary means removing the endometriosis and conserving as much of the ovary as possible. Small areas of endometriosis on the surface of the ovary can be cauterised. Chocolate cysts (Figure 5.2, page 45) inside the ovary can be removed with an operation called a *cystectomy*, and adhesions around the ovary can be divided. However, this surgery may be very technically challenging, and sometimes the endometriosis recurs.

Removing one or both ovaries, if they are seriously affected by endometriosis or adhesions, decreases the chance that you will need more surgery in the future, but can affect your fertility, and cause an earlier menopause. If only one ovary is removed, the other will take over the job of both ovaries, but if both ovaries are removed menopause will occur.

Whether or not your ovaries should be repaired or removed depends on several factors including your age, your plans for future pregnancy, and your personal preference. There are advantages and disadvantages with both treatment plans.

However, if your ovaries *are* to be removed, then the endometriosis should be removed too. You can then use the hormonal medications that you (as a young woman) need to feel well, with a lower chance that the endometriosis will recur. Once you reach the normal age of menopause (45 years of age or older), you can decide whether or not to continue your hormonal therapy, just as women who have never had endometriosis do.

Every woman's situation is different, but this is a guide to how I manage decisions about ovaries in my practice:

A young woman having her first laparoscopy

A young woman not only needs her hormones, but also does not know what her future plans for pregnancy may be. Personally, I never remove an ovary in a young woman at her first laparoscopy. I am usually able to remove all her endometriosis, with a cystectomy if necessary. If I am unable to treat all her endometriosis myself, I will remove those areas I can treat completely. If necessary, I will arrange a second laparoscopy performed together with a bowel or bladder surgeon. I do not remove ovaries in young women who are not expecting to have their ovaries removed.

A woman less than around 35 years of age, who has had a laparoscopy before and knows that she has severe endometriosis affecting her ovaries — or a woman over 35 who plans future pregnancies

The ovary can almost always be conserved, but this type of surgery requires specialised laparoscopic surgical skills. I always try to conserve as much normal ovary as possible. Occasionally, there are women whose pain is unlikely to improve without removal of a very severely damaged ovary. If so, after careful discussion, she may decide that the most severely affected ovary should be removed, and the least affected ovary be conserved. However, this is quite uncommon. Young women need their ovaries.

Before removing an ovary, I need to be sure that there is no other useful option available, that her pain is truly coming from that ovary, and that other causes of pain have been excluded. Remember that endometriosis is not a life-threatening condition, so there is time to consider what you want done.

A woman of approximately 35 to 45 years of age, with no future plans for pregnancy

Where healthy, I believe that the ovaries should still be conserved. They will provide hormones until menopause.

However, when the ovaries are seriously damaged by endometriosis or adhesions, I will occasionally remove one ovary if she has explained beforehand that she would be happy with this choice.

Some women are happy to leave the decision on whether or not to remove one ovary (if damaged) to my judgement at the time. Neither she nor I know exactly what will be found during her operation. We agree that I will not remove either ovary if they look healthy, but that if they are badly damaged by endometriosis, scar tissue or adhesions, I may remove one of them. I will repair and conserve the better of the two ovaries, and remove the one that looks most damaged. I will, of course, remove any other areas of endometriosis present, wherever possible.

Some women want both ovaries kept, regardless of whether or not they are severely damaged while others want both ovaries removed even if they look normal. They may have suffered repeated ovarian cysts or have cancer of the ovary in their family. It is always a question of balancing the different priorities.

A woman over 45 years of age

As normal menopause usually occurs between the ages of 45 and 55 years, removing the ovaries in this age group, and therefore hastening menopause, is less important from a medical point of view. Of course it may still be important for her body image. If a laparoscopy is needed, some women *choose* to have their ovaries removed, even if they look healthy, to decrease the chance of developing cancer of the ovaries in later life (see Chapter 8, page 136). This is a personal choice. If both ovaries are removed, then hot flushes usually start within a few days. Hormone replacement therapy (HRT) is available, if desired, to treat these symptoms.

A woman who is already past menopause

The ovaries are now no longer making estrogen hormone. Few women in this age group need a laparoscopy, but if they do I offer to remove their ovaries to decrease the risk of ovarian cancer in later life.

It is important to be sure *before* your laparoscopy, that both you and your gynaecologist understand what surgery will be done if severe endometriosis involving the ovaries is found.

No matter how damaged they are, whether or not an ovary is removed remains your choice. Different women make different decisions. This is why it is important that your doctor knows what your preferences are before your surgery begins.

Will menopause cure my endometriosis?

No, but your symptoms should improve.

After menopause, when estrogen levels fall, endometriosis usually becomes much less active. If your main problem has been period pain, you will probably find menopause a relief. Other symptoms associated with a normal monthly cycle such as menstrual migraine, hormonal mood swings and premenstrual syndrome should also resolve.

However, occasionally endometriosis does cause troublesome symptoms after menopause, even in women who do not use hormone replacement therapy. Scar tissue can affect nearby organs such as the ureter or bowel.

Using estrogen replacement therapy (HRT) after menopause can stimulate any endometriosis that remains to become active again and cause symptoms. Your body likes the estrogen replacement, but so does the endometriosis! This does not always happen, but it can make whether or not to use HRT an even more difficult decision than usual.

If your menopausal symptoms are severe, you may choose to start HRT, but stop it if your pains return. If you are already on HRT, it may be worthwhile reviewing it with your general practitioner every year or so, to see if a lower dose would be enough for you.

Endometriosis blocking the ureter after menopause

Katherine is a 53-year-old mother of three grown-up children a few years past menopause. In her forties a hysterectomy for heavy but not painful periods had been unexpectedly difficult. Her gynaecologist found many adhesions throughout her pelvis for which no cause was known. Several years later, Katherine developed pain on the right side of her pelvis. Katherine rarely complained, but this pain had been difficult to cope with. A laparoscopy showed that the right ovary was very firmly stuck to the side wall of the pelvis, just where the ureter lies. A large part of the right ovary was removed, but a piece that lay over the ureter was left to avoid damaging the ureter. Review of this tissue by a pathologist showed it to be endometriosis. We now had a reason for the scar tissue found at her hysterectomy many years before. Katherine had had severe endometriosis without pain, without any effect on her fertility and without realising it.

The pain on her right side improved for a few months, but then returned, higher up, near the kidney. An investigation called an IVP showed that the ureter on her right side was partially blocked. Urine could not pass easily from the kidney to the bladder. Katherine had another laparoscopy, this time with a kidney doctor (urologist) present to help. The blockage was caused by the remaining piece of scarred ovary pushing on the ureter. The rest of the ovary and all the surrounding scar tissue were removed through the laparoscope and her pain went away. We thought that would be the end of her problems, but a year later, the pain was back and another IVP showed that the ureter was again blocked. An operation through a large cut removed a golf-ball-sized amount of endometriosis from over the ureter and the ureter was re-attached to the bladder in a different position. Katherine has stopped her HRT to decrease the chance of more endometriosis. Will it come back again?

We don't know.

I have had a hysterectomy for endometriosis. What is the best form of HRT for me?

There is no one 'right' answer to this question, so I will explain what the issues are.

Most women on HRT take two hormones: an estrogen that makes them feel well and a progestogen that protects the uterus from cancer. After a hysterectomy, the uterus no longer needs protecting, so taking a progestogen becomes unnecessary. Estrogen can be taken by itself. This 'estrogen-only HRT' is very popular as it is the progestogen that makes some women feel 'premenstrual' and the progestogen that may increase the risk of heart disease and breast cancer. So, for most women who choose to take HRT after a hysterectomy, including those with mild endometriosis, an estrogen without a progestogen is probably the best choice.

The difficulty comes in women who have had severe endometriosis in the past, especially those whose endometriosis has not been removed. Taking estrogen without a progestogen *might* increase the chance that the endometriosis becomes active again after menopause and *might* increase the small chance of cancer in the endometriosis that remains. Then again, it might not. Until we know more about how endometriosis responds to both these hormones, it is impossible to say what is the best HRT for women who have had severe endometriosis after hysterectomy.

Will my endometriosis become cancer?

Usually, no. Endometriosis is a benign condition, which means that it is not a cancer. So, for almost all women, the answer is *'No'*.

However, there are two less common types of ovarian cancer that are more common in women with endometriosis. These two types of cancer are called 'endometrioid' and 'clear cell' cancers.

The words 'endometrioid' and 'clear cell' describe what the cancers look like under a microscope.

If these cancers are found, it may be impossible to know whether the cancer started in an area of endometriosis, in the ovary, or in the peritoneum near the ovary. As these cancers usually develop in older women, it has usually been many years between the diagnosis of endometriosis and the diagnosis of ovarian cancer. This is one reason why it is has taken such a long time for doctors to realise that there is any link between endometriosis and ovarian cancer at all.

Although this information is disturbing for women with endometriosis, it is not all bad news. Developing cancer in an area of endometriosis is still unlikely, and, cancers that do form in an area of endometriosis have a higher survival rate than other ovarian cancers.

Cancer of the ovary is difficult to diagnose as there are no good screening tests for it, and it usually causes few symptoms until it is quite advanced. This is why some older women who are having pelvic surgery (for whatever reason) sometimes choose to have their ovaries removed at the same time, even if the ovaries are normal. Removing the ovaries does not completely remove the risk of cancer, but it does make it much less likely.

How common is cancer of the ovary?

In Western countries, approximately 1 in 70 women develop cancer of the ovary during their lifetime. However, this risk may be around 1 in 40 for women with severe endometriosis affecting their ovaries (see References 18 and 19).

The risk of ovarian cancer is also increased in women with a close family history of ovarian or breast cancer. Some of these women have a particular genetic abnormality found on blood testing. Women with this type of genetic abnormality sometimes choose to have both ovaries removed once they have completed their family to decrease their risk.

What happens if cancer is found at my laparoscopy?

In rare cases, a woman having a laparoscopy for what is thought to be a benign (not cancerous) cyst is found to have what looks like a cancer. The gynaecologist must then decide what surgery to do. In my practice, if abnormalities are found which could be a cancer, I choose to take a biopsy (very small piece) of the abnormal area for a pathologist to check under a microscope, and do no further surgery that day. My patient wakes up having had a very short laparoscopy, from which she recovers quickly. We wait for the pathologist to decide whether or not it truly is a cancer, and if so, what type it is. If it is a cancer, then depending on what it is, the appropriate treatment is offered and the woman can contribute to the decision making herself.

Cancer in an area of endometriosis

Elizabeth is a 59-year-old teacher who had a hysterectomy and removal of both ovaries 20 years ago for management of her endometriosis. Her gynaecologist planned to remove both ovaries and any endometriosis, but there were so many adhesions present, and her operation was so difficult, that a small piece of ovary with some endometriosis was left behind on the left side.

Twenty years later, Elizabeth noticed a pain in her back on the left. She thought it was backache, but a scan of her spine looking for arthritis found a 7 cm lump in the left side of her pelvis.

The lump was removed and found to be an 'endometrioid' type of ovarian cancer. There was no evidence of any cancer spread at her operation. Whether the cancer developed in an area of old endometriosis or in the small piece of remaining ovary is impossible to tell. Elizabeth had chemotherapy, which she tolerated well, and has returned to teaching. She is well.

What about complementary therapies?

Many women ask me this question. I have no training, nor experience, in complementary therapies so my opinions are those of a scientifically trained person who knows that modern medicine does not have all the answers, and remains open to new treatment options. This is why I am so pleased that Dr Margaret Taylor, a very experienced complementary therapist, has written Chapter 12.

Many of my patients tell me of the benefits they notice with complementary therapies, especially with regard to the hormonal changes they notice during the month. I am pleased for them, and happy with their choice. However, I feel nervous about recommending things I do not understand, so leave advice on these options to their natural therapist.

Do I think complementary therapies work?

Just like surgery and the medications that I might prescribe, I think they work for some women and for some problems. Complementary therapists see women for whom modern medicine has failed, and I see women for whom complementary therapies have failed. By working together, there is a good chance we can help most women. At our clinic we offer surgery, medications, counselling, lifestyle advice and links to complementary therapists we feel comfortable with.

For a doctor to say that any treatment 'works', we are required to have 'proof'. What does 'proof' mean? It means different things to different people, but I will try to explain what it means to a doctor.

Basically it means that large, well-designed trials have proven that the treatment is both safe and effective. In medicine we have been through times when it was enough for one or more doctors working with a medication to say that they thought it worked. This is no longer acceptable for medical treatments. Trials investigating the old claims have shown some to be true and others false. The improved knowledge the trials have provided has allowed us to move forward to better and more effective treatments over time.

Trials of any treatment usually divide a group of women into two groups. Half the women are given the herbal (or other) treatment and half are given a dummy treatment that looks the same (called a placebo). Neither group knows whether they are taking the real treatment or the dummy treatment. At the end of the treatment period, the number of women who feel better (or have had side effects) in each group are compared. The more women involved in the trial, and the more carefully the trial is run, the more reliable it is likely to be. Using a dummy tablet (placebo), allows for the fact that some women will get better by themselves over time with no treatment at all.

Trials such as these also look for side effects and safety issues for any treatment. If a herbal therapy can change the body enough to improve health, then it may also be able to cause side effects, even if these only affect very few people. To believe otherwise seems naïve, especially as throughout history some herbs have been used as poisons.

Have any herbal trials been done so far?

Yes. More and more herbal and diet therapy trials are being done, although as yet few involve treatments for endometriosis. These trials have shown a mixture of results. Some have shown clearly that herbal treatments are both effective and safe. For example, the nausea of pregnancy *is* less in women who use ginger supplements. The symptoms of arthritis *are* improved with Glucosamine.

Cranberry juice *has* been shown to decrease urinary tract infections and Evening Primrose Oil *can* improve sore breasts.

Other trials have shown no benefit for some treatments. For example, a Chinese herbal formulation was found to be no more effective than placebo for the hot flushes of menopause (see Reference 20).

What is more concerning is that some herbs have been linked to serious illness. For example, lead poisoning has been reported after the use of Ayurvedic (Indian) herbs; and black cohosh, despite its widespread use, has been associated with severe liver damage in very rare cases.

This is why the advice of an experienced herbal therapist is so important. For now, it is the personal advice of your herbal therapist and the quality of the place they source their herbs from that you will be relying on. The value of the care you receive will depend on their expertise and commitment to continued learning.

Whether it is surgery, medications or complementary therapies, we must all be honest with women about what we can and cannot achieve for them. If complementary therapies can improve our success in managing pelvic pain, then whatever they are, they are welcome. I look forward to any new ideas that improve the suffering of women with endometriosis. However, proof of effectiveness and information about side effects is the standard we should expect from whatever health care we choose. The challenge for complementary therapists is to work out which treatments (or combination of treatments) are truly effective and which are not, just as we have done in medicine. Once proven, these treatments will be rapidly accepted just as cranberry juice and glucosamine have been.

Over the next few years, the management of endometriosis will continue to change. New options for treatment will emerge and others will lose favour. Some of these new treatments may well come from areas considered as alternative today.

Which complementary therapies do I prefer?

As a scientifically trained person, before I can accept a new treatment, I need to understand how it *might* work, even if few details are available now. As I believe herbal therapies to be medications, I find it easy to accept that some herbal therapies do help endometriosis and the pain it causes. Equally, acupuncture and dietary therapy are based on sound principles. However, I find it very difficult to see any logical basis for homeopathy, where ingredients are diluted so extensively that no original product remains.

Then again, I have many friends (all dedicated to their homeopathic remedies) who will laugh at me for saying this!

Chapter 9

. . . .

What else could the pain be?

NOT ALL PERIOD OR PELVIC PAIN is endometriosis. Some women realise this when their laparoscopy shows a normal-looking pelvis with no endometriosis, and they are left wondering what to do about their pain. Their pelvis may *look* normal but it still hurts!

Others realise it after their endometriosis has been removed. Some of their symptoms improve, while others do not. Endometriosis was only one of their problems.

It is now time to look at other causes for your pain. Although these are common, you are now in a difficult position. Some of these conditions have only recently been shown to cause pain. Medical knowledge on how best to diagnose and treat them is improving, but is not yet complete.

In addition, no area of medicine covers all the possible conditions you may have, so there is no single professional who can offer everything you need. Some women spend years looking for the cause of their pain and a way to manage it. Distressingly, many never find the answers they need.

I suggest that this is where *you* may be able to help yourself. Each of the common causes of pelvic pain has its own fairly distinctive features. You are the one living with your symptoms every day, so with some information on what to look for, *you* may be able to work out what the problems are more quickly than your doctor can. You can at least bring up possibilities for discussion.

Recognising your pain from among those described in this chapter may point you in the right direction for the help you need, always bearing in mind that not every woman fits the normal picture for each condition. Once you have an idea about what your problem may be, then your general practitioner is the person who can help you put together a plan. Your general practitioner knows what services are available in your area. They can also help if your symptoms don't quite fit anywhere.

When thinking about your pain, consider what time of the month you get the pain, what makes it better, and what makes it worse. Your pain might be *cyclical*, which means that it occurs each month at a particular time of your menstrual cycle. Ovulation pain or period pain fit this pattern. Alternatively, your pain may be *chronic*, which means that it is long-term pain present on most days of the month. Remember that you may have more than one cause for your pain.

Some examples

Women with severe *period* pain after their endometriosis has been completely removed might have prostaglandin pain, adenomyosis, clot colic or pelvic congestion syndrome. None of these conditions show at a laparoscopy.

A woman with *chronic* pain after her endometriosis has been completely removed might have adenomyosis, neurogenic pain, interstitial cystitis, irritable bowel syndrome, adhesions, a pelvic infection or a mixture of these.

A woman with pelvic pain *after* a hysterectomy and removal of both ovaries might have neurogenic pain, more endometriosis, adhesions, interstitial cystitis, an ovarian remnant, or bowel pain.

The causes of pain described in this chapter include:

1 Pain from the uterus — adenomyosis, prostaglandin pain and clot colic
2 Pain from the bowel — irritable bowel syndrome, bloating, food intolerance and constipation
3 Pain from adhesions
4 Pain from nerves — neurogenic pain
5 Pain from muscles or joints — myofascial pain
6 Pain from the bladder — interstitial cystitis
7 Pain from ovaries — ovulation pain, functional ovarian cysts and ovarian remnant syndrome.
8 Pain from veins — ovarian vein syndrome and pelvic congestion syndrome.
9 Pain from the appendix
10 Endosalpingiosis
11 Pelvic infections — pelvic inflammatory disease.

It is easier to understand the different types of pain if you understand how we feel pain and what *referred pain* is, so this is described first in the section 'How we feel pain'. This background information is especially useful if you have chronic pain.

Is my pain just stress? Am I just weak?

No. You will notice that stress was not included as a cause of pain. We all know that stress can worsen a pain that already exists, but it is rarely the cause of the pain. A headache when you are happy and rested is a headache. A headache after a bad day, when you are tired and unhappy is unbearable.

Almost everyone nowadays has stress of some kind. Stress is a part of being human, rather than a weakness that should be hidden or denied. A certain amount of stress is useful. It keeps us motivated and active. Stress becomes a problem when it becomes overwhelming or impossible to resolve. Women with endometriosis have many reasons to be stressed.

How we feel pain

Imagine your finger touching a hot stove. The nerves in your finger notice the pain quickly and send pain signals from your finger to the brain. To reach the brain, the pain signal travels along a nerve to a part of the spinal cord called the *dorsal horn*. It then travels along another nerve up the spinal cord to the brain. It is when the pain signal reaches the brain that we feel pain.

Whether or not you notice the pain depends on how strong the pain signals are. A burn hurts a lot. It sends strong pain signals up to the brain, which acts rapidly to move your finger away from the stove.

There are always calming signals coming down from the brain telling us to ignore unimportant sensations such as clothes against our skin, or the normal function of body organs. A burn hurts so much that it quickly overcomes these calming signals and we feel pain. The normal filling and emptying of the bladder is an example of a slower, less urgent type of pain.

We do not notice our bladders filling until they are reasonably full because of the calming 'ignore bladder' signals coming down from the brain. Once there are more 'full bladder' signals going up to the brain than 'ignore bladder' signals going down to the bladder, we realise it is time to empty our bladder, but know that there is no hurry to do so. If we are doing something interesting at the time, we can still ignore our bladder, at least for a while. As the bladder fills even more, it becomes increasingly difficult to ignore, and the urge to empty the bladder becomes even stronger.

If there is a urine infection in the bladder, it becomes more irritable and sends 'full bladder' signals up to the brain even when it is not very full. The calming 'ignore bladder' signals are overcome much earlier than normal and the urge to pass urine comes more quickly. Because of this, women with a urine infection go to the toilet more often than usual. Equally, if you are anxious, there are fewer calming 'ignore bladder' signals going down to the bladder and the need to pass urine also comes earlier. Most women need to go to the toilet more often if they are anxious.

This is a good example of the interplay of emotions and pain. Anxiety does not cause a full bladder, but means that we notice the full bladder more. This is true of any unpleasant sensation. Our brain is more able to ignore it when our general physical and emotional health is good, and we send more calming signals down from our brain to whatever part of the body is painful.

Referred pain

Referred pain is pain felt in one part of the body, when the cause of the pain lies somewhere else. Why does it happen?

The spinal cord is divided into levels, one for each segment of the spinal cord. These segments have a name according to their position on the spinal cord (cervical, thoracic, lumbar or sacral) and a number within that area. For example, the first level in the lumbar part of the spinal cord is called L1, and the second level in the sacral part is called S2.

At each level of the spinal cord, two nerves feed into the dorsal horn. One of these nerves comes from an area of skin or muscle, and the other nerve comes from an organ inside the body such as the uterus, heart or diaphragm. For example, at the 10th thoracic level (T10), the dorsal horn receives one nerve from an area of skin and muscle over the lower abdomen, and one nerve from the uterus.

If a pain signal passes through either one of the two nerves that enter the spinal cord, it spreads to the other nerve as well. The brain becomes confused and cannot decide where the pain came from. Was the pain from the skin and muscle, or was it from the organ inside the body? If the brain cannot decide, it feels pain in both places, or sometimes just in the area that is actually normal and pain free. Pain felt in the area that is normal is called 'referred pain'.

There are several examples of this. During a heart attack, many people feel pain in their chest (via the nerve from the heart) *and* pain down their left arm (via the nerve from the skin and muscles of the arm). Both these nerves go into the spinal cord at the same level. There is nothing wrong with the skin and muscle of the arm, but the brain is confused and feels pain in both areas.

Another example of referred pain is the shoulder pain some women get for a few days after a laparoscopy. There is a segment of the cervical spinal cord in the neck (C4) that receives nerves from both the diaphragm *and* an area of skin over the shoulder. If a small amount of the gas used during the laparoscopy settles near the diaphragm and irritates it, pain is felt just below the ribs where the diaphragm is, but also in the shoulder. There is nothing wrong with the shoulder but the brain becomes confused and feels pain in both places. Sometimes the pain is only felt in the shoulder. When the gas near the diaphragm disappears, both pains go away.

Levels T10, T11, T12, L1, and L2 of the spinal cord receive nerves from both the abdominal wall over the lower abdomen or thighs *and* the pelvic organs. This means that pain in an area of the abdominal wall can cause referred pain deep in the pelvis. Equally, a pain in the pelvis can cause referred pain in the muscle wall of the abdomen or the thighs.

Other types of pain

Whether we feel 'touch' or 'pain' depends on how strongly the nerves in an area are stimulated. Light stimulation is felt as touch, and strong stimulation felt as pain. When pain has been present for a long time, structural changes in the nerves can affect the way a nerve sends pain signals. Eventually even light touch becomes painful, as the nerves that notice pain become more sensitive. In the pelvis this means that sensations that are not usually painful, such as normal bowel function become painful. This process is called *allodynia*.

Long-term pain can also cause *hyperalgesia*. This means that things that have always been painful become even more painful. The nerves that carry pain signals send more signals than usual when something painful happens. Once again, this is due to structural changes in the nerves.

Severe pain can also cause *wind-up* pain. This means that pain signals coming into one part of the spinal cord spread to levels of the spinal cord above or below that level. The brain then finds it even more difficult to know where the pain is coming from. Several levels are involved and the pain spreads to a larger area than before. For pelvic pain, this means that pain sometimes spreads above the navel on days when the pelvic pain is severe.

Wind-up pain

Lesley is a 38-year-old woman from the country. She had always had painful periods, but things were getting worse. Lesley had pelvic pain on most days, but the first day of her period was particularly painful. On these days she had a burning pain above her navel as well as her normal pelvic pain. Lesley agreed that the higher pain only happened on the days that her pelvic pain was severe. Burning pain often means neurogenic pain (see page 177).

When Lesley had a laparoscopy, endometriosis was found in her pelvis, but her upper abdomen was normal. Yes, she had pain from the endometriosis in her pelvis, but when this was bad, the pain impulse spread to nearby areas of her spinal cord (wind-up pain) and she felt the pain above her navel as well. To manage her pain, Lesley will need treatment for her neurogenic pain as well as her endometriosis.

1 Pain from the uterus

Adenomyosis, prostaglandin pain and clot colic

Pain from the uterus itself is the reason why removing endometriosis from around the pelvis does not always help period pain. Women who expected all their period pain to go after their surgery are often disappointed. They (and possibly their doctor) did not understand that before their surgery they had two types of pain: endometriosis pain *and* uterine pain.

What sort of pain is uterine pain?

Uterine pain occurs on the first one or two days of a period. The uterus is a hollow organ made of muscle. When the muscle tightens (contracts) at period time, it causes a cramp-like pain that comes and goes every few minutes. Between these contractions there is little pain. The pain may be referred to the thighs (but not past the knee) or into the lower back when it is severe. Uterine pain is felt across a large area in the centre of the lower abdomen. If your pain is felt in one small area, or on one side of the pelvis then other causes for your pain are more likely.

Pain during the month is less common but possible. If it is uterine pain, then it should worsen as a period comes closer and go away in the week after your period.

Some women with bleeding between periods notice that whenever they bleed, they get pain that feels like a period. As the lining of the uterus bleeds it stimulates the muscle of the uterus to contract, which sometimes causes pain. If the irregular bleeding from the uterus can be stopped, these pains usually improve.

> **There are three main causes of uterine pain: adenomyosis, prostaglandin pain and clot colic.**

Adenomyosis

Adenomyosis might be new to you. While many women have heard the word endometriosis, few know about adenomyosis even though the two conditions are similar. While endometriosis is lesions that look like the lining of the uterus lying *outside* the uterus, adenomyosis is lesions that look like the lining of the uterus lying in the *muscle wall* of the uterus (see Figure 1.1, page 6).

Just like endometriosis, women with adenomyosis have painful periods. Some have pain through the month that worsens as the period comes closer. Others have heavy periods or pain with intercourse. The uterus is often a little enlarged, and your doctor may have described this as 'bulky'. A uterus may be bulky for other reasons, but adenomyosis and a bulky uterus often go together.

Endometriosis usually forms during a woman's teens and twenties, while adenomyosis usually forms during her thirties and forties. However, like most things in medicine, this is not always true. Occasionally quite young women are found to have adenomyosis, and certainly older women can develop new endometriosis. If your symptoms are like endometriosis, but none is found, then adenomyosis is a possible cause for your pain. Remember that you could have both conditions.

How is adenomyosis diagnosed?
Adenomyosis is difficult to diagnose because it lies in the muscle wall of the uterus between the inside and outside surfaces.

- A *hysteroscopy* (an operation through the vagina to look at the inside lining of the uterus) is usually normal, but will occasionally show tiny gland openings.
- A *laparoscopy* to look at the outside surface of the uterus is usually normal too, but will occasionally show an uneven texture in a bulky uterus. The major benefit of a laparoscopy is to exclude other causes of pain such as endometriosis or adhesions.
- An *ultrasound scan* done using a probe in the vagina on a high quality ultrasound machine may show a pattern of mottling in the wall of the uterus that is described by doctors as a 'rain in the forest' appearance. Even so, most ultrasounds are normal. If the adenomyosis forms a round lump in one part of the muscle wall it is called an *adenomyoma* and may look like a fibroid (see Chapter 8, page 128).
- *Histology* is the only reliable way to diagnose adenomyosis. Histology means that a pathologist has checked the uterus with a microscope. As this is only possible once the uterus has been removed it means that some women decide to have a hysterectomy for their symptoms without knowing whether they actually have adenomyosis or not.

What can I do about my adenomyosis?

The treatment of adenomyosis depends on your priorities. Putting together the right treatment plan for you means thinking about all your symptoms, your plans for future pregnancy and your personal preference.

Possible treatment options include:

- *No treatment.* Adenomyosis is not life threatening, so any treatment is optional.
- A *levonorgestrel releasing intra-uterine device (IUCD)* (see Chapter 6, page 82). This device makes periods lighter, and

sometimes improves the pain. If, once inserted, it does not suit you, then your doctor can remove it.

- *Progestogen* tablets or a progestogen injection to stop periods (see Chapter 6, page 80).
- *Anti-prostaglandin medications* (see Chapter 6, page 70) for period pain.
- *Danazol* in a low dose of around 200 mg daily. This makes periods lighter and less painful but is not a long-term solution (see Chapter 6, page 64).
- *The Pill*, taken continuously to avoid periods (see Chapter 6, page 77). If you do use the Pill, then choose one that is low in estrogen or with a slightly higher progestogen dose.
- *Laparoscopic surgery* to remove an adenomyoma. This is only suitable *if* the adenomyosis lies together in an easily found lump. The operation can be done through a laparoscope, but it is a much more difficult operation than a hysterectomy.
- *Natural therapies.* As described in Chapter 12, these aim to reduce estrogen dominance to make the adenomyosis less active.
- *Hysterectomy.* Most women with adenomyosis are over 35 years of age. Many have no further plans for pregnancy, and may have other gynaecological problems such as fibroids (Chapter 8, page 128) or heavy periods. For these women a hysterectomy to remove the problem permanently is a common and very reasonable choice. Obviously this is not suitable for young women, or those planning a future pregnancy.

If you are very close to menopause, you may decide to wait. When menopause arrives your estrogen levels will fall and any adenomyosis will probably become less active. For most women, their symptoms improve substantially at this time. Then again, if you choose to use HRT after menopause, your estrogen levels will not fall, and the adenomyosis will enjoy the hormones just as much as the rest of your body.

Who can help me with adenomyosis?

- Your gynaecologist. All gynaecologists can insert an intra-uterine device, prescribe medications for you, or do a hysterectomy. However, it takes a skilled laparoscopic surgeon to remove an adenomyoma without doing a hysterectomy.
- Your general practitioner can prescribe medications for you and may be able to insert an intra-uterine device.
- A natural therapist may be able to help some of these symptoms if they have expertise in this area.

A levonorgestrel IUCD for adenomyosis

Diane is a 34-year-old single woman who would love to have a baby one day. Her periods were painful and heavy. A laparoscopy showed no endometriosis but a larger than normal uterus. A high quality ultrasound showed some 'mottling' in the wall of her 'bulky' uterus. Adenomyosis was the most likely diagnosis. Diane had always felt sick on the Pill, and was definitely not ready for a hysterectomy. She decided to try a levonorgestrel-releasing IUCD. Six months later her periods were light. The pain had improved too. Diane still used pain medications each month but was now confident that she could manage her pain. The IUCD can be removed when she is ready to have a baby.

Adenomyosis and hysterectomy

Saskia is a 40-year-old mother of two, working in an engineering office. Looking back, she had been very unsympathetic to friends with painful periods. Periods were never a problem for her, and she couldn't see what all the fuss was about. However, over the last two or three years her periods had become both painful and heavy. The pain was now severe, and an unexpectedly heavy bleed during a meeting with her male colleagues had left her embarrassed. Adenomyosis seemed much more likely than endometriosis.

Saskia had completed her family. She wished to spend time with them, without the pain and inconvenience of her periods. She chose a hysterectomy with conservation of her ovaries. Her ovaries will continue to make hormones for her so no hormone replacement is needed, but she knows there will be no bleeding and no period pain.

Prostaglandin pain

Prostaglandins cause the cramp-like period pain that makes a teenager's life so difficult on the first day of her period. They cause pain in some older women too, especially if they have never had children.

If the prostaglandins affect the nearby bowel, there may be bowel cramps or diarrhoea. If they spread to the rest of the body they may cause fainting, a slight temperature or nausea. Prostaglandin pain is better on the Pill or normal period pain (anti-prostaglandin) medications.

Just as the lining of the uterus (endometrium) can make prostaglandins, so can endometriosis lesions. This may be one of the ways in which endometriosis causes pain.

How is prostaglandin pain diagnosed?

There is no special test for prostaglandin pain. Prostaglandins do not change the appearance of any pelvic organ, so there is nothing unusual to see on an ultrasound scan, a laparoscopy or a hysteroscopy. These investigations only exclude other conditions such as endometriosis, adhesions or ovarian cysts. No blood tests are helpful.

However, if you have pain on the first day of your period that improves or goes away with anti-prostaglandin medications then they are the likely cause.

Why were my periods painless for the first few years?

When a girl first starts her periods, they are usually irregular. This means that they come at unpredictable times. Her body is mature enough to have periods, but not mature enough to release an egg from the ovary each month (that is, ovulate). These irregular periods are called *anovulatory cycles*. Over the next one to four years, as her body matures further, she will begin to ovulate each month and change to *ovulatory cycles*.

Ovulatory cycles are more painful than anovulatory cycles because more prostaglandins are released. So, as a girl's body matures, her periods become more regular but also more painful. As the Pill stops ovulation in most women, it usually helps this pain.

There are some women who never develop a regular cycle. They ovulate some months, but not others. The months where an egg is released are painful, while other months have no pain.

What can I do about prostaglandin pain?

Some medications prevent prostaglandins being made, and so treat the cause of the pain. They include:

- *Anti-prostaglandin medications* (see Chapter 6, page 70). Anti-prostaglandin suppositories work better than tablets but must be prescribed by a doctor.
- *An oral contraceptive pill.* A Pill that is low in estrogen but higher in progestogen is best for period pain. Using the contraceptive pill to skip periods (see Chapter 6, page 77) means fewer periods and less pain.

- *Progesterone only contraceptives.* Contraceptives that use only progestogens usually work well. These include the 'Mini-pill', Implanon®, and Depo-Provera®.
- *A progestogen releasing intra-uterine device* (see Chapter 6, page 82). This provides a progestogen directly to the uterus with only a small amount absorbed to the rest of your body.
- *Other pain tablets* such as paracetamol, codeine and Tramal®. These do not treat the cause of the pain. They make your brain less conscious of it. Tablets that include doxylamine, such as Mersyndol® are useful for night-time pain relief. They should not be taken during the day if you will be driving or operating machinery in case they make you sleepy.
- *Acupuncture.*

Although having a baby does help some women with prostaglandin pain, there are other treatments for prostaglandin pain, and there is no guarantee that your pain would improve.

Fainting and severe pain once periods became regular

Ashleigh is a thin, fine boned, 19-year-old dancer. She had her first period at 14, and for two years her periods were irregular but not painful. Once her body matured and she began to ovulate each month, she suffered severe period pain especially on the day that bleeding began. The pain came suddenly, with little warning. With the pain came fainting so severe, that twice strangers had to call an ambulance when she collapsed. Ashleigh felt sure she must have endometriosis but a laparoscopy showed a normal pelvis. Although relieved that her pelvis was normal, her 'prostaglandin pain' needed management. Anti-prostaglandin medications work best if taken 12 to 24 hours before the pain starts and continued until the pain has settled. Ashleigh felt unable to time this reliably, so decided to use the Pill and have periods only every three months. This at least cut down the number of periods per year from twelve to four. Using the Pill, she could plan when her period would be, and take her anti-prostaglandin medications at the right time.

Who can help me with prostaglandin pain?

- Your general practitioner.
- A gynaecologist.
- An acupuncturist if they have expertise in this area.
- A natural therapist if they have expertise in this area.

Clot colic

Clot colic is a special type of period pain found in women with *heavy periods*. With the heavy bleeding come clots of blood and cramp-like pains. Once a clot is passed the pain improves, just as the pain of labour goes away once a baby is born. Clot colic only happens on the days you have clots. Pain on days when you bleed lightly is not clot colic.

A similar type of pain that is much *less* common can occur in women with a very narrow opening through their cervix. This is called *cervical stenosis*. Menstrual blood cannot pass through to the vagina easily and the uterus contracts forcefully to push it out.

What can I do about clot colic?

Any treatment that makes periods lighter will help clot colic.

In the past, women with heavy periods had few choices. Once their family was complete, many had a hysterectomy to solve the problem. Hysterectomy is still an option for women who have no future plans for pregnancy, but your gynaecologist now has other options to offer you. These newer techniques include:

- *Tranexamic acid.* This tablet is only taken during the heavy days of your period. It makes periods lighter by closing some of the blood vessels in the uterus, preventing them from losing as much blood. The best dose varies — 2 tablets, taken 4 times daily on the heavy days of your period gives the best results, but can make some women feel nauseous. A lower dose of 1 tablet 3 times daily is better tolerated if nausea is a problem. Women with a history (or family history) of blood clots in the legs or lungs should not take this medication.
- A *levonorgestrel-releasing intrauterine device (IUCD)* (see Chapter 6, page 82). This releases a small dose of progestogen medication to the lining of the uterus every day. This thins the lining of the uterus making it less able to bleed. It can be removed later if you wish to become pregnant
- *The contraceptive pill.* This makes periods lighter.
- *An endometrial ablation.* This operation destroys the lining of the uterus, making it less able to bleed during a period. It is *not* suitable for women who wish to become pregnant in the future.

Who can help me with clot colic?
- Your general practitioner.
- Your gynaecologist.

2 Pain from the bowel

Irritable bowel syndrome (IBS), bloating, food intolerance and constipation

There are many causes of bowel pain, but the commonest are irritable bowel syndrome (IBS), bloating, food intolerance and constipation.

What type of pain is bowel pain?

The bowel is a hollow muscular organ (like the uterus), so one type of bowel pain is a cramp-like pain that comes at regular intervals. The bowel contracts forcefully, much as it does if you have diarrhoea. If it is the lower bowel (called large bowel) that is affected, then the pain is felt below the navel. If it is the upper bowel (called small bowel) that is affected, then the pain is felt around the navel or sometimes above it.

Another type of bowel pain is a constant aching pain, often in the lower left side of the abdomen (near sections of bowel called the *sigmoid colon* or *rectum*), or in the lower right side of the abdomen (near a section of the bowel called the *caecum*). These types of pain are especially common in women with constipation. This type of pain is easy to confuse with ovarian pain, adhesions or endometriosis.

The most typical feature of bowel pain is that the pain improves once a bowel action has been passed. There are usually other bowel symptoms too, which might include diarrhoea, constipation, a need to strain to open your bowels, a feeling that the bowel is never empty, an urgency to use your bowels, the passage of mucus from the bowel, excessive wind or bloating.

Bowel pain occurs at any time of the month, not just with periods, but some women do find that their bowel symptoms are worse before a period.

Irritable bowel syndrome (IBS)

You may have already realised that IBS and endometriosis are easy to confuse. They cause similar pain in similar places. Many women who thought for years that their pain was due to an irritable bowel get better once the endometriosis they never knew they had is removed. Others who thought that all their symptoms were due to endometriosis feel much better once their IBS is treated.

IBS is a 'syndrome', which means that it is a collection of any of the bowel symptoms described above, all loosely put together under one name. Some women with IBS have a tendency to diarrhoea, while others tend to constipation. Very few women have all these symptoms, so your IBS symptoms may be different to those of your friend's.

What causes IBS symptoms?

There is still a lot to learn about IBS, but it may be due to a change in how the nerves in the bowel work. Some of these nerves are 'motor' nerves that control how the bowel *moves*. A change in these nerves causes constipation, diarrhoea or a combination of the two. Other nerves are 'sensory' nerves that control how the bowel *feels*. A change in these nerves causes bloating, excess wind, a feeling that the bowel is never empty or urgency before the bowels are open.

Do some foods affect IBS?

Yes. For some women, there are particular foods that make their symptoms worse. Some of these foods are described on page 165. Other women never find a particular food to which they are sensitive, but know that eating a healthy, low fat, low salt, low caffeine and high fibre diet suits them best. This is, of course, the type of diet we should all eat for many reasons, not just our bowels. However, women with IBS respond to food in an exaggerated way, so while a large fatty meal can upset anyone's stomach, it will upset a woman with IBS more.

Even women without IBS often find that a healthy diet improves some aspects of their pelvic pain. If you have endometriosis, then the last thing you need is bowel pain too, so diet is important.

How is IBS diagnosed?

IBS is really common, so if you have any of these bowel symptoms then it is likely that at least *some* of your pain is due to IBS.

However, before presuming that *all* your symptoms are IBS you should realise that it is what doctors call a 'diagnosis of exclusion'. This means that IBS can only be diagnosed after all other causes for the symptoms have been excluded. In young women, this may mean excluding endometriosis with a laparoscopy, or excluding other bowel conditions with blood tests, breath tests, X-rays, an endoscopy or a colonoscopy.

A laparoscopy cannot diagnose IBS as an irritable bowel looks the same as normal bowel through a laparoscope. Remember that many women have endometriosis *and* IBS.

What are a colonoscopy and an endoscopy?

The letters *-oscopy* in a medical word mean to have a look inside something with a telescope. A *lapar*oscopy means to look inside the abdomen and an *arthr*oscopy means to look inside a joint (often the knee). To check the bowel, a bowel doctor (gastroenterologist) uses slim, flexible telescopes. When they are passed through your mouth into the stomach and upper bowel, the procedure is called an *end*oscopy. When they are passed through the anus into the lower bowel, the procedure is called a flexible sigmoidoscopy or a *colon*oscopy. Both tests can be done with a light anaesthetic, so you need remember nothing and have no pain. Ask your doctor which technique they use.

Important symptoms to tell your doctor

Some symptoms should always be reported to your doctor straight-away. These include any bleeding from the bowel, bowel inconti-nence, getting up in the night to empty your bowels, unexplained weight loss, or malabsorption of food. Your doctor will also want to know if anyone in your close family has had bowel cancer.

Malabsorption of food means that food travels through your bowel without being digested properly. The bowel actions (faeces) are pale, smelly, and float. These are not the symptoms of irritable bowel, and may mean a serious bowel disorder. They need investigation.

Women over 50 hardly ever develop IBS for the first time, so if you are over 50 and your bowel habits have changed, you should see your doctor straight away. There are many innocent conditions that can cause this, but a cancer of the bowel needs to be excluded.

What can I do about IBS?

First, make sure that it actually *is* IBS:

- *Tell your doctor about any of the important symptoms on page 162.*
- *Consider whether you could have coeliac disease, fructose intolerance or lactose intolerance.* See page 165.
- *Check your medications and herbal supplements.* Antibiotics, antacids, laxatives, thyroid supplements or some blood pressure tablets can worsen diarrhoea. Amitriptyline, iron tablets, painkillers, tranquillisers and other blood pressure tablets can worsen constipation. Many herbal therapies affect the bowel. Your doctor or herbal therapist may have an alternative medication you can use.

Then try some of these suggestions. They won't all be right for you, but some will:

- *Lifestyle changes.* This means avoiding things that make your symptoms worse, like alcohol and stress. Eating regular meals in an unhurried way and getting enough sleep are good for your bowel. The nicotine in cigarettes irritates the bowel, so if you smoke, then now is always a good time to quit.

- *A better diet.* Just as you have more to lose from a bad diet than other women, you have more to gain from a good diet. Your bowel likes a healthy, low fat, low salt, low caffeine and high fibre diet.

- *Diet advice for particular symptoms.* If you have indigestion or burping, then avoid chocolate, alcohol or coffee. If you have an easily irritated stomach, then tomatoes, citrus fruits, alcohol, and spicy foods are best avoided.

- *Eat more fibre.* A Western diet rarely has enough fibre for our bowels. Most women (but not all) feel better eating more fibre, but you should start it slowly.

- *Care for your bowel bacteria.* It is the bacteria in our bowel that help us digest our food. Some foods contain live bacteria and may help some symptoms. However, there is still a lot to learn about which bacteria help which symptoms. These bacteria enjoy a high fibre diet so increasing the amount of fibre you eat will encourage them to work better for you.

- *Complementary therapies.* Herbal teas, and slippery elm are commonly used for IBS symptoms. Peppermint oil capsules taken 3 or 4 times daily half an hour before meals often helps abdominal pain and bloating, but can aggravate indigestion.

- *Manage your stress.* This is an important part of your care. Stress aggravates IBS and bowel symptoms are particularly common in women who have suffered physical or sexual abuse in the past.

- *Medications.* Most women with IBS don't need medications. There is no medication that treats all the symptoms of IBS and no medication that will 'cure' IBS. The right medication for you will depend on your particular symptoms.
  - Fibre supplements help constipation, bowel pain and sometimes diarrhoea.
  - Antispasmodics such as mebeverine, or 'tricyclics' such as amitriptyline improve painful bowel contractions.

- Laxatives avoid constipation but are rarely necessary on a high fibre diet.
- Loperamide helps diarrhoea.
- Medications that treat the muscles and nerves of the bowel themselves include Tegaserod® (if you tend to be constipated) and Allosetron® (if you tend to get diarrhoea).

Some of these suggestions (lifestyle changes, a generally healthy diet and more fibre) will help almost anyone with bowel problems. Others (like checking for food allergies or intolerances) will only help some women. If possible, change only one or two things at a time, so you will know what helps you most.

Finally, you do not have to treat IBS. If your symptoms are mild, then maybe just making the diagnosis and knowing that it is nothing more serious is enough for you.

Why is JBS worse with stress?

No-one really knows why stress makes some IBS worse. However, the chemicals our brain makes when we are stressed are similar to some of the chemicals that affect the bowel. Stress chemicals may change the way our bowel moves or feels. It is also possible that stress chemicals alter the way our brain feels pain.

Food intolerance and food allergy

Could your diet be aggravating your bowel symptoms? Cutting out anything at all that could possibly affect you may help (at least in the short term), but we all need to eat. We also need to feed our families and eat the right food to keep our body healthy long term. By finding out which foods bother you most, which ones you can eat in small quantities and which ones cause you no problems at all, you can usually avoid excessively strict or restrictive diets.

There are two main ways that food can cause problems: food intolerance and food allergy.

Food intolerance means that the bowel cannot digest certain foods easily. Eating a little of a particular food may cause no problems at all, as the bowel can cope with small amounts. However, eating larger amounts of that food overloads the bowel and causes cramps, diarrhoea or bloating. The common causes of food intolerance are lactose (in milk products), and fructose (see page 167).

Food allergy means that the body's immune system reacts to a particular protein in a food. Sometimes the immune system reacts quickly causing a life-threatening condition called *anaphylaxis*, but usually it reacts slowly causing a variety of problems that may be hard to pick as a food allergy. The commonest foods to cause food allergy are milk, eggs, fish, nuts, shellfish, soybeans and gluten (wheat). Food allergies are less common than food intolerances.

Lactose intolerance

Women with lactose intolerance find it difficult to absorb foods containing lactose such as milk, cheese or ice cream. This is not a food allergy: the body just finds it hard to digest. Lactose intolerance can be diagnosed with a 'breath test' arranged by your general practitioner. If you are found to be lactose intolerant, it is important that you see a dietician for expert advice on how to cut down on milk, while still getting the calcium you need for your bones. Most women with lactose intolerance have mild symptoms that are easily treated by cutting down on how much milk, or milk products they eat at any one time.

Some people who have never shown food intolerance develop a type of lactose intolerance if they cut out lactose for a period of time. For example, Western people who travel to Asia and live on a traditional Asian diet (very low in milk products), then return home and drink a milkshake or eat a large amount of cheese should expect an upset bowel. They are not allergic to milk products, but until their body adjusts back to their old diet, they have temporary lactose intolerance.

Fructose intolerance

Fructose is a sugar found in fruit, but also found in food compounds called *fructans* that release fructose as they are digested. It is normal to absorb fructose slowly from the bowel but if you have a sensitive bowel, what is normal for other women may cause you to suffer bloating, pain or diarrhoea. This is not a food allergy. A small amount of fructose or fructan causes no problems at all, but a larger amount taken all at once is more than the bowel can cope with and diarrhoea, bloating or pain result.

Fruit is an important part of everyone's diet, so a fructose-free diet is not sensible. However, if you cut down on fruits or foods that are high in fructose, and replace them with fruits or foods that are low in fructose, you may suffer fewer bowel symptoms. Fructose is also absorbed more easily from the bowel if another sugar called 'glucose' has been eaten at the same meal.

- *Foods that are high in fructose or fructans include:* wheat-based products (bread, pasta, biscuits), onions, sucrose-sweetened fizzy drinks, apples, pears, honey, and corn syrup (a sweetener in some foods). These foods are best eaten in small quantities or spread across the day if you have an irritable bowel.
- *Foods that are low in fructose or fructans include:* bananas, apricots, plums, berries, oranges, lemons and glucose-sweetened fizzy drinks.

Coeliac disease

Around one in 200 people have coeliac disease. When they eat a protein called *gluten*, their body's immune system makes antibodies that attack their bowel. The damaged bowel can no longer absorb iron and vitamins from food. Gluten is found in wheat, rye and barley, but not in rice, corn or potatoes. Some coeliacs have weight loss and diarrhoea, so their condition is diagnosed when they are very young, but many coeliacs have few symptoms and it is found during investigation of an unexpectedly low iron level, or mild bowel complaints.

Nowadays most coeliac disease can be diagnosed with a blood test. The most reliable tests measure endomysial or transglutaminase antibodies. A test for gliadin antibodies is less reliable. While the blood tests are useful, if they are positive you may still need an endoscopy to be completely sure of the diagnosis. Remember that neither the blood tests, nor an endoscopy can diagnose coeliac disease if you have already cut gluten out of your diet, so it is very important to have the tests done *before* changing your diet.

What is the difference between coeliac disease and gluten intolerance?

There are many people, both men and women, who don't have coeliac disease but feel better on a low gluten or low wheat diet. These people are called 'gluten intolerant' although it may be that they feel better because their new diet is low in fructans rather than because it is low in gluten (see page 167). Certainly most women with bloating feel better when they cut down on bread, cakes and biscuits.

While people with coeliac disease should eat *no* gluten whatsoever for the rest of their life, a person with gluten intolerance (or fructan intolerance) can eat *small* amounts of gluten without problems.

Whatever food issues you have, a special diet is difficult to stick to, a lot of trouble and can be expensive. Then again, if it helps your symptoms then the effort may be worthwhile. If you do plan to cut down on lactose, fructose or gluten, a dietician can help you plan a diet that still provides the nutrients your body needs.

Bloating

Doctors often think of bloating as an inconvenience rather than a major problem. This is because bloating rarely means a serious illness, but also because it is poorly understood and there are no easy answers to the problem. But if you ask women about their bloating, they see it as a major problem: possibly their worst symptom. Bloating makes women feel unfeminine, unattractive and uncomfortable. It also makes any other pelvic pain worse.

So what is bloating?

There are two types of bloating:

- *Bloating where the abdomen swells due to excess wind.* This may be due to swallowing excess air when you talk or eat, or to certain foods in your diet. If your body can't absorb some foods, they stay in the bowel for longer. Bacteria in the bowel ferment these foods, making gas. Unless you have coeliac disease, you are not allergic to these foods, but you may need to eat them in smaller quantities.
- *Bloating where the abdomen looks normal, but feels bloated.* This is usually due to IBS. In women with IBS, the bowel does not move normally so wind doesn't pass through easily. The nerves in the bowel are hyper-sensitive so the bowel feels uncomfortable too. This type of bloating gets worse during the day and is best first thing in the morning.

What can I do about bloating?

We are all different and what causes you to bloat may cause your friend no problems at all. This list describes some of the problems that can cause bloating. It is very unlikely that they will all apply to you, but one or two of them may.

- *Are you swallowing too much air when you talk or eat?* This is more likely if you eat in a hurry, chew gum, drink fizzy drinks or smoke cigarettes. Chewing gum also contains sorbitol, a poorly absorbed sugar that causes bloating and diarrhoea. Chewing gum is best avoided.
- *Are you wearing tight-waisted clothes or panty hose often?* These make you feel more uncomfortable.
- *Do you spend a lot of your day sitting down?* A brisk walk at lunchtime will help your bowel work well and the wind pass normally.
- *Do you eat a lot of fermenting vegetables?* It is normal for foods such as beans, lentils, brussels sprouts, cabbage and legumes to make gas during their digestion. These are not bad foods, but in large quantities they do make gas.
- *Do you have a food intolerance, or coeliac disease?*

So what can I eat?

We all need to eat. We all have lives to live as well. Very few of us have the time to spend finding special food or preparing compli-cated menus. If you are confused after reading all the dietary advice, remember that a simple healthy diet that is low fat, low sugar, low caffeine and high fibre will suit most women well. This diet is suitable for your family too.

Food should be enjoyed. While it is useful to look at foods and how they affect you, they should not rule your life. Even if you have a food intolerance, most women can still enjoy most of the foods they like, but in smaller quantities and not all at once. It is only when someone has a food allergy that it means a food should never be eaten.

Constipation

Almost no-one in Western countries eats enough fibre for their bowel to work well. Constipation is common. It causes a cramp-like pain that improves once the bowels have been opened well. Mild constipation may be one reason why a healthy diet improves some bowel pain. It treats the constipation no-one knew was there.

As well as eating a low fibre diet, many women do not place a high enough priority on their bowel function. Life is busy. Women tend to rush in, strain, and then if no bowel action occurs quickly, give up and hope something happens later in the day. They have lost an opportunity.

The best time to open your bowels is in the morning after breakfast because this is when the bowel contractions are strongest. They start while you are asleep — about an hour or so before your bowel actually opens.

These contractions begin high up in your bowel, move the bowel action around to the lower bowel and then out through the anus. They can open your bowels much more efficiently than you can by straining your pelvic floor muscles, but they do take time. Stress or anxiety can interfere with them — or with your awareness of the need to open your bowels. Straining is harmful to the pelvic floor and should not be necessary if you have a normal bowel, give them time and have enough fibre in your diet.

How can J increase the fibre in my diet?

There are two types of fibre: soluble fibre and *in*soluble fibre. Soluble fibre is found in fruits and grains. It is digested in the bowel, and keeps both the bowel wall and the bacteria in the bowel healthy. Insoluble fibre is found in the outside shell (husk) of grains. It holds water, makes your bowel action larger and helps food pass through the bowel faster.

You can increase the fibre in your diet by eating more high fibre food (multigrain breads, high fibre cereals, fruit etc.), or if necessary using a fibre supplement. Either way, you should always increase the fibre in your diet slowly to avoid bloating.

When starting a fibre supplement, start with 1 teaspoon each morning with plenty of water. This can be increased to 2 teaspoons daily after a week, and then 3 teaspoons daily, if necessary, a week later. Sterculia (Normafibe®) causes less bloating than most other fibre supplements.

What can I do about my constipation?

Before seeing your doctor, there are several things you can do yourself:

- Eat enough fibre
- Eat breakfast every day
- Give yourself enough time to go to the toilet each morning
- Drink enough fluid. No fibre will work well unless you drink enough water. Two litres of fluid, mostly water, is best
- Do regular exercise such as brisk walking each day.

If you still have problems:

- Talk to your general practitioner about your general health. Low thyroid hormone levels can worsen constipation.
- Check the medications you use. Amitriptyline, strong pain medications, some tablets for mental health problems and the long-term use of strong laxatives can all slow the bowel.
- See a pelvic floor physiotherapist to improve your pelvic muscle function and bowel habits.
- See a dietician to review your diet.
- See a bowel doctor (gastroenterologist) if your problems continue.

My constipation is very severe.
Nothing works for me.

A small number of women have severe constipation even when they eat a high fibre diet. They suffer abdominal pain or bloating and use laxatives or enemas frequently. If this is you, then you should see a gastroenterologist. Severe constipation may be due to a very slow bowel or a bowel that is partly blocked. Special medical tests are needed to work out the cause of the problem and how best to treat it.

IBS, bloating, food intolerance and constipation are the problems that bother women with pelvic pain or endometriosis most, but there are others. If your symptoms change over time you should go back to your doctor to discuss them again. You may have developed a new condition, or what was thought to be irritable bowel syndrome may turn out to be something else. If you are unsure, your general practitioner or bowel doctor is the best person to see.

Who can help me with bowel pain?
- Your general practitioner.
- A bowel doctor (gastroenterologist).
- A dietician.
- A physiotherapist with a special interest in pelvic conditions if you have constipation or tight pelvic floor muscles.
- A natural therapist.

3 Pain from adhesions

You may have been told that there are adhesions in your pelvis. So what are adhesions? Adhesions are areas where organs have become stuck together. Just as an adhes*ive* is another name for a glue, an adhes*ion* means a point where organs have become 'glued' together (see Figure 2.1 on page 16). Adhesions can affect fertility if they are near the ovary or the fallopian tubes.

What sort of pain can adhesions cause?

Adhesions around an ovary cause pain felt on one side of the pelvis, that is particularly severe during ovulation. Ovaries are sensitive organs. They like to move freely (just like testes) and become painful if tied down by an adhesion. At ovulation, the ovary changes in size. There is more tension on the ovary at this time and the pain worsens. If the ovary is stretched even further by a 'functional cyst' (see page 195), then the pain becomes even more severe. As women who are on the Pill do not usually ovulate, they have less pain from adhesions affecting the ovary.

Adhesions in other areas of the pelvis are less likely to cause pain than ovarian adhesions. If they do cause pain, it is always felt in the same part of the pelvis. It may be worse with sudden movement or intercourse. A tender area in a pelvic muscle may cause a similar type of pain (see page 182).

Adhesions between loops of bowel rarely cause pain unless they block the bowel, or prevent normal bowel function.

What causes adhesions?

Anything that irritates the lining of the abdomen (peritoneum) can cause an adhesion. The common causes include endometriosis, a pelvic infection, an operation (especially if it is done through a large cut), or severe appendicitis where the appendix has ruptured. However, in some women, no cause for the adhesions can be found. If you have had pelvic surgery in the past, then you should expect that you have at least *some* adhesions, but as most adhesions do not cause pain, they may not require treatment.

How are adhesions diagnosed?

Unfortunately, only a laparoscopy will reliably show if you have adhesions, and whether or not they involve the ovary. Even women who have many reasons why they *might* have adhesions do not. Equally, some women have more adhesions found during a laparoscopy than expected. Adhesions do not show on an ultrasound scan.

Can adhesions affect my surgery?

Yes. Adhesions make any operation more difficult because:

- They block the surgeon's view of the pelvis through the laparoscope. Dividing the adhesions to allow a better view makes the operation longer.
- They may mean less room for the laparoscopic instruments. This makes the operation slower.
- Organs that are stuck together are more easily damaged when the adhesions are divided.
- They may hide important organs like the ureter under scar tissue. This makes them easier to damage during an operation.

For all these reasons, adhesions make the chance of a hole (perforation) in an organ higher than usual (see Chapter 5, page 55).

Can adhesions be prevented?

Sometimes, yes.

Safe sexual practices mean fewer sexually transmitted disease and less risk of pelvic infection. Treating endometriosis early and effectively may decrease the chance of adhesions. Surgery through a laparoscope, rather than a larger cut, is less likely to cause adhesions. This is one of the strengths of laparoscopic surgery. Gentle handling of tissues by your surgeon, and care to control any bleeding are important, and an adhesion barrier placed near the ovaries during surgery may keep them apart during the healing phase. There are many different types of adhesion barriers, but most dissolve over one or two weeks. None are perfect and none will avoid all adhesions, but they may make them less likely.

Unfortunately, one factor that cannot be changed is your own skin type. Some women have tissues that make lots of adhesions even after minor surgery. Others have many operations yet form few adhesions.

What can I do about the adhesions that I have?

- *Do nothing*. Adhesions only matter if they cause pain. No treatment may be necessary.
- *The contraceptive pill*. This helps ovulation pain because it prevents the ovary changing shape at ovulation.
- *A laparoscopy to divide the adhesions*. When the organs are loosely tied together, this is not difficult. The adhesions lie like fine curtains between the pelvic organs and are easily cut using scissors or laser (see Figure 2.1, page 16). However, dividing organs that are firmly fixed together is one of the most difficult areas of laparoscopic surgery. It is very easy to make a hole (perforation) in one of the organs involved. This hole then needs to be repaired. (See Eleanor's case study in Chapter 5, on page 55.)
- *Surgery to remove one or both ovaries*. This only applies to older women with completed families.

The difficulty with dividing adhesions is that even when separated beautifully, the adhesions often reform. This is less likely after a laparoscopy than a laparotomy but it can still happen.

Who can help me with adhesions?

- A laparoscopic surgeon (gynaecologist) if surgery is required. Almost all adhesions can be divided through the laparoscope, but not all gynaecologists perform this type of surgery.
- A dietician if your adhesions affect your bowel and he or she has a special interest in this area.
- Your general practitioner if you would like to use the contraceptive pill.

4 Pain from nerves – neurogenic pain

Neurogenic pain is different to other pain. The endometriosis is gone, no other problems have been found, but there is still pain. This is the pain described by women who say, 'Nothing seems to work for me.' Neurogenic pain is easier to understand if you have read about how we feel pain in Chapter 9, on page 146.

What type of pain is neurogenic pain?

Neurogenic pain is constant pain, not just pain with periods. It is present on most days. The pain may be burning, with occasional sharp, stabbing feelings. There may be unusual sensations such as hot or cold feelings, a mild pricking of the skin, or a different feeling when the skin is lightly touched in that area. Many normal activities such as moving, stretching, or opening your bowels cause pain. Neurogenic pain symptoms vary from day to day. It is a 'wearing' pain that often disturbs sleep.

Your abdomen may not *look* swollen, but *feels* swollen in the same way that your lip feels swollen after an anaesthetic at the dentist. This is especially common in women who have scars on their abdomen that are numb to touch. There may be allodynia, hyperalgesia or wind-up features to your pain (see page 149).

Women with neurogenic pain often wake up after an operation with no pain, overjoyed that their pain has gone. This is because the medications used by the anaesthetist to put you to sleep treat neurogenic pain very effectively. Unfortunately, the pain often returns over the next few weeks or months once the effect of the medication wears off.

What is neurogenic pain?

Neurogenic pain is pain that starts in the nerves themselves at some point on their pathway from the pelvis to the brain. For any one of many reasons, the nerve pathway from the pelvis to the brain has become 'sensitised' and well established. The nerves have learned to transmit pain very well, and cannot unlearn it. The original cause of pain may be gone, but the nerves are unable to forget the pain they knew before.

The idea of neurogenic pain as a cause of *pelvic* pain is fairly new, but it has been recognised as a cause of pain in other parts of the body for some time. Examples of this type of pain include nerve damage from a prolapsed intervertebral disc, diabetes or a genital herpes infection. For each of these conditions, the reason for the pain is different.

A prolapsed disc puts pressure on a nerve. Even when an operation takes pressure off the nerve, the nerve may remember the pain and continue to send pain signals. Long-term diabetes can chemically damage nerves, which then transmit pain. Men or women with genital herpes have small ulcers like cold sores on the scrotum or labia caused by the herpes virus. Over two weeks the ulcers heal completely but the pain may continue. In all these examples, a condition has injured, upset or irritated a nerve, and the nerve has continued to transmit pain even when the cause of the pain has gone.

Neurogenic pain affecting the pelvis is diagnosed if the symptoms fit and no other cause for the pain has been found. The exact reason why the nerves have become sensitised may never be known, but endometriosis, surgery or long-term pain itself can all cause permanent structural changes to nerves.

What can I do about neurogenic pain?

Like endometriosis, it is only in the last ten years or so that much has been known about how to manage neurogenic pain effectively. This does not mean that treating neurogenic pain is easy, but there is much more available now.

Of the many ways of treating neurogenic pain it is unlikely that any one of these will magically provide a complete cure. Once chronic pain becomes established, it may be not be possible to eliminate it completely. The best results are achieved with a mix of medications, and lifestyle changes. The good thing is that even if your pain is not completely cured, you *can* expect a big improvement.

Medicines that can help neurogenic pain

The medicines used include:

- *Anti-prostaglandin medications* taken regularly (see Chapter 6, page 70). An irritated nerve makes large amounts of prostaglandins that irritate it even more. Anti-prostaglandin medications improve the chemical environment around the nerves and allow them to work better.
- *Tricyclic medications* such as amitriptyline. These medications increase the calming signals sent down from the brain, so that fewer pain signals get through. It is especially useful if the pain is aching or burning in quality.
- *Anti-arrhythmics* such as mexiletine. These are normally used to settle irregular heart rhythms. They are useful for sudden episodes of sharp pain.
- *Anticonvulsants* such as gabapentin or valproate. Anticonvulsant medications are normally used to treat epilepsy. In chronic pain they stabilise the nerves and make them less irritable.
- *Tramadol.* Tramadol is an opioid pain medication that acts in a similar way to morphine, but has other actions too (see Chapter 6, page 73).
- *Ketamine or magnesium.* These medications stop the spinal cord making a substance called NDMA that irritates nerves.
- *Local anaesthetics.* These block nerves for a short time.
- *Corticosteroid medications.* Steroids settle down inflamed nerves.

Normal pain medications such as codeine or pethidine do *not* work well for neurogenic pain. You may have worked this out already.

Treatments that don't involve taking medicines

- *Exercise.* Neurogenic pain feels better after rest because there is less activity in the nerves. However, long-term rest is a trap. You cannot rest forever and in the long term, you will have much less pain if your body is fit and active. It is important that you see daily exercise and increased muscle strength as part of your pain management program. The endorphin chemicals made during exercise improve wellbeing too.
- *Maintain your interests.* This gives your brain other things to think about apart from your pain. Are there things that were important to you before your pain? Are there activities that you enjoy? Are there goals you *can* achieve despite your pain?
- *Get enough sleep at night.* Tired nerves are more irritable.
- *Avoid being overweight.* A heavier body weight overloads your muscles and joints. You do not need a new cause of pain (see page 182).
- *Manage your stress.* A relaxed brain sends more 'ignore pain' signals to balance your pain better.

Gabapentin for neurogenic pain

Isobel is a 35-year-old teacher whose severe endometriosis had been removed at an extensive laparoscopic operation by an experienced endometriosis surgeon a few years before. The endometriosis had been removed, but she still had pain that bothered her every day and often at night. She was worn out and worried that she just wasn't herself. When the pain was particularly severe in her pelvis, she felt pain above her navel too.

This was 'wind-up' pain. She also suffered constipation, ovulation pain, and a pain in her **urethra**. Isobel no longer had endometriosis, but she certainly had several causes of pain.

Isobel started gabapentin to treat the part of her pain that was neurogenic. She described the first month on her treatment as 'liberating'. The pain above her navel and most of her pelvic pain had gone. She slept well. Her friends felt that they needed whatever had made her look so obviously well!

Gabapentin will not treat her ovulation pain, (due to adhesions around an ovary), her constipation pain, or her urethral pain (see page 188). They will need to be managed separately, but at least she now has the energy to work on her other pains. A doctor who uses medications to treat brain, spine and nerve conditions (neurologist) will continue the management of her neurogenic pain.

So which treatment mix is best for me?

Working out the best combination of these treatments for your pain may be too difficult for your gynaecologist. Fortunately, there are now pain specialists who manage a wide variety of chronic pain conditions in both men and women. Pelvic pain is just one of the conditions they see. Such specialists work in 'pain clinics' and have a lot to offer. If you have neurogenic pain, a pain specialist is the best person to advise you on which mix of treatments will suit you best.

Before going to a pain clinic, it is important that any endometriosis lesions have been completely removed. Pain clinics do well for women with neurogenic pain, but are less successful if you still have endometriosis present. If it has been a long time since your last operation, it may take another laparoscopy to be sure that other causes of pain have been excluded.

A pain clinic uses what is called a multi-disciplinary approach to pain management. This means that professionals from many areas of medicine work together to get the best result possible for each individual person. The pain clinic team might include doctors (a pain specialist, an anaesthetist, a psychiatrist and a rehabilitation specialist), as well as physiotherapists, occupational therapists, psychologists and others. It is this mix of skills that makes pain clinics so successful. If you go to a pain clinic, it is unlikely that you will see all of these people, but they are there if needed.

As most women with endometriosis have been told at one time (or many times) that their pain was psychological, it is not surprising that some are suspicious when asked to see the psychologist or psychiatrist who works in the pain clinic. There is no need to be. If your pain specialist recommends psychological help it is not because they think your pain is imaginary. It is because your recovery will be slower if you are stressed, depressed or anxious.

The only good thing about neurogenic pain is that treatments are improving. What was once almost untreatable is now manageable. However, it will take effort on your part, a mixture of treatments and good advice.

Who can help me with neurogenic pain?

- A pain clinic gives the most complete care.
- Your general practitioner.
- Your gynaecologist may be happy to prescribe some of these medications if he or she has an interest in this area.
- A neurologist.

5 Pain from muscles and joints – myofascial pain

Muscle pain is not something many women think of when they have pelvic pain. Tender points in the neck and shoulders have been known about since the 1940s, but it is only recently that similar points in pelvic muscles have been recognised as a common cause of pelvic pain in women.

These tender points cause pain that feels as if it comes from the pelvic organs (uterus, ovaries, bladder or bowel). This is because the nerves that carry pain signals from the muscles of the abdomen, back, thighs or pelvis join the nerves that carry pain signals from the pelvic organs when they reach the spinal cord, and before they reach the brain.

What type of pain is muscle or joint pain?

Muscular pain is described as dull, aching or deep pain. It is worse on some days than others, but felt on most days. It may be aggravated by changes in position, and made either better or worse with exercise. Muscle or joint pain is difficult to diagnose because it is often 'referred' to other areas of the pelvis. Some examples of this include:

- A tender point in the muscle of the abdominal wall on one side felt as pain coming from the ovary on that side. The ovary itself is normal.
- A tender point in the muscles of the lower back felt as pain in the uterus or bladder. The uterus and bladder are normal. Other lower back conditions such as a prolapsed disc or strained ligaments cause a similar pain.
- The pain from a cut in the abdomen after an operation referred to pain in the pelvis.
- Tender points in the muscles of the inner thigh referred to the vagina. This pain is worse if the thighs are spread apart, making some sexual positions painful.
- Tender points in the muscles lining the pelvic bones, causing pain that seems to come from the uterus or ovaries.
- Tender, over-active pelvic floor muscles causing pelvic pain and painful sex.

How can I tell if I have muscle or joint pain?

There is no blood test or scan that can prove your pain is muscular. It is diagnosed from your description of the pain, and the finding of tender spots during a physical examination that when pressed cause your particular pain. Joint pain is uncommon in young women, but can be investigated with an X-ray, or CT scan if it seems likely.

Think about when you get your pain. Is the pain worse in some positions, after certain movements or with exercise? If so, then at least part of the pain may be muscular. A 'pain diary' is useful. Episodes of pain are written down each day, together with your other activities, any emotional stress and the stage of your menstrual cycle. Over time, a pattern of pain at certain times or with certain activities may become obvious.

Muscle or joint pain is especially common if:

- You have injured your back, pelvis or knees.
- You have problems with posture, such as a lordosis ('sway back'), a scoliosis (curved spine), a short leg, a stiff or unstable sacroiliac joint, or generalised poor posture. The two sacroiliac joints are found on either side of the bottom of the spine at the back.
- You have recently been inactive or gained weight.
- You do excessive exercise or have muscle strain.

Before presuming that your pain is muscle or joint pain, it is important to exclude other conditions. Conditions that are easily confused with this pain include a prolapsed vertebral disc, a nerve caught in scar tissue, or medical conditions like fibromyalgia, arthritis, multiple sclerosis or systemic lupus erythematosus (SLE). Your general practitioner can help you exclude these conditions. Fibromyalgia has generalised muscle tenderness rather than isolated tender spots.

What can I do about muscle or joint pelvic pain?

Recognising which factors have caused your pain is a large part of managing the problem. If your pain is due to poor muscle tone from inactivity, then exercises and improving your general health are important. If your pain is due to too much activity with muscle fatigue, then rest and modifying or avoiding the aggravating activity helps. Whatever the cause, you have developed tension and irritability in a group of muscles or a joint.

The best treatment for you will depend on the cause of the problem. A physiotherapist with an interest in pelvic conditions or trigger point therapy is a good person to see for this problem. The treatments that they may recommend include:

- *Specific work on your tender areas*. This includes therapeutic massage, pressure therapies, myofascial release therapy, heat therapy and ultrasound treatment.
- *Exercises* to improve your posture, stretch tight muscles (this decreases trigger point activation) and improve the strength in weak muscles around the joints.
- *Consider your general health*. Low levels of B-group vitamins, low thyroid function and low blood sugar levels can all aggravate muscle irritability.
- *A 'TENS' machine*. This is a small machine the size of a pack of cards. Two small sticky pads are placed over the tender area, and electricity passed between the two pads. This blocks pain impulses going to the brain from that area. It should be set at a level where you notice a gentle tingling sensation and should not be painful.
- *Cool and stretch technique*. A physiotherapist uses a cooling spray to decrease pain around the tender point, and the muscle is then stretched to its full length. This treatment can be repeated daily, usually for one or two weeks, and should

provide rapid results. It is only suitable for muscles on the exterior of the body. If the muscles become sore, the treatment should be stopped for a few days.

- *Needle injection of the tender area with an anaesthetic.* It is actually the needle in the tender point rather than the anaesthetic that helps the pain, but without the anaesthetic, the procedure would be too painful. Needling brings pain relief, but must be repeated weekly for around six weeks. If you don't improve over this time, there may be other factors contributing to your pain.

- *Acupuncture.* Acupuncture has been used to treat pain for centuries. However, it should be seen as an opportunity to manage the pain while you correct the underlying problem, rather than as a complete treatment in itself.

- *Treatment for anxiety or depression.* Both anxiety and depression cause muscular pain by increasing muscle tension. They may not have caused your pain, but they can slow your recovery.

- *Medications.* Some tender areas in muscle are due to irritation at the place where the nerve joins the muscle. There are some features in common with neurogenic pain. Anti-inflammatory medications (see Chapter 6, page 70) and low dose amitriptyline (see page 74) often help muscular pain. Botox will relax overly tense vaginal muscles for up to 6 months.

If treatment is effective and an active tender point settles, then your pain should resolve. However, unless the original cause of the problem is fixed, the tender point, *and the pain* may return. This means that some long-term changes in posture, exercise or general condition are needed. An excellent book for anyone with muscle or joint pain is *Explain Pain* written by D. Butler and G. Moseley (see Reference 22).

Arthritis as a cause of pelvic pain

Sita is a 45-year-old doctor who had developed chronic pelvic pain over two years. She had always had some pain with periods and suspected that she had adenomyosis in her uterus (see page 151). Her pain was worse at period time, but could come at any time of the month.

Sita had a hysterectomy, but was disappointed to find that although her period pain had gone, her other pelvic pain continued. After many tests, Sita was found to have early onset arthritis in her spine with pain 'referred' to her pelvis.

Four different causes of pain

Misha is an 18-year-old university student, referred for removal of endometriosis found at a laparoscopy. On discussion, Misha had four separate causes for her pain! Removing her endometriosis would only treat one of her pains and leave her disappointed. Her four pains were:

- Muscular pain referred to her pelvis. After horse riding, or working with a hoe in local vineyards, her period pain was much more severe. During a few months of study for her exams, where she neither rode horses, nor worked in the vineyard, her period pain improved.
- Bowel pain. At any time of the month, bloating and pelvic pain could occur. After passing a bowel action, her symptoms improved. A change in diet, investigation of possible food intolerance, and review by a gastroenterologist were advised.
- Prostaglandin pain. This was the pain felt on the first one or two days of her period. The contraceptive pill or an anti-prostaglandin medication would help.
- Endometriosis pain. The endometriosis should be removed.

Who can help me with muscular or joint pain?

- A physiotherapist with an interest in pelvic conditions.
- A pain clinic.
- Your general practitioner if he or she has an interest in this area.
- A sex counsellor if you have tight vaginal muscles.

6 Pain from the bladder — interstitial cystitis

You may know all about cystitis. If so, you probably mean *bacterial cystitis* which is the medical word for a bladder infection. Bacteria get into the bladder, grow there, and irritate the bladder wall. A bladder infection gets better with antibiotics because they kill the bacteria that cause the infection.

The word 'cystitis' really only means an inflammation (irritation) of the bladder. It does not say what caused the inflammation. Interstitial cystitis (IC) is different from bacterial cystitis. There is irritation of the bladder wall but no infection. Antibiotics don't help because there are no bacteria present.

IC is a poorly understood condition. What *is* understood is that it can cause long-term pelvic pain and that it is more common in women with endometriosis. Although some men get interstitial cystitis, it is ten times more common in women.

Even though IC is not a bacterial infection, women with IC often get more bladder infections than other women. Any IC symptoms usually worsen during and after a urine infection.

For reasons that are not well understood, women with IC often *also* have an irritable bowel (see page 160), fibromyalgia (generalised muscle pain), vulvar vestibulitis (a painful area near the opening of the vagina), migraines or allergies as well as their IC. They may also have endometriosis. This makes the pain of IC complicated to both diagnose and manage.

Like endometriosis, many women with IC suffer pain for years before the correct diagnosis is made. This is very distressing. Just like endometriosis, IC is now receiving more attention than before. There have been significant improvements in the way IC is treated, and it is diagnosed much more frequently now than in the past.

What type of pain does interstitial cystitis cause?

The pain may be a burning pain, a shooting pain, a pressure feeling or a spasm. It is felt in the pelvis, in the bladder itself or in the urethra (the tube carrying urine out of the bladder). Commonly, the *pain* worsens as the bladder fills and improves as the bladder empties.

Women with IC usually have other bladder symptoms such as *frequency* (wanting to go to the toilet often), *urgency* (needing to go the toilet in a hurry), and *nocturia* (needing to get up to the toilet at night). Intercourse may be painful, especially in positions that put pressure on the bladder.

The pain may be aggravated by intercourse, periods or foods that are high in acid or potassium. Stress does not cause IC, but it can certainly make it worse.

How is IC diagnosed?

There is no one good test for IC. Really it is what doctors call a 'clinical diagnosis'. This means that if the symptoms fit IC and no other cause for the symptoms is found, then the diagnosis of IC is made.

To exclude other causes of pain you may need:

- One or more urine tests to exclude a urine infection or the presence of cancer cells.
- A bladder diary, which records how much urine you pass, and how often you pass it over a few days.
- An ultrasound of the kidney, pelvic organs and bladder.

- Review by a urologist to check that other conditions are not present, and,
- A short operation called a **cystoscopy** where a telescope is inserted through the urethra into the bladder. A cystoscopy looks at the inside surface of the bladder.

A cystoscopy done in women with IC usually looks normal, but can be useful to exclude other problems such as endometriosis inside the bladder (uncommon) or other causes of bladder irritation such as bladder stones or bladder cancer.

How can I treat my IC?

There are probably several types of IC currently put together in one group, so it is not surprising that no one treatment helps everyone. For some women, dietary changes are enough to manage their symptoms, while others need the experience of a doctor who specialises in bladder and kidney problems (urologist) to work through the treatment options until a suitable option is found. As more becomes known about IC over the next few years, it will become easier to fit the right treatment to the right person.

Usually it is a matter of working through a number of treatments with your doctor until you find one that works for you. No treatment works in everyone and unfortunately no treatment usually works forever. Luckily about 10 per cent of women spontaneously get better over time.

There is more information on IC at www.ichelp.com

For now, the treatment options include:

- *Dietary changes.* Drinks that are high in potassium, acid or caffeine such as fruit juices (including cranberry juice), fizzy drinks, coffee, tea or alcohol should be avoided or drunk in smaller quantities. Particular foods may be a problem, too. An IC diet to help you work out which foods might be a problem for you is available at http://www.ichelp.com/TreatmentAndSelfHelp/ICAndDiet.html

- *Drinking the right amount of fluid for you.* This may mean drinking more (to dilute the urine and avoid bladder irritation), or drinking less (if the extra fluid aggravates your symptoms). The best fluid to drink is water.

- *Lifestyle changes* that include exercise or stress reduction all improve symptoms. IC is not due to stress, but stress makes it worse. Some women find meditation, hypnosis, massage and relaxation therapies useful. Hot or cold packs placed between the legs, warm baths, wearing loose clothing, cotton underwear and avoiding tight belts may also help.

- *Bladder retraining.* Learning to hold on longer is worthwhile. A continence nurse or physiotherapist can show you how to retrain your bladder and improve your pelvic floor muscle function.

- *Amitriptyline* (see Chapter 6, page 74). This helps frequency, urgency, pain and the number of times you pass urine at night. Only low doses are needed.

- *Pentosan polysulphate sodium* (Elmiron®). This is the only tablet medication specifically used for IC. It helps about 40 per cent of women with IC but is expensive and may take up to six months to work.

- *Other medications.* These include Resiniferotoxin® (made from peppers), Botox® injections into the bladder wall (to decrease bladder pain), anti-prostaglandin medications, anti-spasm medications and muscle relaxants.

- *Hydrodistension of the bladder.* The bladder is over-filled with salty water (saline) to stretch its wall. It is done under a general anaesthetic because otherwise it would be painful. After the bladder has been stretched in this way, 90 per cent of women with IC will show a special pattern of bleeding in the bladder wall. Around 60 per cent of women will have fewer IC symptoms for some months after a hydrodistension.

- *Bladder instillations.* These are medicines mixed with fluid and put inside the bladder. They aim to settle bladder irritation, or decrease pain. These medicines include dimethyl sulfoxide (DMSO) usually given as weekly treatments over six weeks, and Chlorpactin® given as one treatment while you are under an anaesthetic. Steroid medications, heparin, local anaesthetics, and hyaluronic acid have all been used for IC.

- *Transcutaneous Electrical Nerve Stimulation*. A TENS machine, acupuncture or biofeedback may improve bladder pain in some women. These machines are sometimes used for pain relief in childbirth.

- *Sacral nerve neurostimulators*. These devices stimulate the bladder electrically. They are implanted in the buttock and stimulate nerves to the bladder.

- *Urethral dilatation*. This is rarely done now, but was much more common in the past when stretching the urethra was thought to be helpful.

- *Major surgery*. Surgery to remove part of the bladder is *rarely* used in severe situations where all other treatments have failed.

If there are times when your pain or urgency comes on quickly, drinking 500ml of water mixed with 1 teaspoon of bicarbonate of soda may help. This should be followed by 250ml of water every 20 minutes over the next few hours. If pain persists, try ibuprofen or paracetamol. If no better, have a urine test for infection and only take antibiotics if an infection is found.

Pelvic pain due to interstitial cystitis and endometriosis

Niamh is a 26-year-old whose endometriosis was diagnosed and removed at a laparoscopy four years ago. Her period pain improved, but over time she developed a new type of pain. This pain was above her pubic bone, worse if she delayed passing urine, and better once some urine had been passed. It was also worse after intercourse, whenever she was anxious or after drinking fruit juice, soft drinks or red wine. She passed urine frequently and could not 'hold on' as well as before.

A urine sample showed no sign of infection, but did show tiny amounts of white blood cells. A cystoscopy done by a urologist was normal.

Niamh worked on her diet, stress and the type of drinks she chose. She started a small dose of amitriptyline taken each night (see Chapter 6, page 74).

Six weeks later, her pain was 50 per cent better, but she still passed urine often. Her urologist recommended a small dose of oxybutynin to slow the bladder muscle. This improved her symptoms even more. Niamh still has some pain, but it is now manageable.

Who can help me with bladder pain?

- A urologist.
- A physiotherapist with an interest in pelvic conditions and bladder function.
- Your general practitioner if he or she has an interest in this area.
- A gynaecologist if they have an interest in this area.
- A pain clinic if other treatments have failed.

7 Pain from the ovaries

Ovulation pain, functional ovarian cysts and ovarian remnant syndrome

Anything that stretches or ties down an ovary can cause pain. Ovaries are important and sensitive organs and they don't like it!

What type of pain is ovarian pain?

This depends on whether or not your pelvis is otherwise normal, or you have a pelvic condition aggravating one or both ovaries.

If you have a normal-looking pelvis, you have not reached menopause and you are neither pregnant nor on the contraceptive pill, then normal ovulation pain is common. You may notice a deep ache on one or other side of the lower pelvis lasting from a few hours to a day that happens each month almost exactly 14 days before a period arrives. As the ovaries usually take it in turns to ovulate, normal ovulation pain swaps sides most months. If one of your ovaries has been removed, then the ovary that remains will ovulate each month and the pain will be on the same side each month. Not all women with a normal pelvis get ovulation pain.

If you have a pelvic condition, such as adhesions or endometriosis, affecting an ovary then your pain will last for longer, and be more severe in the months when it is that ovary's turn to ovulate. Anything that ties down the ovary makes ovulation pain worse, because the ovary is not free to change size and shape freely. The pain will still be worst around ovulation time, but may bother you at other times of the month too. If both ovaries are affected, then the ache will affect both sides of your pelvis.

Functional ovarian cysts and ovarian remnant syndrome cause slightly different types of ovarian pain.

What can I do about normal ovulation pain?

- *Do nothing.* Ovulation pain is not dangerous.
- *Take anti-prostaglandin medications* (see Chapter 6, page 70). Prostaglandin chemicals are released at ovulation, so these medications help, especially if they are taken before the pain is too severe.
- *Use a contraceptive pill.* Most Pills stop ovulation, but some of the newer very low dose Pills do not.
- *Use a progestogen only contraceptive* such as Implanon®.

Functional ovarian cysts

Functional cysts are cysts that form as part of the function of the ovary. It is normal for an ovary to make small, round, fluid-filled cysts from time to time in women who are neither pregnant nor on the contraceptive Pill. Most are not painful, but some are.

If they do cause pain, it is a constant ache, felt most of the time on one side of the pelvis. It may last a few weeks or a few months, but ultimately goes away by itself. As functional cysts can make hormones, periods become irregular and some women notice tender breasts. If the cyst pops (ruptures), there is a sudden pain that goes away a few hours later. Functional cysts don't cause long-term pain so they are rarely confused with endometriosis.

Importantly, there is another condition that can cause a sudden pain in one side of the lower pelvis, irregular periods and breast tenderness: *an ectopic pregnancy.* An ectopic pregnancy is a pregnancy in the fallopian tube rather than in the uterus. It is a dangerous condition and easy to confuse with a functional cyst. If you are unsure, see your doctor. A good quality pregnancy test will be positive in women with an ectopic pregnancy and negative in women with a functional cyst.

How can I know if I have a functional cyst?
- An ultrasound scan shows a cyst that looks like a round balloon filled with clear watery fluid. It should be less than 5 cm across and have no solid pieces inside it. If it has ruptured, then the ultrasound may be normal or show a small amount of fluid in your pelvis, and
- *Your pregnancy test is negative.*

What can I do about functional cysts?
- *Do nothing.* Most functional cysts go away within two or three months. You may wish to have another ultrasound scan two or three months later to ensure that it has resolved.

- *Start the contraceptive pill.* This may not remove your cyst, but will help prevent more functional cysts in the future.
- *A laparoscopy with removal of the cyst.* This is only necessary if your doctor is unsure what type of cyst it is, or your pain cannot be managed. Even if the cyst is removed, this does not prevent other cysts forming.

Ovarian remnant syndrome

This syndrome describes pain or a pelvic mass in a woman who has had both her ovaries (and often her uterus) removed in the past. A small piece of ovary has been left behind *unintentionally* at her operation, and has enlarged and become painful. It usually occurs in women who have had a lot of pelvic surgery in the past and had many adhesions in their pelvis. The gynaecologist who did their operation did not intend to leave behind any ovary at all, but scar tissue or endometriosis made removing the ovary difficult. Over time, even a tiny piece of ovary can respond to hormonal signals from the brain and grow or make cysts.

What type of pain does it cause?
Ovarian remnants cause pain that is felt on one side of the pelvis. In younger women, the pain is worst about once a month, when ovulation would have been, but in older women it can cause chronic pain. Not all ovarian remnants cause pain, but those that do, start to cause problems within a few years of surgery.

How is it diagnosed?
Your description of the pain is the most useful way to diagnose an ovarian remnant. Other ways include:

- *A blood test for estrogen or FSH.* If you have had both ovaries removed, and are not using HRT then you should have low levels of estrogen and high levels of FSH (a hormone made by the brain). If your estrogen levels are normal or your FSH is low then it is likely that a small piece of active ovary remains.

- *An ultrasound scan* may show a cyst in the pelvis that has formed in the remaining piece of ovary.
- *A laparoscopy.* The ovarian remnant looks like white, often cystic, scar tissue. Sometimes a medication called clomiphene citrate is used before surgery to make the remnant larger and easier to find.

What can I do about an ovarian remnant?

Any treatment that removes the ovarian remnant or makes it less active will help the pain. These options include:

- *No treatment.* At menopause the remnant will become less active, just as a normal ovary does, and your pain *might* improve.
- *Medications to make the ovarian remnant less active.* The Pill, a GnRH analogue (see Chapter 6, page 66) or a continuous progestogen medication (see Chapter 6, page 80) usually help.
- *An operation to remove the ovarian remnant.* This surgery can be difficult because most remnants are small and trapped among scar tissue. They lie close to the ureter, which is easily damaged during surgery. The good thing about removing the remnant is that the pain usually resolves.
- *Radiotherapy.* The same radiation treatment used to treat some cancers can be used to make the ovary inactive. This is an uncommon treatment nowadays.

Who can help me with ovarian pain?

- Your general practitioner (for ovulation pain or functional cysts).
- Your normal gynaecologist (for ovulation pain or functional cysts).

- A laparoscopic surgeon (gynaecologist) for removal of an ovarian remnant.

8 Pain from veins

Ovarian vein syndrome and pelvic congestion syndrome

Just as some enlarged (varicose) veins in the legs ache, varicose veins in the pelvis can ache too. If it is the ovarian vein that is enlarged, then the condition is called ovarian vein syndrome (OVS), whereas if it is the veins around the uterus that are enlarged, it is called pelvic congestion syndrome (PCS). Both conditions are commonest in women who have had children and are aged in their twenties and thirties.

What type of pain can veins cause?

The commonest pain is a generalised dull ache felt in one or both sides of the pelvis. It is worse after standing for long periods of time, straining to pass a bowel action or walking, because these activities encourage congestion in the pelvic veins. Sometimes just changing position is enough to bring on the pain.

As a period comes closer, the pelvis becomes even more congested, the pain worsens and a painful period follows. Painful intercourse on deep penetration is very common, as is an ache after intercourse. Other symptoms include a low backache and, in some women, occasional sharp pains.

Lying down reduces the pelvic congestion and improves the pain, just as it does for varicose leg veins, so most women with pelvic congestion still sleep well.

Why does it happen?

In the past, pelvic congestion syndrome was thought to be more common in women who found orgasm difficult. Nowadays, few doctors believe this theory. Changes in the way veins carry blood are a more likely cause.

Veins are thin-walled blood vessels that carry blood back from the pelvis to the heart. To help them do this, they have valves that allow blood to move forwards but not backwards. This helps the blood travel upwards when you stand up. If the valves don't work, the blood does not return to the heart as efficiently and it collects in the veins of the pelvis. The pressure from this blood causes congestion in the pelvic organs and stretches the wall of the vein. The vein becomes enlarged and 'varicose'.

How are varicose pelvic veins diagnosed?

- *Examination* of the labia, thigh or buttocks *may* show enlarged veins in these areas too.
- A *doppler ultrasound scan* shows an enlarged vein and poor vein valve function. The left ovarian vein is affected much more commonly than the right.
- A *venogram* is an X-ray test that shows the size and position of the veins in the pelvis. A dye is injected into the pelvis and an X-ray picture taken. Where doppler ultrasound is available, a venogram is rarely necessary.
- A *laparoscopy* may show enlarged veins in the pelvis.

Just having enlarged pelvic veins does not mean that they are the cause for your pain. An Israeli study (see Reference 23) looked at women with pelvic pain and an enlarged left ovarian vein, who were already booked for surgery to donate one of their kidneys. During this operation it is usual to divide the ovarian vein. It was a good opportunity to see if dividing the vein also helped their pelvic pain. After the operation, half the women were better, but half were not. This suggests that some of them had pain due to their enlarged ovarian vein, but for others their pain had another cause.

What can I do about enlarged ovarian or pelvic veins?

The best treatment for you will depend on which veins are varicose and whether these veins are truly the cause of your pelvic pain.

- *No treatment.* Unless your pain is severe, this may be your best option. The enlarged veins may not be the cause of your pain.
- *Treat other health problems.* By treating other conditions such as heavy periods (see Chapter 9, page 158), emotional distress (see Chapter 11, page 219), and premenstrual tension, you may find your pelvic pain improves or becomes easier to live with.
- *Surgery to divide (ligate) an enlarged ovarian vein.* The best operation depends on which veins are enlarged and whether or not you have completed your family. If it is the ovarian vein that is enlarged, it can be divided by removing the ovary on that side, or by dividing the vein and leaving the ovary. Dividing the vein and leaving the ovary is a much more difficult operation.
- *Surgery to ligate enlarged pelvic veins.* This involves removing the uterus (a hysterectomy). An operation to divide the veins and leave the uterus is currently impractical. A hysterectomy will also treat pain from the uterus itself, and heavy periods.
- *Embolisation of the enlarged vein.* An X-ray doctor (radiologist) inserts a small tube through a blood vessel in your groin and passes it through to the enlarged vein. A substance is injected into the vein to block (embolise) it.

Even women who choose a hysterectomy with both ovaries removed do not always find that their pain goes completely. There are many unanswered questions about pelvic congestion syndrome and the best way to manage the pain it causes. All these procedures have risks, so you should discuss them carefully with your doctor. He or she will know what services are available in your area, and what they would recommend for your individual situation.

Who can help me with vein pain?

- Your gynaecologist, particularly if they are skilled at laparoscopic surgery. It requires laparoscopic skills to exclude other conditions such as endometriosis, remove an ovary through the laparoscope, divide the ovarian vein and remove the uterus through small cuts if you choose a hysterectomy.
- A radiologist working with your gynaecologist.

9 Pain from the appendix

If you have had *appendicitis* you will know that you became sick quite quickly, over a few days. You had a high temperature, pain on the right side of your lower abdomen, looked sick to those around you, and then had an operation to remove your appendix. This is the common way in which an appendix causes pain.

But can the appendix cause long-term pain without ever developing actual appendicitis? This is something that doctors disagree on. Some believe it can, but most believe that unless the appendix is infected, it does not cause pain.

A recently reported American study (see Reference 24) studied 300 women who had chronic pain on the right side, no abnormality found at a laparoscopy and a normal-looking appendix removed. Of these women 10 per cent found that their pain had gone after their surgery. This, of course, also means that 90 per cent of these women were no better.

Would their pain have gone away even without surgery, or did removing the normal-looking appendix actually help them? It is difficult to know.

Certainly if the appendix is affected by abnormalities that can be seen, such as endometriosis, then it is best removed.

What pain might the appendix cause?
It might cause pain in the lower right side of the abdomen.

What is the appendix?

The appendix is part of the bowel. It is a hollow tube, closed at one end and opening into an important part of the bowel called the *caecum* at the other end. The appendix is about the same shape and size as a woman's little finger. If it becomes blocked and infected with bacteria this causes *appendicitis*. An operation to remove it is called an *appendicectomy* or an *appendectomy*. Acute appendicitis is not a cause of long-term pain.

What treatment is available for appendix pain?

As no useful role for the appendix has been found in humans, if it causes problems, then it is removed. This can almost always be done through a laparoscope.

Treating actual appendicitis, or removing an appendix that lies in a difficult position requires a bowel surgeon, but in other situations a gynaecologist skilled in laparoscopic surgery may be able to remove it for you.

Removing the appendix usually goes smoothly, but complications are possible, and many gynaecologists are not trained in this type of surgery. For this reason, it is only done in women who have symptoms that could fit with appendix pain, or in women where abnormalities of the appendix (such as endometriosis) are seen at their surgery.

Who can help me with appendix pain?

- A laparoscopic surgeon (gynaecologist) as part of your endometriosis surgery.
- A laparoscopic surgeon (bowel surgeon).

10 Endosalpingiosis (serous change)

Sometimes a white lesion that was thought to be endometriosis is found to be endosalpingiosis when checked by a pathologist.

So what is the difference between endometriosis and endo-salpingiosis?

Endometriosis is tissue that looks a little like the lining of the uterus.

Endosalpingiosis is tissue that looks a little like the lining of the fallopian tube.

The two conditions are similar but certainly not the same. Just like endometriosis, it can only be diagnosed with a laparoscopy. It may look just the same as endometriosis, but once it is sent to a pathologist, they can pick the difference when they look at it through a microscope.

Doctors disagree as to whether or not endosalpingiosis causes pain.

A German study looked at over 1000 women having a laparoscopy during one year. They found endosalpingiosis in 7 per cent of these women. It was just as common in women with pelvic pain, as in women without pelvic pain (see Reference 25).

However, many laparoscopic surgeons have treated women whose pain has improved after removal of endosalpingiosis. It may be that tiny areas of endosalpingiosis are normal and painless, while larger areas might be painful. There is more to learn about this condition.

Who can help me with endosalpingiosis?

- A laparoscopic surgeon (gynaecologist). These operations require the same skill as endometriosis surgery.

11 Pelvic infection (pelvic inflammatory disease)

It is normal for a woman to have bacteria in the vagina and cervix, but not in the uterus, fallopian tubes, around the ovaries or in the abdominal cavity. A pelvic infection means that these areas have become infected. The infection may be *acute*, which means that it came on quickly and has only been present for a short time, or *chronic* which means that it has been present for some time. Some women have repeated acute infections, never completely recovering between bouts of infection.

There may be a mixture of bacteria present. Some, such as gonorrhoea or chlamydia, are transmitted sexually while others are just the normal bacteria living in our bowel or vagina all the time.

What type of pain do pelvic infections cause?

An acute infection can cause a wide variety of symptoms. Some women become very sick quite rapidly. They have a high temperature, severe pain across both sides of their lower abdomen and may vomit. They look sick. There may be an increase in the vaginal discharge or abnormal vaginal bleeding. Other women have mild pelvic pain, but nothing severe enough to cause her to see a doctor. This type of infection can easily go unrecognised.

Over time, infection can damage the fallopian tubes and cause adhesions. If the fallopian tubes become blocked, they fill with fluid and enlarge. This is called a *hydrosalpinx*. Infection and adhesions around the fallopian tube and ovary on one side may form a tender mass called an abscess. These long-term problems can cause chronic pelvic pain.

Some women only find out that they have had a pelvic infection in the past when they have a laparoscopy to investigate why they have not become pregnant easily. The infection had blocked their fallopian tubes.

Occasionally, there is pain and tenderness over the liver in the upper right segment of the abdomen. This is due to adhesions around the liver and has a special name (Fitz-Hugh-Curtis syndrome).

Can pelvic infections be prevented?

Safer sexual practices including the use of barrier contraception (condoms and diaphragms) decrease the risk of catching the sexually transmitted infections that commonly cause pelvic infections.

Vaginal douching should be avoided.

How is a pelvic infection diagnosed?

- *A doctor's examination* of the pelvis may show tender areas on both sides of the lower abdomen, an increased vaginal discharge, and tenderness on vaginal examination when the cervix is moved from side to side. Occasionally a hydrosalpinx or abscess near the ovary is found.

- *Swabs* taken from the cervix may show infection with chlamydia or gonorrhoea. Nowadays, a urine specimen can check for chlamydia infection too. To do this, the laboratory needs the first few drops of urine you pass in the morning, rather than the 'mid-stream' urine specimen that checks for a bladder infection. If you are told that a sexual partner of yours has chlamydia, you need to be checked for infection too.

- *Blood tests* for white blood cells, C-reactive protein and ESR may show high values. These tests look for infection or inflammation anywhere in the body.

- *An ultrasound* may be normal, but may show a dilated tube, ovarian cyst or ovarian abscess.

- *A laparoscopy.* This is the most reliable test. It shows red inflamed pelvic organs and sometimes pus, as well as a hydrosalpinx or abscess if they are present.

A laparoscopy is not always necessary but if there is any doubt about whether or not you have a pelvic infection, it can be very useful. Without a laparoscopy, many women have their pain labelled as PID, which may or may not be true. From then on any pain they have may be considered as just another infection.

While a laparoscopy is useful to *diagnose* a pelvic infection, it is best to leave any major surgery until the pelvic infection has been treated. If surgery is done during an infection, there is a high chance that severe pelvic adhesions may form.

How is a pelvic infection treated?

A pelvic infection is treated with antibiotics. Which antibiotics are used will depend on how sick you are, what type of bacteria you have, and whether or not you have been admitted to hospital. Most women have more than one type of bacteria causing their infection, so they need more than one antibiotic. You may be prescribed:

- One antibiotic for a group of bacteria that include chlamydia (as well as similar bacteria that are not sexually transmitted)
- One antibiotic for a group of bacteria called 'anaerobes', and
- One antibiotic for other bacteria.

Your partner may need antibiotics too. If so, it is important that you both take the antibiotics at the same time, to avoid re-infecting each other

If you are very sick, you may be admitted to hospital so that your antibiotics can be given to you through an intravenous (IV) drip. Whatever you need, it is important that your infection be treated. The longer it is there, the more damage it can do, and the more likely it is that your pain could become chronic.

Who can help me with a pelvic infection?

- Your general practitioner.
- A gynaecologist.

Is a vaginal infection the same as a pelvic infection?

No. Vaginal infections are common. There are always bacteria in the vagina, but most are 'good bacteria' and quite healthy. When other bacteria, or the fungus 'candida' spread from your bowel into the vagina, the healthy bacteria leave and the vaginal discharge changes. These infections are not sexually transmitted, and almost all women will get a candida infection (thrush) at one time or another.

Chapter 10

. . . .

You and your gynaecologist

IF YOU FEEL NERVOUS at the thought of seeing a gynaecologist, you are not alone. Most people do. Not only does your visit concern a private part of your body, but also the outcome of your visit is important to you. If it goes well, you may be on the path to less pain.

How to choose a gynaecologist

Obstetrics and gynaecology cover a large field: too large for all gynaecologists to be expert in all areas. We all specialise to some degree. Some doctors specialise in laparoscopic surgery and endometriosis.

Your general practitioner (GP) knows the services available in your area, and if you have a choice will try to refer you to a gynaecologist who suits your personality and needs. If you will be attending a public hospital, ask which hospital has a good reputation for laparoscopic surgery. This increases the likelihood that the doctor you see will have a good understanding of endometriosis. There is very little endometriosis surgery that cannot be done through a laparoscope, but these skills are not available everywhere.

What is an Obstetrician and Gynaecologist?

An obstetrician cares for women when they are pregnant.
A gynaecologist cares for women when they are not pregnant.
To become an Obstetrician and Gynaecologist (O and G) in Australia and New Zealand requires a minimum of a six-year medical degree, a one-year internship and then a six-year specialist qualification. After completing specialist training, some O and Gs specialise further in a particular area of gynaecology, while others continue to work in both areas. So a gynaecologist is also an obstetrician, but may or may not still deliver babies.

Endometriosis surgery is difficult surgery. There are great benefits to be had, but there are also risks. No surgeon seeks to hurt their patients and no surgeon likes complications. It is important to us that our patients are happy with the care we provide. Because of this some gynaecologists choose *not* to do endometriosis surgery because it is not their area of expertise. This is a very reasonable and responsible choice.

All gynaecologists in Australia and New Zealand spend time each year in training. This is compulsory if we wish to continue working as gynaecologists. However, there are many areas of training we can choose, so we all develop different areas of interest. Most gynaecologists in Australia are able to diagnose endometriosis by laparoscopy, but only some are able to do the more complicated surgery necessary to remove the endometriosis completely.

Learning and maintaining the skills necessary for modern endometriosis surgery is a heavy commitment for a gynaecologist. It requires time away from work, and significant expense. Operating close to delicate organs on a regular basis also adds that extra stress to a surgeon's life that some doctors wisely decide they do not need. If your current gynaecologist has areas of expertise outside endometriosis he or she may refer you to another gynae-cologist, especially if your endometriosis is severe. If, after reading Chapter 9, your pain may be due to something else apart from endometriosis, then you should see one of the professionals recommended in that section rather than your endometriosis surgeon.

If the gynaecologist you are considering is a friend or relative of yours, you may be better to consider a different doctor. Your doctor friend will want everything to go smoothly for you; yet can provide no more guarantee of this than for any other patient. It is very difficult to be both doctor and friend, and your non-medical relationship may suffer. In some circumstances there may be no other suitable alternative, but if there is a choice, you can always ask him or her whom they would recommend.

Finally, it is important that you feel some rapport with your doctor. If problems occur, a good relationship will help both you and your doctor through a difficult time. If you don't feel com-fortable with your gynaecologist, ask your GP or gynaecologist for a second opinion. Your doctor will not be offended. We all have patients with whom a useful relationship develops easily, and others with whom it is more difficult.

You should also ask for a second opinion if you believe that your pain is not being taken seriously.

> **It is sometimes said that there is a doctor for every patient and a patient for every doctor, but no doctor who suits everyone.**

I have had pain for SO long and I am SO angry

You may have a lot of reasons to be angry. Severe pain, disappointments, having your pain ignored or being treated badly is enough to make anyone angry. You may be angry because a treatment failed, and life seems unfair, even when you know that those who cared for you did their best. Anger can be a positive thing if it helps you keep going, but it is not helpful if it prevents you moving forward to recovery.

A new doctor is a new opportunity to look at your pain afresh. Difficult though it is, it is important to give a new doctor the opportunity to do *their* best. To you, he or she may be just another doctor. To them, you are a new person and a new challenge.

Some women only feel able to express anger to those doctors who listen most and treat them well. They feel unable to tell those they dislike how they feel. It is important that you are able to explain how you feel about past treatments, but where anger runs deep it can interfere with your new professional relationship. More importantly, it can interfere with your care and treatment. This is not in your interest.

If you feel unable to move forward due to fear, disappointment or anger, then this needs to be resolved. A counsellor may be the best person to talk to about your feelings. He or she is someone who is not part of your medical care, not a member of your family and not a friend. You can talk freely.

Preparation for your visit, and what to ask

Your first visit to the gynaecologist is a first for both of you. He or she does not know the type of person you are, nor what you are looking for. Time must be spent talking about your pain, any previous treatments, and going through the options you have now.

I find that two women with exactly the same symptoms may make completely different treatment choices. Some wish to avoid surgery at all costs, even if that means living with pain, whereas others think of surgery as their first choice.

Something as complicated as pelvic pain takes time to work through. If you are well prepared for your visit, then less time is spent going through the basic information your doctor needs, and more time can be spent learning about your condition, and considering which options would suit *you* best. After all, the most important thing to come away with is a plan with which you are happy.

Being prepared for your visit means thinking about the questions you may be asked beforehand. In my practice we ask women to fill in a short questionnaire at home before their appointment. This allows them time to think about the answers and look up any information if necessary. If all the things they wish to discuss are written down, then they are unlikely to be forgotten on the day. Your gynaecologist will appreciate the care you have taken.

The questions a gynaecologist usually asks might concern:

- *Your periods.* Are they regular? How long is it between the first day of one period and the first day of the next period (cycle length)? Are they heavy or light? Are they painful? Do you have bleeding between your periods?
- *Your pain.* When do you get pain? Is it related to periods, and if so, during which days? What makes it better? What makes it worse? Does it wake you at night? Where is it? Does the pain move to any other areas?
- *Your bladder and bowel function.* Are these normal? Do they cause pain? If so, do you think the bladder or bowel pain is related to your periods?
- *Your sexual relationship, if relevant.* Does intercourse hurt? If so, where do you think the pain is? What contraception are you

using? Are there any other sexual problems you wish to discuss?

- *Treatments you have tried.* Do any medications help your pain? Have you had any surgery in the past? If so, when was this, what was found, what was done, and did it help?
- *Any plans for pregnancy, if relevant.* Are you currently trying to get pregnant? Do you plan a pregnancy in the near future? Have you had a problem becoming pregnant in the past?
- *Your medical history.* Do you have any illnesses? Have you had any other surgery? Were there any problems with anaesthetics? Do you have any allergies?
- *Your family history.* Does anyone else in your family have endometriosis? Is there a history of gynaecological conditions, bleeding disorders, blood clots or drug allergies?

What is a 'normal' period?

Although periods vary widely between different women, they are remarkably similar for each person. Women with *regular* monthly periods usually know how many days they will bleed, how many pads or tampons they will need and when the next period will be. They notice when something is different.

Normal regular periods last between one and eight days (usually five days), occur every 24 to 35 days (usually 28 days), and lose less than 80 ml of blood (usually 50 ml). Whatever cycle length you have, it should be the same, or almost the same each month. If not, then you have irregular periods. Irregular periods are much less predictable. The time between periods varies, periods may be long or short, and the amount of blood lost varies widely.

A period is considered 'heavy' if it is common to pass clots of blood, have 'flooding' or 'accidents' on sheets or clothing, or change pads during the night.

It is not normal to bleed between periods, although sometimes a tiny amount of blood passed only at ovulation time may be normal for you. Bleeding between periods should be reported to your doctor.

Your gynaecologist will be especially pleased to see details of any pelvic operations you have had in the past. This information might include photos from your surgery, an operation sheet describing what was done, or a copy of the letter sent to your general practitioner. The more information your gynaecologist has about your previous surgery, the better they can advise you on future treatment.

It is easy to forget to ask the questions you want answered during your visit. It is best to write your questions down before you go, and check your list before you leave. I do this myself whenever I see a doctor.

If a laparoscopy is planned, ask what type of surgery would be done if endometriosis is found. If your doctor can only offer cautery or laser ablation, then that narrows your options if you are found have endometriosis. These treatments suit some endometriosis, but not all. If you don't feel you have enough information, ask more questions. Frequently, there are different types of surgery possible according to your wishes and individual needs. Be sure that your doctor understands what surgery you want in different situations. They will not be able to ask you while you are asleep.

No-one remembers all that is said during one appointment, especially if they are anxious or in pain. Taking your partner, parent or friend with you is a good idea. Your special person may remember things you missed, and it is good to have someone who heard the same advice you did to talk to later on. You could ask your doctor to list the options you have on a piece of paper to take with you and consider later on.

If, after you leave, you cannot decide what to do, you may need more information or just some time to think about it. You could look at the websites listed in the appendix on page 276, talk to your general practitioner, talk with your family, or make another appointment with your gynaecologist to discuss it further.

> **In the end, there is always the option of 'do nothing' and live with it. Remember that it is your pelvis, and your choice. It is also your responsibility to accept the consequences of the choices that you make.**

Vaginal examinations

No-one enjoys vaginal examinations. This is the time when women say to me: 'Why in the world did you become a gynaecologist?' From a gynaecologist's viewpoint, a vaginal examination is just a way of obtaining information you can't get from questions alone. I appreciate that this is not the way that most women see it!

Embarrassment, although very understandable and probably unavoidable, is unnecessary. As gynaecologists, we examine women every day. Whatever your body shape, tattoo preference or body piercing, it is the person underneath who matters, and with whom we have a professional relationship. Your doctor will not think less of you after a vaginal examination.

J am a virgin. Will the gynaecologist want to examine me?

Probably not, but your doctor may not realise that you are a virgin unless you tell him or her.

Cervical smear tests are not necessary in women until they have been sexually active for at least 12 months. As a virgin you will not be pregnant, and a sexually transmitted disease is unlikely. So if you have never had intercourse there is less need for your doctor to examine you vaginally. He or she may still wish to check your abdomen, because this shows where your pain is. Your parent or support person can stay with you during the examination if you wish. However, if there is private information you wish to tell the doctor, this is a good opportunity to speak to them alone. An ultrasound can show whether or not your uterus or ovaries are enlarged. If your gynaecologist feels that a vaginal examination *is* important, they can discuss this with you, and explain what will be done.

If you have your period at the time of your appointment, you may choose to re-schedule it to another day. However, your gynaecologist is used to the sight of blood and provided that you are comfortable, will be happy to see you for most conditions regardless. Generally they have spare sanitary pads or tampons if needed, and an examination during a period does help in isolating exactly where the period pain is coming from. Some tests, such as cervical smear tests are not reliable when done during a period, so if you are unsure it is best to ring and ask if your appointment should be changed.

There are two parts to a vaginal examination. The first part is called a *speculum examination*. It involves inserting a vaginal speculum into the vagina so that the cervix and the walls of the vagina can be seen. A vaginal **speculum** is an instrument that holds the vagina open. It is used if you are due for a smear test, if you may have endometriosis of the upper vagina, or to look for other gynaecological problems.

The second part is called a *bimanual examination* because both hands are used. Two fingers of one hand are inserted into the vagina and the other hand is placed on the lower abdomen. A bimanual examination allows your doctor to check the size, tenderness and position of the uterus and ovaries. It is more difficult in larger women. Sometimes lumps (nodules) of endometriosis can be felt along the uterosacral ligaments at the top of the vagina, or in the area between vagina and bowel. You should tell your doctor which parts of your pelvis are tender as this may be where your endometriosis lies.

Vaginal examinations may be especially traumatic for women with a painful pelvis, or those who have been sexually assaulted in the past. If you are anxious about being examined, you should tell your doctor. He or she may be unaware of your feelings and there may be another alternative. No doctor wants to cause pain or emotional distress.

Yes, it is possible.

Amber is a 32-year-old woman who had suffered 17 years of severe chronic pelvic pain. Most nights she was woken by agonising, nauseating pain in her back and pelvis. She had given up on men, sex and smear tests. Any attempt at vaginal examination caused excruciating pain. Her vaginal muscles were overly tense and she had vaginismus (see Chapter 2, page 19). Amber had pain in her pelvis after passing urine, bladder frequency and painful bowel actions at period time. A laparoscopy done a few years before had found 'no endometriosis'.

When we met, she was using very high doses of depo-provera as well as the contraceptive pill to stop her periods altogether. Even so, she had severe pelvic pain day and night. Amber was very courageous, but pain for so long had made her wonder if life was worth living. There were so many aspects to Amber's pain that no single treatment would be enough.

We worked though several treatments:

- 10 mg of amitriptyline at night helped her neurogenic and bladder pain. She could now sleep at night without disturbance.
- A laparoscopy showed that she did indeed have endometriosis, but it had an unusual appearance that is commonly missed. Her back pain improved substantially.
- Amber stopped her depo-provera and contraceptive pill. She did not need contraception, they had not helped her pain and her mood was better without them.
- A Mirena® IUCD was inserted to treat pain from her uterus and take over from the depo-provera when it wore off and her periods returned.
- Amber realised herself that fizzy drinks and coffee aggravated her bladder pain so she cut them out.
- Review by a urologist and starting ditropan improved her bladder pain even further.
- Counselling for the emotional distress she suffered over many years continued.
- A sex therapist continues to work through the vaginismus with her.

Amber still has some pain, but in her own words she 'has her life back' and the pain is '95 per cent gone'. This process has taken four months to achieve. She is not ready for a relationship yet, but who knows?

Chapter 11

. . . .

Coping with endometriosis

Jane Marsh, RN

EVEN THOUGH ALL THE WOMEN I see have endometriosis, their needs vary. Some women have few problems. Their endometriosis can be treated easily, their general health is good and they feel positive about their life. Other women have had a difficult time with endometriosis over many years. They may have other health problems, or personal issues that seem overwhelming.

We discuss practical ways to cope with the effects of endometriosis on their day-to-day lives. Like all of us, women with endometriosis have stresses in their lives that are nothing to do with their disease. We look at practical ways they can help themselves.

This chapter includes a few of the common situations women with endometriosis talk to me about. It provides ideas for working through them. It is divided into ways you can support yourself and ways in which others can support you. Luckily, very few women have all these problems!

Supporting yourself

Coping better with the pain

Pain is a very personal thing. No two women have the same pain and no-one else can experience *your* pain as *you* do. Your doctor can explain medical ways to manage and sometimes cure your pain, but the changes you can make yourself are important too. Even when your medical treatment has been successful, you may still have some pain. Looking after your general health and emotional wellbeing can help you cope better with whatever pain remains.

- *Learn more about your pain.* For some women, finally knowing what it is that has caused them pain for so long, and learning what endometriosis is, helps a lot. The worry that went with an unknown pain is gone, even if the pain itself is still there. Even a laparoscopy that finds no endometriosis can be reassuring. Yes, the need to investigate the pain remains (see Chapter 9) but it is good to know that the pelvis looks healthy. If there are things about your care, or your pain, that you don't under-stand, ask lots of questions.
- *Prioritise your life.* You may find that you can't do *everything* you want to do, so decide what is actually important and what is not.
  - Leave household chores undone if you are not well. At these times, you need to *rest* and look after yourself. You needn't feel guilty – any dust will wait!
  - Avoid taking on more projects or social plans than you can comfortably handle. Pick the important ones and say 'No thank you' to the rest.
  - Make health and being happy together a priority for your family. Your family will function best if you are *all* well, so your needs are important too.

- Where you can, avoid those activities that upset or stress you.

- *Make time for exercise that you* can *do, despite the pain.* Exercise releases chemicals called endorphins that decrease pain. It also distracts your mind from the pain, improves strength, helps with weight loss and makes you feel well. There may be days when you are not well enough to exercise, but do what you can when you can. You can start with gentle exercise, and do more as your strength and endurance improves. Walking, swimming and aquarobics are good exercises to start with.

- *Avoid negative thoughts.* You may have difficult memories of a friend or relative who had serious gynaecological problems. You are an individual and your experience needn't be the same as theirs.

- *Avoid becoming tired.* Your pain will feel worse if you are tired and worn out.
  - Get plenty of sleep.
  - Eat a well-balanced healthy diet to ensure a good intake of vitamins and minerals (see Chapter 12). Avoid alcohol and caffeine. You don't need any 'morning after' feelings.
  - Drink plenty of water. Around 2 litres of fluid daily, is a good goal. Dehydration makes you tired.
  - Encourage and allow your children and partner to do jobs around the house. You don't have to do everything yourself and it will help your children learn to be capable, independent adults.
  - Realise that you needn't be responsible for sorting out every emotional need or disagreement in your family, particularly if they do not involve you directly. There may be things that your family can sort out for themselves.
  - Look for an easier way of doing things. Your partner or children will still love you if they have bought biscuits

rather than home-made ones in their lunchbox. Maybe it's time for them to make their lunch themselves, particularly if you work too.

- *Consider complementary therapies.* An experienced and well-trained therapist might help you. Most of these therapies need persistence and may only work for you while you use them. They are not intended as a replacement for the medications or surgery that your doctor recommends. They can work together with conventional treatments to give you the best result possible.
  - Acupuncture. Acupuncture uses fine needles inserted in the skin at specially chosen places to provide pain relief.
  - Hypnotherapy can help by improving relaxation; making you less aware of your pain and helping you feel more positive about yourself.
  - Herbal and dietary therapies are discussed by Dr Margaret Taylor in Chapter 12.
- When the pain is bad:
  - Use hot packs on your abdomen for warmth and comfort.
  - Take a hot restful bath.
  - If you have children, use what childcare you can afford so that you give yourself a rest. You will be much better company for your children once you feel better.
  - Spend the evening after work in bed. You will be more tired after a day working with pain and you need rest. Your children can come to you to have a book read, or talk about their day. They might really enjoy this time with a more rested and available mother.
  - If you are able to, do something interesting that takes your mind off the pain.

To gain control of your pain you may need to be proactive in seeking out the best treatment available. You may need to mix natural and conventional treatments with a change in your diet, exercise and lifestyle. These are things over which you *do* have control. Remember, your doctor will not be able to fix everything for you. There will be things that you have to do yourself. Working on your health to benefit your pain can benefit your life in other ways too.

Feeling different to your teenage friends

You may think that you are the only teenager ever to have endometriosis, but you are not. It is actually quite common among teenagers. However, if none of the girls you know have it, it is easy to feel 'different' or isolated. Over the years, you may not have understood why your pain was so bad, or why regular period pain medication didn't work for you. Your teachers, friends and parents may not have understood either. They may not have been as supportive as they could have been.

Your local endometriosis support organisation can help you get in touch with other girls your age who also have endometriosis. It is very comforting to talk to girls with a similar experience. It is your choice who you tell about your endometriosis, but you need not feel alone.

Teenagers in general find their relationships at home stressful. Is there someone you trust to whom you can explain what irritates or upsets you? Is there something in particular that worries you? You may have been prescribed the contraceptive pill, yet worry about what this might mean for weight gain, your long-term health or your reputation among your friends.

At your age you have exams and other school expectations to cope with, a growing sexual awareness, skin problems, body image issues, family conflicts and a lot more.

Maintaining your relationships

Endometriosis can strain any relationship: mothers, fathers, siblings, partners, children, workmates, or friends. To avoid this, it is worthwhile explaining to the people that are important to you what endometriosis is and how it affects you. They may have absolutely no understanding of endometriosis, so it is in your best interest to educate them. They won't want to talk about it all the time, but there are some things it is important that they understand.

You should also remember that some of the people in your life may have their own issues to work through once you are diagnosed with endometriosis.

- *Your parents.* It is a parent's natural response to shield their children from any harm or pain. When they can't do this, they may feel guilty, anxious or angry. They may also be scared for you, yet not wish to show it.

- *Your partner.* Your partner may want to 'fix' any problems you have for you, to save you from worry. If they are unable to do so, they may feel useless and unimportant. Tell your partner that you do not expect him (or her) to fix your endometriosis for you, but that you still need their support. There is nothing to see from the outside in a woman with endometriosis, so your pain may be difficult for a man to relate to. They will never have endometriosis themselves and may not understand the pain you are in. Don't presume they understand your pain, or how you are feeling.

- *Your children.* Your children will notice that you are not yourself at some times of the month. Let them know that it is not their fault and explain what you *are* able to do for them. Children may not ask *why* things happen and presume that it is their fault. This is a burden they should not have to bear. There may be good things to come out of your illness. A mother who rests more and limits her social obligations is more available to cuddle or have quiet times with her children.

- *Your friends.* Over time, your friendships with some people may change. It is hard to maintain every friendship when your pain makes you cancel activities at the last moment, or cut down on some social activities. Your friends may tire of asking how you are feeling. You can surround yourself with a few good friends who will support you no matter what. Be aware that your friends have troubles of their own. They may not have endometriosis, but we all have problems and there may be times when you can help them in some way. Even if this is difficult physically, you can still be a good listener. Friendships work best when there is listening and support on both sides. Your friends may be embarrassed to bring up their own troubles when your problems seem so much more important than theirs.

- *Your workmates.* All workplaces (and bosses) are different, but it may be sensible to tell them what is happening. You may prefer that your employer does not know about your condition, especially if you can cope with all your duties easily. However, if your pain is severe, they will notice your time off work, lack of concentration and inability to meet deadlines. If you have a reasonable boss, he or she will appreciate the effort you are making to get better and manage your pain. Without an explanation they might feel that you are not interested in your work. If you have an unreasonable boss, then you may be better to keep this information to yourself unless it becomes necessary to explain. If you feel that you are being mistreated because of your illness, your workplace representative or the Equal Opportunities Board may be able to help you.

Feeling feminine and attractive

Pain, bleeding, bloating and the side effects of some medications can make you feel unattractive. Some women describe this feeling as 'living in an alien body'. Not surprisingly, your morale and self-worth may suffer. It is time to look after yourself, both physically and emotionally.

- *Talk to your partner if you can.* The longer you feel these things without explaining how you feel the harder they may be to discuss. If you feel uncomfortable doing this, you may prefer to talk to a good female friend.

- *Do activities you enjoy* that allow you to relax and feel good about yourself. A long hot bath with your favourite bath salts, and music, a facial or body massage. A do-it-yourself facial, or manicure can be just as good if your budget is limited.
- *Wear something comfortable* that is not tight around your abdomen and makes you feel attractive.

Involving your family in your care

It is a good idea to take someone you feel comfortable with to your appointments with the gynaecologist. This special person could be your parent, husband, boyfriend, girlfriend, sister, or anyone you choose. Having them there will give you more confidence and will help them to understand what is happening to you. If you need surgery, this special person may be able to come with you when you are admitted to hospital and support you while you are waiting for your surgery.

Involving your family with your care helps in practical ways too. An involved family will be more likely to help rearrange your sport, dance or other commitments according to your menstrual cycle.

Feeling scared of surgery

It's normal to be anxious about an operation, but a pity if that anxiety stops you making good decisions about your health. Finding out as much as you can about what your operation involves may help you feel better. A visit to the hospital before your admission is a good idea. There will be less that is unknown and therefore less to worry about on the day.

Although it is impossible to know *exactly* what your doctor will find at the operation, or *exactly* what treatment you will need, you can find out what the possibilities are. There are many websites on endometriosis and a list of those we find most useful are on page 276. Ask your doctor any questions that are on your mind. You should never feel that your questions are silly. They are about what matters to you. Your doctor may have written information for you to take home and read. When you go into hospital, tell the nursing staff if you are nervous, and don't be embarrassed to ask questions. The nurses are there to help you too.

Finally, while it *is* true that the only reliable way of diagnosing endometriosis is with surgery, *you never have to have surgery.* As explained in Chapter 5 on page 46 endometriosis is not a life-threatening condition. Surgery should be a choice you make after considering the options you have. It may be a good choice in many cases, but it is never your only choice. Some of the choices available to you are explained in Chapter 7.

J am anxious and scared all the time

If you are very anxious or miserable, there may be something more going on. As a woman with pelvic pain, you have probably been through a lot over the last few years. None of this is good for your morale or self-esteem, and all of this can easily add up to feelings of isolation or depression.

If your worries are not being taken seriously and you know something is not right with your body or your emotions, ask for help from the doctor you feel most comfortable with. If you have prolonged feelings of sadness or you cry a lot, you may be depressed. There is no shame in seeking help and you can do so without your friends knowing.

Psychologists are professionals who help you by working out strategies for coping with your own feelings and life stresses. A psychiatrist is a doctor who specialises in the treatment of mental illness including depression. Your general practitioner may be able to help you themselves, but if not, he or she can advise you which type of professional might suit you best. You may also find the book *Coping with Endometriosis* by Robert Phillips and Glenda Motta useful (see Reference 26).

When sex is painful

If period pain was not enough, many women with endometriosis have painful intercourse. This is especially common in women whose endometriosis is near the pouch of Douglas or in the uterosacral ligaments that lie behind the uterus. Although painful sex is a problem for women of any age, it is particularly distressing for young women just starting their sexual life. Intercourse with their partner is an important part of their relationship. To find it painful is a great disappointment. With every attempt at intercourse there may be two or three days of pain, and yet the desire to bond emotionally with their partner remains. Ultimately, it is no wonder that many women avoid intercourse altogether, leaving their partner feeling rejected and unloved.

Removing endometriosis at an operation may cure your pain with intercourse completely, but sometimes the pain remains. If so, it may be due to:

- Anxiety about intercourse itself
- Painful nerve receptors in the pelvis that continue to cause pain even when the original problem has been treated (see Chapter 9, page 177)
- Pelvic muscles that have become painful and tight after years of pain
- Sexual abuse or other traumatic events in your life
- Negative attitudes to sex you may have learned as you grew up
- Seeing scary movies or images relating to sex
- Uncertainty about your sexuality
- Other physical reasons for pain.

A counsellor, especially a sex counsellor, can help with some of these problems, but you should also explain your symptoms to your doctor. Your general practitioner can check for physical reasons for the pain that may be nothing to do with your endometriosis (see Chapter 2, page 19). A sex counsellor can help bring up some of the topics you find most difficult to discuss with your partner, even if you choose to see the sex counsellor alone at first. They can help with:

- Exercises to improve your self-confidence and increase the trust between you and your partner
- Relaxation techniques
- Forms of sexual pleasure that are not painful
- Improving your communication skills as a couple
- Pain management
- Working out what works best for you.

But J just find it SO hard to talk to my partner about sex

Even close couples have some things they find hard to discuss, but it is important that you and your partner can communicate well. Men do not have pain that stops their sex drive, so without an explanation he will not understand. He may feel that you are avoiding sex because you no longer love him, rather than because sex is painful.

Misunderstandings that can damage your relationship happen easily. You may find it easier if your partner comes to your doctor's appointment with you. As your partner learns more about endometriosis and the effects it can have, your discussions about sex may become easier.

- Tell your partner what they do that does satisfy you, rather than presume they know already.

- Tell your partner that you still desire him (or her).
- Discuss your pain and tell him (or her) where it hurts.

A healthy sexual relationship is important for both of you, so it is worth getting it right.

Avoiding pain during sex

Ideas for maintaining your sexual relationship despite pain include:

- *Working out which time of the day or month is least painful for you*, and arranging some special time together then. This often means having intercourse early in the month, just after your period, or early in the day when you are not tired.
- *Slow, shallow and gentle penetration until you say it is OK* allows you to stay in control. You will have more control of the depth of penetration if you are on top of your partner. Knowing that intercourse will not proceed further than you wish, allows you to feel more confident. Your partner will be fearful of hurting you so will appreciate a lead from you. A shorter time of penetration may avoid prolonged pain afterwards.
- *A water-based lubricant* such as KY Jelly®, or Astroglide® may make penetration easier. Natural lubrication only occurs if you are relaxed and pain free. This is a big ask of women with endometriosis, so it is not surprising that many use a lubricant. Many women without endometriosis use lubricants too, so there is no need to be embarrassed.
- *Relaxation techniques before sex*. Gentle and prolonged foreplay helps relax your pelvic muscles as well as giving you time to relax your whole body. Most women appreciate longer foreplay before penetrative sex. A pelvic physiotherapist can teach you how to strengthen your pelvic muscles, relax over-tight muscles or dilate an overly tight vagina.

- *New sexual positions.* The pain of endometriosis is usually worse in some positions than others.
- *Consider a medication* for neurogenic pain, such as amitriptyline (see Chapter 6, page 74). This is particularly useful in women with pain on most days of the month, or a 'burning' pain during intercourse.
- *Hypnotherapy* may be useful.

If penetration becomes impossible, you and your partner may be able to find other ways to pleasure each other. The book *Good Loving, Great Sex* by Rosie King (see Reference 27) has good suggestions for 'outercourse' rather than 'intercourse', as well as good ideas for mismatched sex drives.

Worries that you won't have children

Most women with endometriosis fear infertility. As explained in Chapter 8 on page 119, endometriosis is only one of several factors that can affect a couple's fertility. Endometriosis by itself does not mean you cannot become pregnant. A lot depends on how severe it is, where it is, how old you are, and whether there are other fertility issues present affecting either you or your partner. Almost all women with endometriosis are able to have children, even if some require medical assistance to do so.

If you do have difficulty becoming pregnant and are referred to a fertility specialist, there is usually a counsellor at the clinic with whom you can discuss your particular issues. Remember that your partner may have concerns of their own that they may find difficult to discuss with you. Now, more than ever, is the time when communication between you as a couple is so important. Yes, you are trying for a baby, but your relationship is important too. It is the two of you who matter most and a healthy relationship between you is important when caring for a child.

Not ready for a hysterectomy

Mandy is a woman in her late thirties who, although single, would love to have a child. Mandy has adenomyosis, a condition with pain similar to endometriosis due to changes in the wall of the uterus. Her doctor had offered her a hysterectomy and she was very distressed. Mandy knew that a hysterectomy would cure both her pain and the heavy bleeding she suffered, but she did not want to lose the chance of a pregnancy. We talked about her feelings and her yearnings to have a child one day. To avoid a hysterectomy, she needed strategies to help her cope with the pain.

Mandy decided to take one of the specialist's options and go on the contraceptive pill continuously to stop her periods and hopefully avoid her severe period pain. She would see a complementary therapist to help boost her immune system, and help with her general health and wellbeing. She would improve her diet and start some regular exercise. Just deciding on a plan made Mandy feel better. She felt back in control of her health. She hoped to manage her pain this way until either she met a partner with whom she could form a relationship and try to start a family, or she felt psychologically ready to have a hysterectomy.

Don't let premenstrual syndrome (PMS) make everything worse

Premenstrual syndrome is a collection of symptoms that some women notice in the days before a period. These symptoms may be emotional or physical and include:

- Greasy skin
- Fluid retention
- Decreased libido
- Irritability

- Sore breasts
- Backache
- Fatigue
- Depression.

Severe PMS seems very common in women with endometriosis. This makes the time before a period particularly difficult. Not only is there the pain of endometriosis, but the symptoms of PMS as well. The closer a period comes, the more anxiety a woman may feel. She knows the pain will come soon. Any PMS symptoms are the last straw.

Some women notice PMS symptoms for just one or two days before a period, while others suffer for up to two weeks. Women with mild symptoms may be able to carry on with their day-to-day life well despite their PMS, but for women with severe symptoms it can be debilitating. Severe PMS can contribute to accidents, antisocial behaviour, emotional crisis, and time off work or school. Stress does not cause PMS, but like most things, it makes it worse. In extreme cases, some women may feel suicidal.

While feeling forgetful or reclusive is common, aggression is the symptom that most women, their families and friends relate to most. There is also the guilt that women feel when they think about how their behaviour impacts on those closest to them.

If your symptoms are due to PMS, they will become worse the closer you are to a period. If they come at any time of the month, regardless of when your next period is due, then PMS is less likely, and you should talk to your general practitioner about it.

PMS just part of the problem

Mary and Rod have two small children. Rod worked long hours, with Mary as the main caregiver to their children, 24 hours a day, 7 days a week. Mary battled with her mood swings and her endometriosis pain. Rod suffered the mood swings too. Mary had no outlet and no close supportive family, so she rang Rod at work when she couldn't cope with the pain or the children. Rod's work suffered, as did their marriage. Their problems at times seemed monumental.

Mary and Rod felt better after we discussed what PMS and endometriosis involve, as well as Mary's feelings of loss of self, lack of support and entrapment with the children. Some strategies were put in place. Mary decided to have surgery to remove her endometriosis and lessen her pain. Once fully recovered she would look for a job outside the family. Rod would attempt to get home at a more reasonable hour to help with the children and support her plans to re-enter the workforce.

When I saw Mary again, she had started a part-time job that she enjoyed. She enjoyed her time with the children more now, and so did they. Working in the evening fitted in with both Rod and the children's needs. Her surgery had improved her pain and she felt much more positive about her life. So did Rod.

Ways that you can manage your PMS

- *Explain to your partner and family how your PMS affects you.* If you feel unable to do this, your counsellor or general practitioner may be able to help. An explanation that you have limited control over your emotions at that time, particularly if stressed, will ease family tension. They need to know that you need extra understanding at this time and are not 'putting it on'.
- *Manage your pain.* Your pain has not caused your PMS, but with less pain, you will have more energy to cope with your PMS. You will no longer dread the start of a period.
- *Improve your diet.* A diet that is low in salt (to reduce fluid retention), high in fibre and low in fat (to avoid bowel symptoms), high in fruits and vegetables (to supply the

vitamins and minerals you need) and low in caffeine (to avoid over-stimulation) should suit you best.

- *Practice relaxation techniques* such as yoga, or meditation. Relaxation improves your ability to cope with PMS as well as allowing you 'time out' from the stress of family and work commitments. Time for relaxation allows you to regain control of your emotions.

- *Herbal therapies* (see Chapter 12). Natural therapists believe that PMS is due to an excess of estrogen effect in the body. They use a combination of herbal therapies and diet to decrease the effect of estrogen.

- *Exercise.* Exercise improves mental as well as physical well-being.

- *Consider trying the contraceptive pill.* The Pill improves many of the symptoms of PMS. It doesn't suit everyone, but can certainly help. Your doctor can help you decide if the Pill might suit you.

- *Consider an SSRI medication* (see Chapter 6, page 74). These medications stabilise a substance called serotonin in the brain. They can be useful for mood changes before your period. If your life is severely affected by your mood at this time, you may wish to discuss this medication with your general practitioner.

Remember, if your family is at breaking point because of your PMS, don't feel guilty: see your doctor or a family therapist. Help *is* available.

Coping once your treatment is finished

After you have spent a good deal of time seeing your GP, finding an endometriosis surgeon, having your surgery and working through other treatments, there comes a time when you come out of the treatment arena and return to your normal life. Until now you have been active in your treatment choices, but secure in the knowledge that others were there to care for you and help with decision making when needed. Some women find 'going it alone' a nervous and challenging time. *However, it is also an opportunity to be positive, grab hold of your life and move forward.*

Remember that if you need help your general practitioner is still there. He or she knows you well and is the best person to coordinate your long-term care. The relaxation techniques, dietary changes, exercise program, and whatever else has helped you become well should continue. If your symptoms return, your general practitioner can discuss your options with you and arrange an appointment with your specialist if necessary.

How your partner can support you and themselves

This book has concentrated on *her* needs, but *your* needs are important too. A healthy relationship values and provides support to both partners. At times one partner may need more care than the other, but if possible there should be mutual support. You may feel frustrated and resentful that her illness has impacted so much on your life. Even though your partner is in pain, your feelings are still there and still valid. You could talk to a friend about how you feel, take some time out that is just for you, see a counsellor yourself or plan things together that you *both* enjoy.

Telling other people about endometriosis

Endometriosis can be an embarrassing illness for a woman to have. It is much easier to explain an illness which is visible to the outside world (like a broken leg), an illness that will reliably get better over time (like pneumonia), or an illness that affects men too (like asthma or diabetes). It may be difficult or embarrassing for her to explain what her problem is to some friends, family or workmates. There may be some people she does not want to explain her endometriosis to at all.

Making her feel good about herself

When she feels unattractive, try to make her feel loved and desirable. Remember that she is often as confused about her feelings and the disease she is trying to cope with as you are. Flowers are good, but something practical to make her life easier, like a dinner cooked when she comes home, or an offer to get the kids off to school yourself may be even better. Often just an extra 'I love you' is all that is needed. Men rarely understand why woman need repeated reassurance that they are loved and desirable. It is the way we women are. Be free with your kind comments. It is unlikely you will overdo it.

Deciding on a treatment option

It is difficult to be a partner of a woman with endometriosis. Men traditionally want to fix any problems their partners have. They want to save their partner from worry. You may feel powerless to help her when she has pain, and at a loss what to do. This is where the difference between men and women is an advantage. Most women neither expect nor want their man to come up with an answer to their problems. What they want is the opportunity to talk about and talk around their problems, sometimes at some length. This talking may seem unhelpful to a man, but it allows her to consider all aspects of the choices she has and come up with a considered and thoughtful plan that she is happy with. Listening to what she is thinking and how she feels is something very worthwhile that you *can* do. She will also want to know your views and ideas.

Helping her through her PMS

The lack of emotional control at this time distresses women and their families a lot. Women often say that 'they know they are being awful but just can't help it'. Then again, if you disregard what a woman says because 'it's that time of the month again' she may feel slighted and become even angrier. There is no need to tell her she is being unreasonable. She will feel bad enough later, when she recalls what she has said to those who love her most. Some ways in which you can support but not aggravate her include:

- *Giving her some time to herself*, to allow her to relax and get the things done which are on her mind.
- *Listening* if she wants to talk to you, but don't take insults to heart. During this time unexpected outbursts of anger or tears are common.
- *Encouraging her* to seek help for her symptoms, on a day when she feels well. Offer to go with her when she sees her doctor, counsellor or natural therapist, but allow her to go alone if she would prefer.
- *Helping her* work through any issues that trouble her, to relieve stress.
- *Recognising* that the time before a period is not a good time for her to make important decisions.
- *Avoiding* overloading her daily commitments at this time.

Coping with fertility treatment

For couples who *do* have difficulty becoming pregnant, there are new issues to consider. Certainly there is the grief that goes with not becoming pregnant easily, but there may also be concerns about:

- The lack of privacy over something that is usually so intimate
- The side effects of any medications used
- The expense of fertility treatments
- The increased chance of twins or triplets with some fertility treatments
- The rollercoaster of emotions associated with each pregnancy attempt

- The need to keep working for financial reasons (this may be true for both you and your partner)
- Coping with family, friends or workmates who constantly ask how things are going
- The loneliness of going through treatment that has been kept secret from family and friends
- The jealousy you feel when your partner's desire to have a child overtakes all other interests, including your relationship. You may feel guilty that you feel this way.

If you can, try to find a balance between the demands of your treatment and time for each other. It helps to make special time for each other that is not about baby making. If you have a very hectic working life, this is a good time to reduce your working hours and avoid over-committing yourself. You or your partner may not have the time or energy available to devote to a busy working life, your relationship *and* the demands of fertility treatment.

The desire to have children can be very strong, and even those who don't want to have children may feel distressed if the option to do so is lost. Choosing not to have a child feels very different from knowing that you no longer have the choice.

Some women who had never wanted children before change their mind as they get older. We are all entitled to change our mind over time, but this may be a problem for a couple whose relationship is based on a mutual desire to remain childless. The whole topic of fertility may become so emotional that it is impossible to discuss reasonably. This is where time with a counsellor or your general practitioner can help.

The men's website/newsletter at:

http://www.geocities.com/HotSprings/Spa/8449/eccpartners.html or, www.endometriosis.org.uk/partners

has useful information and support for you.

Not ready for a baby

Zena is a married woman in her mid-thirties. Zena had had painful periods for many years, and was considering a laparoscopy to look for endometriosis. The pain was severe, but Zena's biggest problem was her desire to have children. Up until now she and her husband had chosen not to have children. They had boats, motorbikes, a huge mortgage and two full-time jobs to give them the lifestyle they enjoyed. Their friends were childless by choice. We all change our mind sometimes and now Zena wanted a baby before it was too late.

Hugo had worries of his own. He had taken many years to decide to marry Zena. His previous marriage had failed and he was fearful of his marriage to Zena failing too. He was now fearful of pregnancy, and losing the lifestyle he loved.

Zena decided to have a laparoscopy to find out how severe her endometriosis was, and have it removed. This would help her pain, but also give her a better idea of how easily she might fall pregnant. Zena and Hugo needed help. Trying to discuss their differing needs themselves had only resulted in emotion, and conflict without resolution. Consulting a marriage counsellor could help. Involving a third person, acceptable to both people, might help them come to an arrangement that met both their needs.

Lesbian couples with fertility concerns

Lesbian couples may have similar problems to heterosexual couples, when it comes to fertility treatment. However, they may have other problems too:

- The legal availability of fertility services for same sex couples varies from country to country and state to state. You may need to travel away from home to access the services you need.

- To become pregnant, you will require semen from either a friend or an anonymous donor. You may be uncertain about the history of your donor, their personality, appearance, risk of genetic disease, or desire to contact your child later.
- Other people may not understand your desire for children and distress at infertility when you are in a same-sex relationship.
- There may be a lack of understanding if one of you has chosen to be the biological mother when the other partner is more fertile.
- Finding a support group suitable for your needs may be more difficult.

Then again, it will be easier for you to keep your sexual relationship separate to your quest for a baby.

Therapists and support groups

How to choose a good counsellor or complementary therapist

There is a wide range of therapists available, so this can be a bewildering decision.

The first thing to decide on is the type of practitioner you are looking for. You may be comfortable with some types of therapy but not others. Your general practitioner or specialist may recommend a therapist with whom they work regularly, but not all therapists suit all women so you may need to find a therapist yourself.

The next thing to decide is what you are looking for from this therapist.

- What symptoms do I wish them to treat?
- Does this therapist have recognised qualifications in their special area? Most qualified practitioners will belong to a professional organisation.

- Are they happy to work together with your doctor? If not, you may find yourself with two conflicting sets of advice.
- Will it be a long wait for an appointment? In some cases it will be worth the wait. In others there may be another person you could see instead.
- What are the costs involved, and are these costs covered by Medicare or private insurance? Do they charge for missed appointments?
- What time of the day or day of the week are appointments available?
- Will the possibility of treatment by a person of a different ethnic origin or gender be a problem for you?
- What sort of techniques do they use?
- Will there be a set time for treatment and the opportunity to discuss progress and change track if necessary?

Once you have met with your therapist, ask yourself whether you felt comfortable with that person and the treatment he or she recommended. Did you feel confident that that person had *your* best interests at heart? Did you feel able to communicate with them, and was your point of view listened to and acknowledged? Did the treatment recommended make sense and are you happy to go ahead with it? If not, it is not too late to go elsewhere. Most treatment programs require dedication and commitment, so if you are not comfortable with the treatment offered, it is less likely to be successful.

There are no easy fixes for pelvic pain so it is important that you and your therapist are able to build a good honest working relationship. Whatever treatment path you decide on, ask your practitioner how long it will be before you should see improvement. Some treatments do not work instantly, and may need time, but you don't want to waste time on something that just isn't working for you.

Feel optimistic!

There are many reasons why you can feel optimistic despite the problems that you have. Endometriosis is now recognised as a significant problem for many women. You are certainly not alone. The ways to diagnose endometriosis are improving and treatment options are now more effective. Research into even better ways to manage endometriosis continues. If you have older relatives with severe endometriosis, it is unlikely that you will suffer as they have. A lot has improved. Things are better now.

Finding an endometriosis support group

Most endometriosis support groups are made up of women who have had endometriosis themselves. It is very comforting to be among other women with similar experiences. However, support is a very individual thing and different women look for different things in a support group. You should consider:

- What sort of support do I need?
- Can the support group support me in this way, or should I see a psychologist or psychiatrist?
- Does attending my support group give me a positive experience?
- Is the support group well run?
- Where are meetings held? Is this a convenient place for me and do I feel comfortable with the surroundings?
- Would I prefer anonymous support, possibly by phone or email?

Support groups in Australia and New Zealand

Australia

There are support groups active in all Australian states and several regional centres. Current phone numbers, and email addresses for these groups can be obtained from the Endometriosis Association of Victoria:

Phone:	(03) 9870 0536, (03) 9827 2199 or (03) 9457 2933
Website:	www.endometriosis.org.au
Email:	info@endometriosis.org.au
Support Line:	1800 069 697 (freecall within Victoria)

New Zealand

Contact details are available from the New Zealand Endometriosis Foundation:

Address:	PO Box 1673, Mail Centre, Christchurch
Phone:	03 379 7959
Website:	www.nzendo.co.nz
Email:	nzendo@xtra.co.nz
Support line:	0800 733 277

If you live outside Australia and New Zealand, you can contact your local endometriosis clinic, or key the words *endometriosis support* into your favourite search engine.

Chapter 12

....

Complementary medicine for endometriosis

Dr Margaret Taylor

N ATURAL OR 'COMPLEMENTARY' MEDICINE offers some fascinating ideas for the treatment of endometriosis and these ideas work well in conjunction with conventional medicine and surgery. If the body is well nourished by a healthy and appropriate diet and supplemented with vitamins, minerals and herbs, it will be much better equipped to deal with surgery and medical drugs. It is also better able to deal with side effects from such treatments. That is why natural medicine is now often called complementary medicine, because it complements conventional medicine.

The body always tries to heal itself, and sometimes all it needs to recover from a problem is the correct food and environment. Many people have heard of someone who has unexpectedly recovered from a serious illness, such as cancer for example, and surprised everyone. There is no one reason for such a recovery. It usually means that many elements of the treatment contributed to such a healing. Often the first thing to consider is improving lifestyle and diet, both of which today are a long way from being 'natural'.

The body is an intricate system that relies on all parts for it to work effectively, just as a team does. Relieving a symptom is often not possible unless you fix the underlying problem. This is why complementary medicine takes a holistic approach to illness, looking at the whole system because there is rarely one pill or treatment that will work without the patient changing to a healthier way of life that benefits the whole body.

The complementary approach to endometriosis

There seem to be three important differences between the endometriosis lesions in the abdomen and the normal endometrial lining in the uterus:

- Women with endometriosis have relatively too much estrogen
- Endometriosis lesions contain aromatase, the enzyme that makes estrogen
- There is inflammation around the lesions, which usually means a sufferer will feel pain.

These factors come together in a damaging self-perpetuating cycle where inflammation stimulates aromatase, which produces estrogen, which in turn increases inflammation. Sounds hard? Just look at the diagram (Figure 12.1).

Fortunately there are a lot of natural treatments that slow the cycle down, and most of them you can manage yourself, although some medications need a prescription. In this chapter we will look at the natural controls of this cycle and consider how it can be influenced by foods and natural supplements. There are many

Figure 12.1 The endometriosis cycle

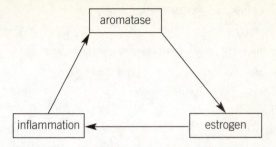

factors involved and it may seem complicated, but taken one at a time they are all quite simple. I find that people like to know why they have to take a particular supplement or food. You generally feel more powerful and in control if you understand why something happens. If it seems too complicated, there is a summary and an eating plan at the end of the chapter.

Estrogen and endometriosis

In complementary medicine it is considered that the main problem in endometriosis is *estrogen dominance*.

Estrogen dominance is a common condition these days, where there is relatively too much estrogen, especially compared to its partner hormone — progesterone. It can result in sore lumpy breasts (fibrocystic breast disease), painful periods (dysmenorrhoea), premenstrual syndrome (PMS) and endometriosis.

The causes of estrogen dominance
- Slow breakdown of estrogen by the liver
- Increased conversion of testosterone to estrogen by the enzyme aromatase
- Decreased plant estrogens (phyto-estrogens) in your diet
- Xeno-estrogens (toxic chemicals that behave like estrogen) in food, air and water.

To reduce estrogen dominance

- Reduce the fat in your diet
- Lose weight
- Introduce friendly (probiotic) bacteria to your gut
- Increase phyto-estrogens in your diet
- Undergo liver detoxification
- Reduce caffeine
- Exercise
- Increase natural progesterone
- Try a herb, Vitex Agnus Castus (also called 'chaste tree')
- Avoid xeno-estrogens
- Block aromatase with zinc, herbs or chrysin.

How can J know if J have too much estrogen?

You might have painful, swollen or even lumpy breasts, nausea, fluid retention and abdominal bloating, heavy periods, fatigue, weight gain, craving for sweets and/or premenstrual irritability and depression.

Reducing the fat in your diet

Estrogen is normally broken down in the liver and then excreted into the bowel. However, eating saturated animal fats encourages the growth of intestinal bacteria, which produce an enzyme called beta-glucuronidase. This enzyme converts it back into a form that can be reabsorbed. So estrogen can cycle round and round between the gut, the bloodstream and the liver many times before it is finally excreted!

This means that women (and men) who eat more animal fat have significantly higher levels of estrogen than those on low fat diets. A high animal fat intake has been linked with benign breast cysts, breast cancer, heavy menstruation, endometriosis, fibroids and prostate enlargement in men. All these conditions are thought to relate to high estrogen. Other research has actually shown that reducing your fat intake leads to lower estrogen in the body.

How do I reduce the fat in my diet?

A low fat diet means reducing foods such as butter, margarine, ice cream and cheese as well as the visible fat on meat. Fried foods are particularly high in fat. Don't reduce the good fats, which are found in foods such as avocado, olive oil, nuts and seeds.

What is Calcium D-glucarate?

Calcium D-glucarate is a special supplement that stops the beta-glucuronidase in the bowel from remaking estrogen after it has been broken down in the liver and, in my clinical experience, it can be effective in lowering estrogen. It is available in the USA (500 mg capsules) and can be imported into Australia for personal use. It is also found in small amounts in spinach, carrots and apples.

Lose weight

Fat cells contain the enzyme aromatase, so people who are obese make more estrogen. The type of obesity may be important. Apple shaped women with a high waist measurement, tend to have high *insulin* levels. Insulin regulates the amount of sugar in the blood and is discussed on page 260. They have more free estrogen than pear shaped women with the weight in the thighs. Apple shaped women (with most of the weight around the middle) probably won't be able to lose weight on a low fat diet. A low carbohydrate diet which reduces insulin would be much more effective. (This is discussed in insulin reduction on page 260.) Regardless of the diet you follow, it is essential to eat lots of vegetables, which are mostly low in carbohydrates and high in fibre and antioxidants. (See the Eating Plan on page 268.)

Why should J eat more vegetables?

A diet high in fibre and low in fat can reduce the activity of the enzyme beta-glucuronidase and so less estrogen is able to re-enter the bloodstream. Foods such as vegetables, fruit, legumes (beans and lentils), muesli, wholemeal bread and wholemeal pasta are high in fibre and low in fat.

Introducing friendly (probiotic) bacteria to your gut

Yoghurt contains special bacteria like lactobacillus acidophilus, which reduce the production of beta-glucuronidase, that enzyme that remakes estrogen. Researchers have found that eating these foods is associated with a lower incidence of breast cancer (see Reference 28) possibly by reducing the re-absorption of estrogen or by enhancing the immune system. If this is true, then it should also be good for endometriosis. It must be yoghurt with a live culture, rather than just any yoghurt. If you are allergic to milk, soy yoghurt has the same bacteria in it (see allergies page 259), or you could take capsules of acidophilus.

Eating more phyto-estrogens

Phyto-estrogens are plant hormones that behave just like weak estrogens. All cells have estrogen receptors — brain, skin, uterus, and even endometriosis cells. A receptor is like a lock and estrogen is the key that fits in the lock and turns on certain processes in the cell. Phyto-estrogens are amazing substances — they act like estrogen but are hundreds of times less active than estrogen. When they occupy the estrogen receptor they prevent some of the normal estrogen from affecting the cell. This means that where there is too much estrogen, such as in endometriosis, phyto-estrogens can reduce the effectiveness of normal estrogen; but where there is not enough estrogen, after menopause for example, they can behave like weak estrogen and help prevent hot flushes and loss of bone density.

Most traditional diets, for example Mediterranean, African and Asian diets, contain many more phyto-estrogens than the Western diet and it is thought that this is why those people have less estrogen-related cancer. Phyto-estrogens are found mainly in legumes, such as soy products (tofu, tempeh, soy milk), beans, lentils, peas, and chickpeas, that are commonly deficient in a Western diet. To increase phyto-estrogens in your system, add foods such as baked beans, bean salads, lentil soups and patties, hummus, as well as soy linseed bread to your diet. Try adding tinned beans to all your curries and casseroles. If you are worried about wind, start slowly. Eat only small amounts at first and gradually build up, having a little each day. As the bacteria in the intestines get used to these foods, the problem should settle.

Linseed – another natural estrogen blocker

Linseed contains high amounts of lignans, which block estrogen receptors in the cell and reduce its effect. Three teaspoons a day of ground linseed, or a mix often referred to as LSA – ground linseed, sesame seeds and almonds – on your vegetables or cereal should be enough.

The cabbage family and estrogen

The cabbage family vegetables should be consumed regularly by women who have estrogen-related conditions. They include all cabbages, broccoli, kale, bok choy, cauliflower, brussels sprouts and radicchio. Substances called 'indoles' found in these vegetables seem to increase the breakdown of estrogen in a way that reduces breast cancer cell growth. These indoles are available as supplements of di-indolyl methane or indole-3-carbinol from natural practitioners if there is a problem eating enough of these vegetables. The herb rosemary also helps in this way. You could make a weak tea and drink it three times a day.

Liver detoxification

Foods high in sulphur, like beans, legumes, onions and garlic help the liver break down estrogen. The same processes that are used to excrete toxic chemicals also break down estrogen, so there can be a bottleneck at times, and naturopaths describe this by saying the liver is 'stressed'. The diagnostic methods used by naturopaths can often pick this up before a blood test for liver function test (LFT) is abnormal, because the LFT picks up liver cell damage, not poor function. Some herbs are useful for improving liver function. These include St Mary's thistle, dandelion and globe artichoke. Many liver detox formulas combine the above herbs with some anti-oxidants to protect the liver cells. A good liver formula would also have some sulphur-containing amino acids such as methionine, choline, inositol, and taurine.

Additional vitamin C is also useful — 1000 mg per day or more and it can be continued long term.

Cutting down on caffeine

Drinking 4–5 cups of coffee a day increases estrogen by nearly 70 per cent. Tea has about half as much caffeine. Decaffeinated tea or coffee or herbal tea would be a good alternative to help keep estrogen as low as possible.

Exercise

Exercise helps with estrogen clearance, and women who exercise tend to have lower estrogen levels, lighter and less frequent periods. It also reduces insulin resistance, which makes it easier to lose weight (see page 260). The exercise doesn't have to be extreme — walking, cycling or swimming for 20–30 minutes, four or five times a week, is sufficient, and exercising in the morning is even better. If small children or other responsibilities prevent you getting out for a walk or to the gym, an exercise bike can be useful. Put it in front of the TV and pedal away, or turn on the early morning television aerobics program. For those suffering pelvic pain, the bike may be less painful than other exercises because the pelvis does not bounce when you use the bike.

Natural progesterone

This is probably the most important natural treatment for endometriosis. Progesterone is produced by the ovary after ovulation and naturally balances the effects of estrogens. Some women don't produce enough. This can happen because of stress, or perimenopause, or from toxic chemicals called xeno-estrogens (see page 256).

Progesterone has some pleasant effects. It is probably the reason that women look and feel so good in later pregnancy. It matures the endometrium each month to prevent heavy periods, and has many effects all over the body that include:

- Helping us use fat for energy
- Helping thyroid hormone
- Being a natural anti-depressant
- Being a natural diuretic
- Normalising blood sugar levels
- Restoring libido (sexual appetite)
- Protecting against breast fibrocysts and helping prevent breast cancer

- Helping prevent endometrial cancer
- Being necessary for the survival of an embryo
- Stimulating the cells that make bone.

Natural progesterone cream rubbed into thin skin is well absorbed. It can only be obtained with a prescription from a doctor. Look around for one who is familiar with its use. In the USA you can buy progesterone cream over the counter as it is very safe. Progesterone in the body can be monitored by measuring levels in saliva, as it is not detected on a blood test when administered in a skin cream.

The normal progesterone script is either a 1.5 or 3 per cent cream. Higher doses may be required for pain management in endometriosis. In fact, levels around about 54–60 mg (5–6 per cent progesterone cream) may be necessary and appear to be well tolerated. Symptoms of excess progesterone are sleepiness and sluggishness and most women will find that they can or should reduce their dosage of progesterone after a few months. However, attempts to go below, say, 4 per cent progesterone (40 mg/gm cream) may allow symptoms to recur. You may get *estrogenic* symptoms at first, so it helps to have a doctor who can guide you, so you don't give up too soon. It can be used in conjunction with the Pill as it does not interfere with the contraceptive effect, and it should help with some of the side effects as well as possibly reducing the endometriosis.

I have been unable to find any reliable research on the results of using natural progesterone in endometriosis, but one doctor who is using it has said that 75 per cent of his endometriosis patients get some relief (Reference 29). Dr John Lee, who popularised natural progesterone cream, stated that it is very effective for mild to moderate endometriosis, but further solid research is needed to prove it one way or the other.

What is the difference between natural progesterone, wild yam extract and progestins?

Natural progesterone is made in the corpus luteum of the ovary after ovulation (20–25 mg per day) and by the placenta during pregnancy (up to 300–400 mg/day — an astonishing increase). Wild yam extract is not a progesterone. It actually has an estrogenic effect! Progestins are sometimes referred to as progesterone, but they are only synthetic versions of it. Although, like progesterone, they are useful for preventing heavy bleeding in the uterus, in other areas of the body (such as the brain) they can interfere with natural progesterone and can cause PMS or depression.

Vitex agnus castus (chaste tree)

Vitex is a useful herb for many women as it encourages the ovary to ovulate more effectively and produce more of its own natural progesterone from the corpus luteum after ovulation. Many research studies in Europe have shown its effectiveness for simple period pain and premenstrual syndrome, and it's the most important herb for endometriosis. Use 500–1000 mg in the morning. This won't work if you are on the contraceptive pill, because the Pill prevents ovulation.

Avoid xeno-estrogens

Many modern chemicals are xeno-estrogens. They include pesticides, plasticisers, alkylphenols, PCBs, dioxins, cadmium and lead. They are similar enough to estrogen to mimic its action in the body. The difficult thing about these chemicals is that they seem to be everywhere. Reproductive disorders such as sterility are occurring in wildlife, and girls are maturing sexually much earlier than before. These may be effects due to xeno-estrogens. We all have xeno-estrogen in our bodies. For example, nine healthy volunteers in New York in 2003 had an average of 91 industrial chemicals in their body, some of which were xeno-estrogens. These people do not live in a toxic area or work with chemicals. Xeno-estrogens are very difficult for the body to eliminate, and are mainly found in the fatty tissues, and not much in the watery part of the blood, so blood tests don't give a true picture.

Dioxins are contaminants of weedicide 245T and by-products of industrial processes. They are the main toxic chemicals that have been researched for endometriosis. Monkeys who were given dioxin in their food (like us) for four years developed endometriosis spontaneously. Ten years later laparoscopy showed that the monkeys who received higher exposure to dioxins had developed more severe cases of the disease. By then their blood levels had come down to normal human levels (Reference 30). It seems that these chemicals can induce endometriosis and then it keeps going on its own, perhaps because of the self-perpetuating cycle described at the beginning of this chapter. In humans it is impossible to do this sort of research and the dioxins we are exposed to are so numerous that it is difficult to know which ones to measure in the blood. We do know that dioxins are more commonly found in the blood of women with endometriosis than women who don't have it. If you want to read more about xeno-estrogens go to http://www.ewg.org/reports/bodyburden

How can I avoid xeno-estrogens?

Pesticides can be minimised by eliminating them from your home and garden as far as possible, and by buying certified organic foods. If you're in areas commonly sprayed with pesticides (for example golf courses), take care to keep your hands away from your mouth and wash your hands thoroughly after exposure. Pesticides are very easily absorbed through the skin.

Heavy metals such as cadmium and lead are also suspected xeno-estrogens. Blood levels of lead are dropping in most people since the introduction of lead-free petrol, but some old houses have a huge lead burden in the dust and soil, mostly due to old lead paint. Cadmium can be found in superphosphate from Nauru and is now on lots of farmland, but it is also found in areas where industrial waste was dumped. There are apparently over 600 known toxic waste sites in Australia, many of them in areas that are now residential housing, so if you suspect that you have only been ill since moving to a certain house, you could find out the history of your land and/or get your soil analysed.

Plasticisers, for example phthalates, are used to help keep PVC plastic flexible in products such as toys, teething rings, shower curtains, floor coverings, car seats and some food wraps. Avoid them and reduce absorption by having plenty of fresh air in the house and car.

Other xeno-estrogens include alkylphenols (in shampoo and cosmetics), bisphenol (a hardener in paints or lacquers such as the lining in tinned foods), or plastics (such as water pipes or bottle top linings). *Choice* magazine, October 1997, has further details.

Persistent organic pollutants. This group of chemicals has the most hormone-disrupting effects — it includes polychlorinated biphenols (PCBs), dioxins and some pesticides such as DDT. They have a long life, and they're widespread in the environment. Because they're fat-soluble, they're found especially in animal fat, so changing to organically grown meat and dairy foods will reduce exposure.

What if I can't reduce my exposure?

If you can't reduce exposure, the answer is to improve liver function to get rid of them more quickly. See the above section on liver clearance of estrogen (page 252). We use the same processes to get rid of these chemicals. Onions, garlic and eggs have plenty of sulphur, which we need for excreting these toxic substances. (Sulphur is not the same as sulpha antibiotics.) Nature's phyto-estrogens also help to reduce their effects — another reason to eat those beans! There is some research showing that excreting them through the skin by sweating is effective (Reference 31). So, showering after exercise or saunas and washing the skin with soap is worthwhile in conjunction with the liver formula and vitamin C.

Blocking aromatase

Aromatase is the enzyme that produces estrogen from testosterone. As described on page 84 one of the most distinct things about endometriosis lesions is that the cells produce aromatase and normal endometrium doesn't.

Chrysin is a natural inhibitor of aromatase. It is a bioflavonoid from a plant. Chrysin was first used in the 1930s as part of breast cancer treatment and in 1993 (Reference 32) was shown to be similar in effectiveness to an aromatase-inhibiting drug (amino-glutethimide). It is now mainly used by men who want to stop all their testosterone being converted to estrogen as they get older. It does the same in women — slows the conversion of androgens (testosterone) to estrogen.

A great advantage of using plant extracts instead of pharma-ceuticals is that the plant extracts have other health benefits. Chrysin is also a potent antioxidant with vitamin-like effects in the body. It also has an anti-inflammatory effect, possibly by blocking the enzymes that make prostaglandins (see Chapter 6, page 72). These are both useful effects for women with endometriosis. As chrysin is poorly absorbed orally, it is not effective in tablet form. However, it can now be administered in a skin cream with excel-lent results. Chrysin is only available on prescription from a compounding pharmacy. 1 gm/day of 0.5 per cent cream is the correct dose for women.

Other natural inhibitors of aromatase include the herbs *epilobium*, *nettle* and *saw palmetto*, and the mineral *zinc*. They can all slow down the production of estrogen by aromatase.

Inflammation and endometriosis

What is inflammation?

It's just the same as the hot red painful swelling that accompanies the healing of an injury or infection. The inflammation that occurs in the endometriosis lesions may be the cause of the pain of endometriosis. Unfortunately, high levels of estrogen stimulate the COX enzyme to produce more prostaglandins (see Figure 6.1, page 72).

What increases inflammation (apart from estrogen)?

Meat, fat and sugar are the simple answer. Meat and fat contain the arachidonic acid that prostaglandins are made from. Sugar is a problem because the excess amounts that are eaten these days stimulate *insulin resistance*, which is very inflammatory (see page 260). Blood in the peritoneal cavity can cause inflammation and may be why excess reflux of menstrual blood up the fallopian tubes may contribute to endometriosis.

Can food allergies affect inflammation?

Many people have undiagnosed food allergies that cause chronic problems such as sinusitis, tiredness, depression, an irritable bowel, eczema etc. If you have these symptoms as well as your endometriosis, it would help to find out and avoid the foods that are causing it, because they may be increasing inflammation. If your symptoms are mainly in the bowel, ask your doctor for a blood test for endomysial antibodies and gliadin antibodies because gluten in wheat and other grains are commonly the cause. If it's mainly sinus and mucus in the throat, try having *ABSOLUTELY* no milk or dairy products for a week and then have a glass of milk. This technique of eliminating something from the diet and then reintroducing it is the most accurate way of finding an answer, but eliminating the food properly can be difficult. Reading food labels is essential because, for example, bread can have milk in it. A nutritional doctor, naturopath or dietician would be able to guide you.

How can I reduce inflammation?

There are many ways to reduce inflammation:

- Reduce insulin resistance
- Eat more fish oil – more fish in your diet, or 1000 mg three times daily
- Anti-inflammatory herbs
- Other natural supplements such as Bromelain and Quercetin.

Insulin resistance

Eating foods with sugar causes the pancreas to produce insulin. When it happens excessively this condition is called *insulin resistance*. It increases the risk of heart disease and breast cancer. Insulin increases the amount of food going into the fat cells and makes it difficult to get it out again for energy. This is a major cause of putting on weight and leads to diabetes. Fat cells also produce estrogen with the aromatase enzyme. Insulin also strongly increases inflammatory prostaglandins, so one of the most important ways to reduce pain would be to stop eating sugar and other carbo-hydrates such as pasta, rice, potato, many breakfast cereals, white bread, cake and biscuits with a high glycemic index (GI). High GI foods put the blood sugar up quickly which overstimulates insulin to reduce it again.

Insulin resistance can be reversed by exercising and eating like a modern hunter-gatherer. This means plenty of protein and vegetables and less starch and sugar. 10,000 years ago humans had no bread or pasta at all in their diet and were perfectly healthy, so don't worry that you'll miss out if you reduce them substantially. But you do need to eat lots of vegetables to ensure adequate fibre. The Atkins diet would be too inflammatory for women with endometriosis because there is too much red meat and fat and cream. There are other more healthy low carbohydrate diets with more vegetables and healthier fats and oils, for example the Zone diet or Protein Power. Exercise also reduces insulin resistance.

Fish and fish oils

Eat as much fish as possible — say 3–5 times a week. Increasing vegetables and fish increases the *Omega 3 fatty acids* that are nature's anti-inflammatories. The big fish such as shark/flake, ray, swordfish, barramundi, gemfish, orange roughy, ling and southern bluefin tuna accumulate lots of mercury because they are large, live longer, and are at the top of the food chain. You don't need to eliminate them altogether, but it's better to eat other smaller fish most of the time. Freshwater fish in geothermal lakes and rivers in New Zealand may also accumulate higher levels of mercury. Canned tuna has lower levels of mercury than fresh bluefin tuna because the tuna fish used for canning is a different, smaller species and is generally caught when less than 1 year old. Fish oils have Omega 3 fatty acids that inhibit endometriosis in laboratory research. One group of 50 women with endometriosis and gut pain, treated with a diet with less sugar, coffee and cheese and addition of olive oil and omega 3 fatty acids, improved significantly (Reference 34).

Herbs

There are some very effective herbs that inhibit inflammation. *Boswellia, devil's claw, turmeric* and *ginger* have all been shown to possess similar anti-inflammatory activity to NSAIDs in arthritis

(Reference 35). They reduce the production of prostaglandins, so there's no reason why they wouldn't work in endometriosis as well. The quality of herbal tablets and extracts can vary widely so it is better to get herbs from a herbalist, who can access top quality 'Practitioner Only' products (in Australia) from one of the herbal manufacturers who assay their products to make sure they are correct potency. These manufacturers often make a tablet combination of anti-inflammatory herbs that are much easier to take than herbal liquids. On the other hand, the advantage of using herbal liquids is that a good herbalist can combine herbs with different actions for your specific symptoms. The most common ones you might be given include:

- Cramp bark or dong quai for period pain
- Sedative or tonic herbs for stress
- St John's wort for depression
- Pulsatilla for ovarian pain
- Gotu kola or dan shen to reduce adhesions
- Vitex agnus castus to increase your progesterone
- Liver herbs (St Mary's thistle, globe artichoke, dandelion) to assist excretion of estrogen and toxic chemicals
- Grapeseed extract or other powerful herbal antioxidants
- Nettle, epilobium or saw palmetto (pygeum) to inhibit aromatase.

Other natural supplements

Bromelain is an extract of pineapple, which has an anti-inflammatory effect similar to prednisone (a form of cortisone). Sports people use it to reduce bruising. The effective dose is 600–1200 mg per day.

Quercetin is a natural substance in foods especially tea, apples and onions. It is strongly anti-inflammatory and antioxidant. The effective dose would be 200–2000 mg/day. You can get 10–20 mg/day from foods.

Premenstrual syndrome

Will vitex help my PMS?

Probably/almost certainly. Some of my patients report the benefit within days! Almost always within the first month. Before I knew about vitex, I prescribed evening primrose oil and vitamin B6 and magnesium for PMS. They often helped a little, which is what the research says — some benefit, but not much.

- Vitex agnus castus — 1000 mg daily in the morning
- Vitamin B6 — 100 mg in the morning combined with a multivitamin and magnesium 400 mg daily
- Evening primrose oil — 1000 mg capsules 2 or 3 times daily. While vitex helps most women with PMS, evening primrose oil helps some but not others.

If vitex doesn't help you within the first month or two of treatment, your PMS may be related to too many sugar and milk products. Women with PMS eat more dairy products than other women — we don't know why. It would be worth a trial month off sugar and dairy foods to see if it helps you.

Vitamin B6 deficiency makes tissues in the uterus and breast more susceptible to the stimulating effects of estrogen, and in my clinical experience, vitamin B6 deficiency is fairly common. Vitamin B6 should always be taken with other B vitamins and, as it gives some people vivid dreams, it should be taken in the morning. No more than 200 mg per day should be taken as it can cause nerve damage in high doses.

What if I feel as if I have PMS all month?

Tired, depressed, achy, irritable, bloated? If it happens in the first half of the month, it's not (just) PMS. It may be a food intolerance or allergy, especially if you have good and bad days. These foods are very addictive — 'milkaholics' may need milk many times a day, for example in coffee, and after a few days on a completely milk-free diet, they suddenly feel completely different — light, energetic, cheerful. They say, 'I never knew other people felt like this in the morning. It is so great to wake up with energy and enthusiasm for the day. And I'm not craving my coffee (with milk) all the time. I miss the milk in my coffee but it's worth it, to feel this good.' It could be any food you eat often, such as wheat, yeast, egg, tomato, sugar and so on. Find out by strictly eliminating the food you suspect from your diet for 10–14 days and then trying it. The result will be an obvious return of your symptoms if that particular food is causing the symptoms.

What about period pain?

As explained in Chapter 2, on page 13, not all period pain is endometriosis. Ordinary period pain will not respond as well as other symptoms to excisional surgery for endometriosis.

Here is where high tech medicine and natural remedies can work well together. Natural therapies for period pain include:

- Vitex agnus castus. This herb helps period pain because it increases the progesterone that matures the lining of the uterus, so it is released easily at period time
- Zinc 20–30 mg per day
- If these don't prevent it, try magnesium 200 mg every 2 hours while you have the cramps (Reference 36).

This is an email I got from a friend of mine who is a physio-therapist. 'Just a quick thank you for the Vitex tip. Marked improvement this month in my period pain, so THANK YOU!!' She had only been on it 3 weeks!

Zinc

I learnt about zinc from one of my secretaries many years ago. She was typing a letter I'd written about zinc for another problem, which she also had, and decided to try it. She was amazed to find that her next period arrived with no pain. So was I, so I tried it on lots of other women and it often worked. Zinc deficiency is very common in Australian women, and it is important for making hormones. In Australia a study has shown that 85 per cent of women do not get enough zinc in the food they eat (Reference 37) and most women with endometriosis would be in that 85 per cent. Zinc is in oysters, meat, fish, nuts, dried peas and beans. We need 11–15 mg/day when we are healthy, and probably twice that amount if we are not well. Supplements are safe to take even if you are not deficient, as long as you follow the directions. I suggest 30–50 mg/day, for example you might take zinc chelate 220 mg twice a day, because each tablet has about 20 mg of real zinc. In some brands this would be labelled 20 mg zinc (as chelate).

How can I know if I am deficient in zinc?

If you are deficient in zinc, you may have:

- White spots on your nails
- Poor wound healing and wound infection
- Slow growth and sexual maturation (late onset of periods)
- Poor appetite (anorexia) and taste disorder
- Poor resistance to infection.

Magnesium

Magnesium is nature's antispasmodic mineral. People who are low in magnesium can have restless legs, insomnia, anxiety, twitches in muscles, palpitations, leg cramps or period pain. If you are low in magnesium, then magnesium supplementation may help your period pain (Reference 37). But of course if your period pain has another cause, it won't help. Magnesium is in green vegetables, nuts and seeds. It is the middle of the chlorophyll molecule — the green pigment in plants that has the magical property of using sunlight, air and water to make the substance of plants. According to CSIRO research, 39 per cent of Australian women do not eat enough magnesium in their food (Reference 37).

How can I tell if I have magnesium deficiency?

Magnesium deficiency can cause:
- Restless legs
- Insomnia
- Anxiety
- Twitches in muscles
- Palpitations
- Leg cramps
- Period pain
- Heart attack.

Should I be on the Pill?

There is no simple answer to this question. The pain and disability of endometriosis can be significant and any relief possible is a great boon and should not be shunned for minor reasons. In natural medicine, barrier methods of contraception are preferred — diaphragms and condoms, but for some people the only practical contraception is the Pill. My opinion is that the research shows that it is a fairly benign medicine — even the long-term studies show little risk, especially when compared to other risks of modern life. So my suggestion is to use the Pill where necessary for symptomatic relief, and when symptoms improve you may be able to stop using it if you wish, or continue if you want to use it for contraception. The main question is whether you tolerate it well. There are many studies that show that nutrient needs are greater on the Pill, so it makes sense to take a multivitamin as well. The increased risk of breast cancer is *tiny* compared to the greatly increased risk due to smoking, alcohol or not exercising.

What about alcohol?

The effects of alcohol on estrogen metabolism and estrogen-related disorders are complex. Moderate alcohol consumption (one glass of beer, one glass of wine or one shot of spirits daily) has been associated with reduced levels of estrogen (but an increased risk of breast cancer). Women who consume alcohol have a 50 per cent increase in risk of endometriosis. When the pain is bad, women with endometriosis tend to drink more alcohol. This is not the time to drink more alcohol as it increases inflammation and will only increase the pain. At other times a little (perhaps a glass or two a week) is probably OK.

Insomnia?

Do you have trouble sleeping or do you find that winter depresses you? You may be low in *melatonin*. This hormone helps us sleep and is important in preventing cancer. It also inhibits cyclo-oxygenase production of prostaglandins. Being exposed to bright light in the morning causes melatonin to be produced at bedtime. It decreases with ageing and is a popular anti-ageing supplement in the USA. In Australia you are allowed to import it for your own use. Why not make sure your melatonin production is optimal by going for a walk in the morning? Homeopathic melatonin is available over the counter in Australia. (Unfortunately I have not found the homeopathic melatonin to be effective, while natural melatonin is.) If you can't increase your melatonin naturally it is available on prescription from doctors interested in natural hormones. Certain pathologists can measure your level from your saliva.

So, what should I eat?

Well, you now know that coffee, sugar and fatty foods are not good for you, and that fish and vegetables are desirable, so how do you eat as a busy Western woman? It partly depends on your shape. If you are thin or pear shaped with big thighs, you can eat more grains (bread, pasta, rice) than if you are apple shaped and have a big waist.

Apple shaped women can lose some of those waist inches if they get most of their carbohydrates from vegetables. Sugar is *OUT*. Use low GI foods (look up a list on the website: www.glycemicindex. com) or if the food is high GI, don't have too much of it and have it in a meal with protein to slow down its digestion and absorption so it doesn't cause a peak of blood sugar and insulin. *DO* make sure you get enough protein. The recommended daily amount of protein for a sedentary adult is 0.75 gm protein per kilogram of body weight. Children, and adults who are active, need 1 gm protein/kg body weight. For example: one or two eggs, 100 gm tin of fish and a serve of chicken in a day for an average woman. One slice of ham and a salad is not enough protein for lunch. You will be hungry and craving sweet things in an hour or so.

Suggested eating plan for women with endometriosis

I have formulated an eating plan specifically for women with endometriosis using all the dietary factors that research suggests. If you have food cravings on this diet they should settle down after a few days on this eating plan.

Use olive oil for all cooking, rather than sunflower, safflower or canola and definitely do not use mixed vegetable oil. Sprinkle LSA or ground linseed on almost everything. Organic fruit and vegetables with free-range meat and chicken are a good investment.

Breakfasts

- Unsweetened muesli with 2 teaspoons LSA and soy milk or soy yoghurt
- Soy yoghurt and LSA
- Egg and soy linseed toast
- Egg and tomatoes and mushrooms
- 1 or 2 eggs and 2 or 3 of the following: fried Jap pumpkin *or* eggplant slices, *or* mushrooms, steamed broccoli, red capsicum, spinach *or* beet tops
- Miso soup with silken tofu (most Japanese women have this every day)
- Tinned kippers and lemon juice on spinach
- Baked beans on soy linseed toast with fresh tomato

Lunches

- Soy linseed roll with salad and tuna, pink salmon, chicken or turkey *or* omit the roll and have at least 100 gm of the meat or fish with salad
- Smoked salmon and avocado in a salad or sandwich
- Takeaway Asian stir-fry with prawns, squid, other seafood
- Homemade soup with chicken and lots of vegetables
- Lebanese falafel and hummus roll with lettuce and tomato and tahini dressing
- Bean salad and lots of other salads. Try sprouts such as lentil, alfalfa or mixed sprouts. Dressings are OK in small amounts

Dinners

- Vegetables and fish — grilled, curried with tomato or coconut milk. Rice is usually eaten with this, but you will be better off with more vegetables instead if you need to lose those waist inches
- Vegetable curry with tinned beans and rice (use plenty of turmeric, onions and garlic in all your cooking)
- Vegetarian dinners with chickpeas, red kidney beans, dhal or lentils
- Veal, chicken, turkey dishes, always with plenty of vegetables
- Lean red meat once a week or less, and not char grilled
- Egg and vegetable frittata — put semi-cooked vegetables in a frypan with beaten egg. Cook on low heat until the bottom is

done then put under the griller for a few minutes. No more than 2 egg yolks per day, but you can use egg whites freely
- Lentil patties and buckwheat and vegetables
- Seafood marinara pasta (use wholemeal spaghetti or 100 per cent durum wheat as they have a lower GI) *and* vegetables

Desserts
- Fresh fruit and yoghurt (soy preferably)
- Diet jelly and pineapple

Snacks
- Fresh pineapple — eat one per week
- Nuts and seeds. The oil they contain is good for us
- Celery and carrot sticks with Lebanese dips — hummus and baba ganoush (made of roasted eggplant). Most other dips are made of cream cheese or pate, which are high in fat
- Apricots, strawberries, plums, half an apple. Most other fruit has a lot of sugar, which will trigger an insulin spike unless it is in small amounts in with a meal
- If you 'need' sweet things, make sure they are at the end of a meal so the other food will slow its absorption and prevent a peak of blood sugar and insulin. Have only a tiny taste, for example 2 squares of chocolate and then put it away!

Won't all this protein cause inflammation?

This diet does not have excess protein. In this eating plan I have combined the anti-inflammatory effects of fish and vegetables with the insulin-reducing effects of lowering carbohydrate and getting sufficient protein. In most people the reduction of sugar and fat will be effective in reducing inflammation and therefore pain. If after a month you still have lots of pain, reduce the arachidonic acid (which prostaglandins are made from) by reducing egg yolks to one per day and making sure the meat has no visible fat, and marinating any red meat in olive oil and red wine for 24 hours in the fridge. Fish and white meats like pork and veal have much less arachidonic acid than red meat.

But does it work? (Sarah's story)

Sarah, age 29, had had endometriosis for seven years. She had a very large tender scar on her abdomen, which was the result of poor wound healing in several operations. I suspected zinc deficiency. She couldn't lie on her tummy or have any pressure on her abdomen. This made it difficult for sex, which was painful inside as well. Her periods were very heavy and painful and so she was on two-month cycles of an oral contraceptive. When off the hormone tablets her breasts were very sore and she had a migraine for the whole five days. (This suggests too much estrogen.) A previous medication had affected her liver. She had always had chronic flatulence and abdominal discomfort and recently, severe dizzy episodes.

I prescribed progesterone cream, zinc, a liver formula, vitamin C and an organic diet with less bread, and ordered a blood test for iron and gluten intolerance (because of the flatulence and possible zinc deficiency). I also injected the scar with local anaesthetic (lignocaine). This is a treatment from Germany called 'Neural therapy', not often used in Australia, but helpful in chronic pain. After a second treatment she had no more pain in the scar.

After two weeks she was feeling better, even though she was in the premenstrual week. She usually had severe PMS and migraine. As the blood test showed she had antibodies to gluten, I started her on a gluten-free diet (no wheat, rye, oats or barley). A gluten-free diet would not be necessary for most women with endometriosis but in her case it was the reason she was poorly nourished and the aromatase – estrogen – inflammation cycle was perpetuating itself.

At two months she told me that the gluten-free diet had helped immediately with stomach discomfort and she had more energy. Sexual intercourse was no longer painful. I changed the liver formula to one with soy, red clover and black cohosh, to reduce the effect of estrogen and help with cramps and PMS.

After five months she said she'd 'never felt healthier'. She had normal bowel actions and no flatulence or cramps. She had only a small headache and a little period cramp on the day before her recent period. She had no dizziness or white spots on her nails since she had been taking zinc, and cold sores were happening less often. These are all linked with low zinc.

After eight months periods were lighter and not so painful. She prefers to remain on the Pill for contraception. She still uses progesterone cream and the female herbs and says she feels 'fantastic'.

Help! It's all too hard!

Well, let's try to summarise what you need to do and form a practical plan. You certainly won't need to do everything I have talked about. I suggest you make a list of the items you think are important for you and then form a plan of action and talk it over with your doctor. My most successful patients keep a folder or book and record the important changes and thoughts about the process. Apparently keeping a diary of your problems and the resulting feelings helps to resolve emotional problems too.

The first steps to get started

- The diet. This is the most important thing, so sit down and make a shopping list of all those foods you are going to need.
- Increase your progesterone. If you're not on the Pill, get some vitex, if you are on the Pill; get a script for natural progesterone cream from a doctor.
- Supplements of zinc 30–50 mg daily (for example zinc chelate 220 mg twice daily).

- Omega 3 fish oil capsules 1000 mg three times daily.
- A multi-vitamin with 25–50mg of vitamin B6 in the morning. (Actually a multivitamin for men is good if it has the herbs nettle, saw palmetto or epilobium to inhibit aromatase.)
- Perhaps an anti-inflammatory herbal combination.

The next steps

- Find a source of organic vegetables, free-range meat and chicken.
- Plan your exercise program – write it down, tell people about it and ask them to encourage you to keep to it. Have your shower after the exercise.
- If you think you have allergies, plan a visit to a natural therapist to get help to work it out.

That will probably be enough for the first month. If you are not improving by then, you will need to adjust the therapy according to the symptoms you still have.

If after a month you still have too much estrogen, painful periods or new symptoms, you will need to work with your doctor and/or naturopath with the more detailed ideas in this chapter. A trial of chrysin cream, di-indolyl methane, calcium D-glucarate or reduction of progesterone cream may help.

Sadly, there is no one simple pill that will help. Getting the body to resume health is complicated, often needing a significant lifestyle change, but the process is very empowering. You can feel very proud of yourself for being able to make a difference to this complicated condition. Don't forget that in Nature this aromatase – estrogen – inflammation cycle has its natural controls (otherwise everyone would have endometriosis!) so the answer is to use enough of the natural controls to turn down the speed of the cycle. Thank goodness we have the option of conventional medicine as well.

I used to think that natural remedies were weak and inefficient compared to prescribed medicines, but now with modern research we know so much about how diet and herbs work that they can be combined scientifically and the results can be stunningly effective.

Chapter 13

. . . .

Conclusion

W HAT WE HAVE WRITTEN in this book is not the end of the story. It is only where we are now. New ways of managing this disease and the other causes of pelvic pain will be found. Some of these new discoveries will prove to be useful. Others will not.

Many of our current treatments will be overtaken by better surgery, better medications, better complementary therapies and better lifestyle advice. We hope to be able to prevent endometriosis altogether one day.

For now, there is the ability to manage pelvic pain better than it has ever been managed before.

Appendices

Useful websites

The contact details for endometriosis support groups are listed in Chapter 11, on pages 243–44.

In addition, the following websites may be useful for you:

General information on endometriosis

www.ecca.com.au (our clinic website)

www.endometriosis.org.au (Endometriosis association of Victoria website)

www.endozone.org (to receive the latest news on endometriosis)

www.endometriosis.com.au (Epworth endometriosis clinic)

www.endocenter.org (USA based website with free news and support)

www.my.webmd.com/hn/endometriosis (general medical website)

www.endometriosisassn.org (the USA-based international endometriosis association)

Fertility

www.fertility.com/australia

Gay health
www.gayhealth.com (a general website with health issues of interest to gay and lesbian couples)

Support for teenagers
www.endocenter.org
www.kidshealth.org (a USA website with health issues for kids and young adults)

Support for men
www.endometriosis.org.uk/partners
www.geocities.com/HotSprings/Spa/8449/eccpartners.html

Complementary therapies
www.nccam.nih.gov/health/ (for the USA national centre for complementary and alternative medicine. This includes information on the safety, uses and current trials into complementary and alternative therapies.)

Other medical conditions
www.ichelp.com (for interstitial cystitis)
www.physiotherapy.asn.au (and click on the 'Find an APA physio' link. The Australian Physiotherapy Association National Office is on (03) 9534 9400)
www.posaa.asn.au or www.pcosupport.org (for polycystic ovarian syndrome)
www.menopause.net.au or www.jeanhailes.org.au (for information on menopause and hormone replacement therapy)
www.fpq.com.au (This website operated by the Family Planning Queensland includes a list of useful websites covering a variety of conditions.)

Glossary

Abdomen

The part of your body that lies between your ribs and the top of your legs.

Adenomyosis

A condition where cells that look like the lining of the uterus are found in the wall of the uterus.

Adhesion

The place where two organs are attached together.

Anti-prostaglandin medications

Medicines that stop the body making chemicals called prostaglandins.

Bilateral salpingo-oophorectomy

An operation to remove the ovaries and fallopian tubes on both sides of the pelvis.

Catheter

A soft rubber tube inserted into the bladder to collect urine.

Cautery

A surgical operation to burn a lesion.

Chocolate cysts

Lumps of endometriosis that are found in one, or both ovaries.

Colostomy

A bowel operation where faeces pass into a bag attached to the abdomen rather than out through the anus.

Cystoscopy

An operation using a thin telescope to view the inside of the bladder.

Danazol
A medication used to treat pain from endometriosis.

Diaphragm
The thin muscle that separates the abdomen from the chest.

Dysmenorrhoea
The medical name for painful periods.

Dyspareunia
The medical name for painful intercourse/sex.

Dysuria
The medical name for pain when passing urine.

Endometriomas
The medical name for chocolate cysts in the ovaries.

Endometrium
The medical name for the lining of the uterus. This is the tissue that bleeds during a period.

Excisional surgery
Surgery to remove endometriosis by 'cutting it out'.

Fibroids
Benign tumours that grown in the muscle wall of the uterus.

Frequency
Passing urine more often than normal.

Gestrinone
A medication used to treat the pain of endometriosis.

GnRH analogue
A medication used to treat the pain of endometriosis.

Hysterectomy
An operation to remove the uterus.

Incision
A skin cut made during an operation.

Laparoscopy
An operation through small holes used to look inside the abdomen.

Laparotomy
An operation through a larger incision used to look inside the abdomen.

Lesion
Any unusual or abnormal area.

Navel
Belly button or umbilicus.

Opioids
Medications to treat pain from any cause.

Ovulation pain
Pain felt when the ovary releases an egg.

Pelvis
The part of your body inside your hip bones.

Peritoneum
The thin slippery skin that covers the pelvic organs.

Speculum
Instrument placed in the vagina to view the cervix and take a smear test.

Symptoms
Things you notice when you are unwell.

Ureter
The tube that carries urine from the kidney to the bladder.

Urethra
The tube that carries urine from the bladder to the outside.

Uterosacral ligaments
These ligaments pass from the uterus back to a part of the spine called the sacrum at the back of the pelvis.

References

The abstracts for these studies can be found at www.ncbi.nlm.nih.gov/pubmed by searching for the author. For example, to look up reference number 24, type in Agarwala N, then search.

You will need to go to a medical library if you wish to read the full article.

1   Donnez, J. & Squifflet, J., *et al. Typical and subtle atypical presentations of endometriosis.* OG Clinics of Nth America, 2003 Mar, pp. 83–94.

2   Redwine, D.B. *Ovarian endometriosis: a marker for more extensive pelvic and intestinal disease.* Fertil Steril, 72(2): 1999 Aug, pp. 310–5.

3   Husby, G.K., Haugen, R.S. & Moen, M.H., *Diagnostic delay in women with pain and endometriosis.* Acta Obstet Gynecol Scand, 82(7), 2003 Jul, pp. 649–53.

4   Ballweg, M.L. *Endometriosis. The complete reference to taking charge of your health.* Contemporary Books, McGraw Hill, USA, 2004, pp. 354–60.

5   Abbott, J., Hawe, J., Hunter, D., Holmes, M., Finn, P. & Garry, R. *Laparoscopic excision of endometriosis: a randomized, placebo-controlled trial.* Fertil Steril, 82(4), 2004 Oct, pp. 878–84.

6   Demco, L. Mapping of pelvic pain under local anesthesia using patient assisted laparoscopy, *Textbook of Laparoscopy*, eds J. Hulka & H. Reich. W.B. Saunders Company, Philadelphia, 1998, pp. 391–7.

7   Chapron, C., Pierre, F., Querleu, D. & Dubuisson, J.B. *Complications of laparoscopy in gynaecology.* Gynecol Obstet Fertil, 29 (9), 2001 Sep, pp. 605–12.

8   Shaw, R.W. (ed.). *Endometriosis. Current understanding and management.* Blackwell Science, 1995, pp. 195–201.

9   Moghissi, K.S., Schlaff, W.D., Olive, D.L., Skinner, M.A. & Yin, H. *Goserelin acetate (Zoladex) with or without hormone replacement*

therapy for the treatment of endometriosis. Fertil Steril, 69 (6), 1998 Jun, pp. 1056–62.

10 Fraser, I.S. & Kovacs, G.T. *The efficacy of non-contraceptive uses for hormonal contraceptives.* MJA, 178 (12), 2003, pp. 621–3.

11 Bulun, S.E., Zeitoun, K., Takayama, K., Noble, L., *et al. Estrogen production in endometriosis and use of aromatase inhibitors to treat endometriosis.* Endocrine Related Cancer, 6, 1999; pp. 293–301.

12 Vercellini, P., Frontino, G., De Giorgi, O., Aimi, G., Zaina, B., Crosignani, P.G. *Comparison of a levonorgestrel-releasing intrauterine device versus expectant management after conservative surgery for symptomatic endometriosis: a pilot study.* Fertil Steril, 80(2), Aug 2003, pp. 305–9.

13 Fedele, L., Bianchi, S., Zanconato, G., Portuese, A. & Raffaelli, R. *Use of a levonorgestrel-releasing intrauterine device in the treatment of rectovaginal endometriosis.* Fertil Steril, 75(3), 2001 Mar, pp. 485–8.

14 Chatman, D.L. & Ward, A.B. *Endometriosis in adolescents.* J Reprod Med, 27(3), 1982 Mar, pp. 156–60.

15 Abbott, J.A., Hawe, J., Clayton, R.D. & Garry, R. *The effects and effectiveness of laparoscopic excision of endometriosis: a prospective study with 2–5 year follow-up.* Hum Reprod, 18(9), 2003 Sep, pp. 1922–7.

16 Treloar, S. *Genetic influences on endometriosis in an Australian twin sample.* Fertil Steril, 71(4), 1999 Apr, pp. 701–10 and personal communication from S. Treloar.

17 Jansen, R. *Getting Pregnant.* 2nd edn. Allen & Unwin, Sydney, 2003.

18 Van Gorp, T., Amant, F., Neven, P., Vergote, I. & Moerman, P. *Endometriosis and the development of malignant tumours of the pelvis. A review of literature.* Best Pract Res Clin Obstet Gynaecol, 18(2), 2004 Apr, pp. 349–71.

19 Borgfeldt, C. & Andolf, E. *Cancer risk after hospital discharge diagnosis of benign ovarian cysts and endometriosis.* Obstet Gynecol Surv, 59(7), 2004 Jul, pp. 510–11.

20 Davis, S.R., Briganti, E.M., Chen, R.Q., Dalais, F.S., Bailey, M. & Burger, H.G. *The effects of Chinese medicinal herbs on postmenopausal vasomotor symptoms of Australian women. A randomised controlled trial.* Med J Aust, 174(2), 2001 Jan, pp. 68–71.

21 Shepherd, S. & Gibson, P. Unpublished information.

22 Butler, D. & Moseley, G. *Explain Pain.* 2003. Available from www.noigroup.com/ep

23 Belenky, A., Bartal, G., Atar, E., Cohen, M. & Bachar, G.N. *Ovarian varices in healthy female kidney donors: incidence, morbidity, and clinical outcome.* Am J Roentgenol, 179 (3), 2002 Sep, pp. 625–7.

24 Agarwala, N. & Liu, C.Y. *Laparoscopic appendectomy.* J Am Assoc Gynecol Laparosc, 10 (2), 2003 May, pp. 166–8.

25 Hesseling, M.H. & De Wilde, R.L. *Endosalpingiosis in laparoscopy.* J Am Assoc Gynecol Laparosc, 7(2), 2000 May; pp. 215–9.

26 Phillips, R. & Motta, G. *Coping with Endometriosis.* Avery USA, 2000.

27 King, R. *Good Loving, Great Sex.* Random House, Australia, 1997.

28 Le, M.G., Moulton, L.H., Hill, C. & Kramar, A. *Consumption of dairy produce and alcohol in a case-control study of breast cancer.* J Nat Cancer Inst, 77(3), 1986 Sep, pp. 633–6.

29 Hollingsworth, E. *Better sexual health for women.* Nature & Health, 22(3), 2001, pp. 48–52.

30 Rier, S. & Foster, G.F. *Environmental Dioxins and Endometriosis.* Semin Reprod Med, 2003; pp. 145–54.

31 Schnare, D.W., Denk, G., Shields, M. & Brunton, S. *Evaluation of a Detoxification Regimen for Fat-stored Xenobiotics.* Med Hypoth, 9, 1982, pp. 265–82.

32 Campbell, D.R. & Kurzer, M.S. *Flavonoid inhibition of aromatase enzyme activity in human preadipocytes.* J Steroid Biochem Mol Biol, 46(3), 1993 Sep, pp. 381–8.

33 Schellenberg, R. *Treatment for the premenstrual syndrome with agnus castus fruit extract: prospective, randomised, placebo controlled study.* British Medical Journal, 322, 2001, pp. 134–7.

34 Mathias, J.R., Franklin, R., Quast, D.C., Fraga, N., Loftin, C.A., Yates, L., & Harrison, V. *Relation of endometriosis and neuromuscular disease of the gastrointestinal tract: new insights.* Fertil Steril, 70(1), 1998 Jul, pp. 81–8.

35 Mills, S.Y., Jacoby, R.K., Chacksfield, M. & Willoughby, M. *Effect of a proprietary herbal medicine on the relief of chronic arthritic pain: a double blind study.* British Journal of Rheumatology, 35, 1996, pp. 874–8.

36 Wilson, M.L. & Murphy, P.A. *Herbal and dietary therapies for primary and secondary dysmenorrhoea.* Cochrane Database Syst Rev, (3), 2001, CD002124.

37 Baghurst, K.I. & Dreosti, I.E. *Zinc and magnesium status of Australian adults.* Nutr Res, 11, 1991, pp. 23–32.

Women with scientific or medical training who wish to know more about the causes of pelvic pain are referred to the textbook:

Howard, FM. *Pelvic Pain. Diagnosis and Management.* ISBN 0-7817-1724-8 Lippincott Williams and Wilkins 2000.

Index

cyst, 9, 28–9
  chocolate 8, 9, 28, 29, 31, 32
    removal, 44–5
  functional ovarian, 174, 195–6
  ovarian, 1, 29, 57
  rupture, 195
cystectomy, 131
cystoscopy, 190

dairy foods, 250, 257, 263–4
danazol, 33, 35, 63, 64–6, 84, 121, 153
  side effects, 65
DDT, 257
depression, 182, 186, 233, 248, 255,
    263–4
  SSRIs, 74, 235
  teenagers, in, 91
di-indolyl methane, 252, 273
diabetes, 53, 260
diagnosis of endometriosis, 27–30
  bowel, of the, 30
  CA-125, 29
  difficulty, 31
  laparoscopy, with *see* laparoscopy
diaphragm, 25
diarrhoea, 52, 103, 155, 161, 166, 167,
    168
diet, 91, 272
  aromatase, and, 258–9
  Atkins, 261
  bloating, to reduce, 170
  changes, 96–7, 190, 222, 234–5
  coeliac disease, 167–9
  constipation, to avoid, 171–2
  eating plan, 268–70
  estrogen levels, to lower, 248–59
  irritable bowel syndrome, 161, 164
  low carbohydrate, 249, 260, 261
  low fat, 248–9, 250, 268
  reduced fat, 248–9
  therapy, 140, 142, 222
dimethyl sulfoxide (DMSO), 192
dioxins, 115, 256, 257
diuretic, 253
doppler ultrasound scan, 199

dorsal horn, 146, 147
dysmenorrhoea *see* period pain
dyspareunia (painful intercourse),
    11, 19–21, 22, 189, 198, 228–36
dysuria, 12, 24

eating plan, 268–70
ectopic pregnancy, 195
electrocautery, 33–5
embarrassment, 215, 227
emotional distress, 200
emotions, 36
endometrioid cancer, 136–7
endometrioma *see* chocolate cyst
endometriosis, 1–38
  endosalpingiosis, distinguished,
    203
  medications, 94
  ovary, affecting, 194
  post-menopausal, 85–6
  prevention, 77
  remnants, 97
  teenagers with, 88–91
  websites, 276
endometrium, 9, 10, 113–14, 253,
    258
endosalpingiosis (serous change),
    202–3
  endometriosis, distinguished, 203
endoscopy, 168
enema, 51–2, 173
estrogen
  anti-estrogen medications, 84
  cabbage family and, 251–2
  cycle, 248
  dominance, 247
    reducing, 248–59
  endometriosis and, 247–59
  hormone medication for men, 9,
    114
  HRT, in, 136
  lesions and, 84–5
  levels, 64, 66, 81–2, 117, 124, 153,
    196–7, 246, 248, 249
  production, 85

THE
LAST
ADVENTURER

Rolf Steiner

With the collaboration of
Yves-Guy Berges

Translated by Steve Cox

Weidenfeld and Nicolson
London

English Language
First Edition

ISBN 0 297 77363 1

Printed in Great Britain by
Redwood Burn Limited
Trowbridge & Esher

Certain names that appear during the course of this book have been changed. Any resemblance to real names, in this case, is totally fortuitous.

Contents

III   THE SUDAN

MAPS

I
APPRENTICESHIP
AND THE LEGION

1

The Fire
and the Ashes

When I was six years old, maybe seven, I remember my big sister had one of those dolls that talk and move their eyes. I had no interest in it as a doll, but I couldn't see how it worked, and I recall peering at it and feeling annoyed at my failure to understand.

So I carefully cut open its stomach, had a good look, then put everything back in place and sewed it up as best I could.

When my mother came looking for me, with my furious sister in tow, she asked me why I'd done it. To see how the doll worked, I told her, and earned myself a thrashing — for failing to tell a lie. If I'd said that I hadn't done it on purpose, that the doll had slipped, nothing more would have happened. That's how I learned diplomacy — if I did something wrong, I'd say the right words. Life went better, but I felt worse.

I was born on January 3, 1933, in Munich, twenty-seven days before Hitler took power. The doctor soon realized that I had a gastric acid deficiency, because I could not digest milk and kept throwing it up. My condition was critical, but I was sent to a clinic where the doctors put me on a diet of brewer's yeast mixed with apple or carrot juice. It worked: I was, in a sense, brought up on beer.

My parents were comfortably off, as people used to say in those days. My mother, of course, did nothing. My father had inherited some capital from his father, and was a mechanical engineer. When I was four he died of a perforated intestine following appendicitis. I was brought up by my mother and my paternal grandmother. Looking back, I can see that my mother was like any other — meaning that she loved her children — but to me she seemed weak, and I could not admire her. On the other hand I really adored my father. He was my hero. In the First World War he had been a flier in the famous Richthofen squadron, and there were framed medals on the wall, and photos of him standing by his handsome machine. He had shot down twenty-six planes, as well as having been brought down four times himself!

My last memory of him is the thrashing he gave me a week before he died. My godfather had bought me an electric tank for Christmas, with a gun that shot sparks from its muzzle. I got it at five, on the afternoon of Christmas Eve, and two hours later I had it in pieces. My father was furious, though he might have known better: machinery has always been my hobby.

During my early childhood I do not recall ever having playmates in from outside. I was a very solitary boy, and quite happy to be that way, in a household of three women — a kindly grandmother who spoiled me and always stood up for me, a mother who was sweet and good when a little boy like me needed a man to bring him up, and a sister a year older than myself. She played an important part in my life because she was the attractive one, a general favorite, so that while she was being taken to the opera and the theater, I would be left at home.

I grew up a quiet boy with a very ordinary childhood. I had construction sets and an electric train. I disliked rough games, and never got into a single fight all through my adolescence. I liked books, history especially and Roman history above all. Reading and tinkering took up all my time. The Deutsche Museum in Munich was the world's biggest museum of technology. It had everything, including machines that you could operate yourself, complex mechanisms of all kinds, and fascinating experimental demonstrations of physics and chemistry. On Saturdays and Sundays I used to visit it by myself. At the age of ten, I had a season ticket.

In fact I must have suffered a lot from boredom, but without realizing it, since I knew no other existence. Then again, my whole upbringing was distorted by being surrounded by feminine affection, which meant comfort and lots of toys, but also having to behave in the conventional way: "Mustn't tell lies, Rolf"; "Don't do this"; "Mustn't touch that" — always without explanation, because it wasn't done in those days. Keeping up appearances, looking right . . . still, it had its good side: it made me detest hypocrisy.

My father was a Protestant, my mother a Catholic who had married him for love, against her family's wishes. I was baptized and brought up in the Reformed faith, which must always have troubled my mother, who was a devout Catholic. But during my father's lifetime she made no attempt to inculcate her own views, and later on she remained faithful to his memory by refraining from influencing us. On Sundays, when she dressed for Mass, the maid would take my sister and me to chapel.

My one access to the world, and the only contact I had with boys of my own age, was provided by the communal school, the Plinganser Schule. But I had to wait till 1943 to escape the stifling family atmosphere, and that occurred through the *Jungvolk*. Every boy had to join at the age of ten, and remained a member until his compulsory transfer to the *Hitlerjugend* at fourteen.

The *Jungvolk* was a movement conceived and structured with a view to toughening up us future Aryans. We wore the *Hitlerjugend* uniform of black shirt and jacket, khaki shirt with a black neckerchief fastened by a ring, regulation belt, and dagger with swastika. On the surface our organization might seem to resemble the scouts, but we were divided into battalions, companies, and so on, in paramilitary fashion, with leaders chosen from the ranks at each level. We had our own banner and observed strict military discipline. Once a week there were martial songs, marching in step, games and maneuvers, and rifle training. It was hard, but it let me breathe, and although the *Jungvolk* came under the supervision of the Party we as yet received no political indoctrination, unless it was just that at the age of ten I didn't recognize it.

I belonged to the *Jungvolk* from January 1943 to September 1944. After that my mother sent me to the country, and the end of the war saved me from the *Hitlerjugend*. In the *Jungvolk* I was soon promoted to platoon leader — no combat responsibilities, but all the same I commanded thirty-two men, and although they were only eleven years old they took it all very seriously. At the time of the final collapse in May 1945 there were *Jungvolk* children involved in the fighting all over the place. Even the enemies of the Third Reich were moved by the sight of those kids singing as they marched to their deaths, with the game already lost. . . .

For us, too, the war shattered everything. In 1939 I was six years old. I had been at school for two whole years. In 1945, at the time of the German defeat, I was twelve. Between the two dates came the experience of a world collapsing; it was bound to leave its mark.

I was a child, and knew very little about the causes of the war. I lived in a heightened climate that seemed normal to me because it was all I knew. I asked myself no questions; I was a young German who passionately followed his country's victories and suffered from its defeats. With other boys of my own age I would listen to the radio announcements as if to the results of a football championship — we had taken Sebastopol; they were resisting on the Vistula; Stalingrad still held out. I shall always remember the day when France surrendered. I was on my way to school at two o'clock in the afternoon, and all the bells in Munich began to ring. I felt glad.

If we had known nothing of the other side of the picture, the bombing would have reminded us. We didn't like going into the shelters. Children adapt to anything: we played ball in the ruins. When bombs fall, they make a sort of whistling sound. We used to wait for the bombers to pass overhead, then take cover when the time came. We were curious, and eager to watch, because our fighters went up to intercept them and we used to make bets on their victory.

We did not know about the death camps, however, and had never heard anyone mention the extermination of the Jews. We knew that concentration camps existed, but thought they were POW camps. There was one which I knew very well, and where I often used to play when I was twelve. It was at Ganacker, near the village to which I was evacuated. After our house was bombed out in September 1944, my mother sent me to stay with some distant cousins who owned a farm sixty kilometers from Munich. Ganacker showed me another side of Bavaria, a land of peasants, nature, and silence. One day there was the dead town of Munich, the thousands of corpses stacked along the pavements, the noise and the smoke; the next day, fields of potatoes and maize, the smell of bread and manure, frogs in the marshes, crows speckling a white winter. And the time went by at leisure here, measured by the bells of a big clock tower.

The camp was in a small wood between the road and the railway, and I passed it every day on my way to school. It held four or five hundred prisoners — Belgian, French, and German, with an SS guard — who were being used to build an airfield. They worked in groups of twelve, and I often came across crews of them dressed in striped pajamas and pushing truckloads of gravel for the concrete along the rails linking the site to the nearby river.

They were very thin, and the ones who beat them were not the SS but men like themselves, wearing the same dress. The villagers noticed this without interfering. We did not know why the men were detained, and even if we had tried to find out it would have done no good.

I was in that camp on the day I heard that Germany had lost. Discipline had been considerably relaxed there since the advance of the Allied troops, and the fitter detainees had been evacuated a month earlier to a larger camp called Dachau. They had left on foot, because the few trucks still on the road were requisitioned by the army. All that remained at Ganacker were thirty or so detainees too ill to walk, three cooks, four medical orderlies, and two SS guards.

The arrival of the Americans was uneventful. I had hidden in the infirmary because I was stone-cold certain that they were going to kill us all when they came. The GIs tamed me with chocolate, and I saw the two SS men salute the Allied officer and hand over their weapons. Six months later I heard that the Belgian officer had returned, in a major's uniform, to give evidence at their trial, and that they had been acquitted.

Like many young Germans, I was coming out of a dream. The reality of today was not what we had been led to expect; yesterday's expectations were turning into a nightmare. Our upbringing had filled our heads with ideals of the Great Reich: losing was out of the question. They had told us we would fight to the death, and we had been prepared to die, since that was our destiny. Now our marble greatness and our bronze monuments were just a heap of scrap.

The truth was revealed by the gas chambers. No one had ever mentioned all that. It opened my eyes: I wouldn't believe it at first, thinking that it was propaganda. Then came the undeniable facts — Auschwitz, Mauthausen, Buchenwald, Dachau.

Later on, in the Legion, I thought it over a good deal. The shame of the death camps or of Oradour did not make me forget the bombing of Dresden, or the German civilians massacred by the Poles, or Stalin's deportations. Who did not have blood on his hands? In history, the victor is always right. The memories of those years of fire took a long time to sort out, but the shocks I received had sensitized my mind and undoubtedly determined the aims of my life: the protection of the weak and the defense of just causes.

My stay at Ganacker could not last long if I was to get the sort of education my mother thought proper, but most of the schools in Munich were closed, either through bombing or because too many of the staff had been called up. The only place she could find was a Catholic school at Eichstätt, in northern Bavaria, where I was the only Protestant among the hundred and fifty pupils.

The school was in a gloomy old *schloss*, a gray, cold place, standing alone in a pine forest a long way from town. The teachers wore soutanes, and we wore uniforms — gray for class, navy blue for outings, with long trousers in winter, shorts in summer. We attended Mass each morning and went to chapel after dinner for evening prayers. I liked the masculine austerity and dignity which my home life had not provided, and I was fascinated by the religious atmosphere, the statues and paintings in the chapel, the singing and incense, and the light that came through the stained glass windows. Unable to join my schoolmates in Communion, I eventually asked permission to go up on the balcony to pump the organ bellows.

The loneliness I felt was not eased by any special boarding school friendships — no secret societies, midnight feasts, or creeping down to the empty classroom to smoke an illicit cigarette. It wasn't that sort of place, and the discipline was much too strict. I remember once getting six strokes of the cane for running past the rector on my way to the refectory. What I should have done was to stop and say: "Good morning, Father." The punishment was recorded as "for insubordination."

I spent five years at Eichstätt. In class I was a good pupil, and the teachers reported that I was intelligent but undisciplined. I was never rowdy, but I liked arguing and used to be reprimanded for asking too many questions if there was something I did not understand. If anybody had told me I would grow up to be a soldier, I would have been astonished. When I thought about the future I saw myself as an engineer like my father, or else a civil pilot. My hobby was building model planes out of balsa-wood kits, and flying them on Sundays.

As time went by the religious influence of Eichstätt grew stronger. When I had had enough of pumping the organ, I became a choirboy. For an hour every day I followed catechism classes. At evening study I read the Bible. My conversion was a personal matter: none of the teachers or the other boys could have claimed the credit, because I was not that close to any of them. At sixteen I was allowed to make my first Communion, and six months later, because I never do anything by halves, I asked to become a priest. My confessor insisted that I should take three months to think it over, but at the end of that time my decision was the same.

That left me a year before entering the seminary, because I had to take my school certificate first. What I saw in the priesthood was independence. I wanted to be a missionary in Africa, and had been influenced by the stories of our math teacher, a white-haired, sardonic old Jesuit who had spent thirty years among the Papuans in New Guinea. On summer nights, when we lit camp fires, he used to tell us about his life. Some of its simple actions were like exploits to us, like building his own church, making bricks to build a baker's oven, and making yeast with bananas. These attracted me at least as much as bearing the word to the ungodly.

All the same, the worm was in the bud, and the devil soon found a way to obstruct my vocation. Girls had not meant anything to me till my fourteenth year, and sex was a taboo subject. Naturally I noticed the changes in my body, and suffered the ordeals of purity, but the subject was unmentionable, and I was left to my own devices, like many others. Yet my first encounter was at Eichstätt. As well as the teachers, all the auxiliary staff came from the ranks of the Church. There were no civilian employees, only monks and nuns. The Brothers worked in the garden, the Sisters in the kitchens. They also did our washing, and we took turns helping them with the ironing.

One afternoon my turn came around and I found myself alone with a Sister who began trying to catch my eye as soon as I came into the laundry room. Then she smiled at me, left the room, and came back with a generous snack. I blushed, but I ate, and as I did so she came closer and started kissing me and caressing me here and there. I was fourteen and a half, and she must have known that I would be much too tongue-tied to give her away. I couldn't even confess it, because I was still a Protestant then, and now I come to think of it she may have chosen me for that reason.

Sister Maria-Clara was twenty-three, and pretty. The liaison she began lasted for eighteen months, and I still think about her with affection. We used to meet in the laundry room, the cellar, a big alcove she had the key to, and sometimes even in her room. I don't know if I had any rivals among the boys, but I know she liked girls too, because I once surprised her in bed with another Sister. In any case I don't think I would have been jealous. It was a game to me — enjoyable, but that was all. My problem lay elsewhere: all this was happening during my religious crisis, and when I became a Catholic I was leading a double life. That was against my nature and I had to choose, but I found that the game was more serious than I had thought. When I decided to become a priest I suddenly realized there could be no more of that. She had been gone for five weeks, and I missed her terribly. I had become accustomed to her. A few months later I had to face the fact that I could never be a *good* priest because I would not have the strength to deprive myself of that pleasure.

So I gave it up. For me, it was a question of principle. A man who might become Pope ought not to have sexual relations if his rules forbade it. I would not take the risk of betraying my commitment.

The result was a total break with my family. My mother had been overjoyed by my conversion, and still more by my decision to become a priest, especially because she had put no pressure on me to do either. She simply could not take my change of mind, and wrote back that if I persisted I would never set foot in our home again, or see her again. At the same time she stopped my allowance. Without money, I could not continue my studies. My grandmother was dead, my sister still at a college for young ladies, there had been no contact with my mother's side of the family since the scandal of her marriage, and as for my father's side, they were all dead. I was absolutely alone.

I passed my school certificate at seventeen, and took the train to Offenburg straightaway. I had made up my mind to join the French Foreign Legion. I never did see the seminary, near Lake Constance, which I had chosen from a postcard photograph.

2
The Foreign
Legion

The Legion. The first time I saw that name was in a little comic book bought at the Munich station to pass the time on the train back to school at Eichstätt. It was a story about the Rif war in Morocco, in which a company of legionnaires, besieged in an old fort in the desert, was massacred to the last man by a raiding band of rebel nomads. It was a very romantic, absolutely stupid story, but I was fourteen and I lapped it up. So there were men who were ready to die for something other than their own country; for nothing, just like that; for the glory. It was crazy, but it was brave too, and I identified with those heroes. So when I found myself on my own, it was to the Legion I turned. When it came to dying, there had to be a better way than starving to death. It was not a sudden urge or an irresistible attraction; it was simply that there was no alternative.

At Offenburg I presented myself at a gendarme post. I knew that I was in the French occupation zone and I told them that I wanted to join the Foreign Legion. It turned out that I was the fifteenth that day, and I was taken to the barracks that contained the recruiting office, where I gave my name and was assigned a bed. Straightaway there were duties to do — peeling potatoes, sweeping dormitories

— but I didn't mind. If I could not be a good priest at least I would be a good legionnaire.

After four days at Offenburg came the long train journey to Marseilles, where we were marched through the town to Fort Saint Nicholas in the Old Port, sweating like pigs in the hottest weather I'd ever experienced, after an interminable time crammed in with hundreds of other privates.

Two thousand of us were squeezed into the old fort — a lot of Germans, some young, some ex-SS, but also Italians, Poles, Russians, refugees of all nationalities, and a pretty raw sample of humanity — here, like myself, because they had no alternative. Those eight to ten days in Marseilles were very hard. We were confined to quarters, unable to go out, and the NCOs were generous with their boots at assembly and dished out stupid fatigue duties at random. The walls crawled with bugs and the food was practically uneatable — the French themselves hadn't yet sorted out their feeding problems, so the foreigners were getting their leftovers. But we put up with all this quite cheerfully because we would soon be on our way to Africa.

We talked very freely about the war, and yesterday's enemies forgot their hatreds. That is one of the fantastic things about the Legion, even though one of its strengths is the rivalry among the various nationalities. Individual competition alongside collective discipline is the secret. For example take a German — by tradition a good soldier — who sees a Spaniard bring off some sensational feat, or an Italian beating him to some objective. "Not likely!" he tells himself, "I can do better than that." And the Russian at his side wants to go one better still. Psychological pressures of that kind go toward sustaining morale.

Then we were on board the troop transport *Sidi-bel-Abbès*, on our way to Oran, puking into a stormy sea. We reached Oran around six in the morning — reddish cliffs, a few palm trees, gray houses. The sun rose soon afterward, and everything turned golden. Before the boat moored we could see the white-veiled Moorish women on the quay, then the dockers, with their big moustaches and red skullcaps, throwing ropes and jumping onto the deck. All that was new to us.

We were marched to another barracks where we spent the rest of the day in a small courtyard in the sun. We weren't allowed under cover, and stayed there till they mustered us again in the middle of the night to catch a four o'clock train. Three or four hundred of us traveled in livestock wagons, forty in each. After the heat of the day, we felt frozen, but at last we reached Sidi-bel-Abbès, the sacred spot, temple of the Legion! Our troop was convoyed by veterans, of course. They kept up a stream of abuse, but I didn't know what they were saying because I did not yet understand French.

At Sidi-bel-Abbès we were attached to CP3 (*Compagnie de Passage* 3: a CP is a forward replacement group). It was like Fort Saint Nicholas, but a lot cleaner, and we stayed there for ten days, not yet organized but grouped in barrack rooms of sixty, each under a veteran corporal. There were so many volunteers for the paras and the tanks that I wound up with the infantry. We were kept on the run all day — fifteen to twenty assemblies, sweeping the town streets, fetching water for fatigues in the same jugs we used for coffee — with a boot to help you through the door from the veterans posted there for that purpose.

One hundred and twenty of us were posted to Mascara. Back to the cattle trucks, but not a very long journey, and we were met at the station by a band playing the famous Legion tune "*Tiens, voilà du boudin.*" For us it was the first time, and we started to feel part of the family as we marched four abreast through the town.

The barracks stood on a height overlooking the town, and

we entered through the main gate. It was an old brick building built about 1850, a massive four-story rectangle painted yellow on the outside, white on the inside. Everything was kept scrubbed so clean that cement and wood were worn smooth, and we soon found out why: it was we who did the scrubbing.

Each platoon had its own barrack room under a corporal/chief instructor. You had to stand to attention to salute him. Mine was a Russian, a former colonel in the Soviet army, who had already done one tour in Indochina. I never found out what his story was. People don't talk about the past in the Legion.

Next day we finally drew our kit, and stripped off the clothing we had been issued in Offenburg or Marseilles. It was put aside somewhere, probably to be fumigated. Naked, and in single file, we drew our new clothing first of all, then zigzagged from counter to counter to collect the rest of our equipment. Last came our blankets and sleeping bags. It was the white kepi we were really waiting for, and at last it arrived, to be received with feigned indifference. It meant a lot: before we were just rookies, the Legion's rubbish. The white kepi gave us the right to be considered as legionnaires, not as animals to be pushed and prodded at will.

Our stay at Mascara lasted three weeks. During the first week we learned to salute, to tell one rank from another, and to make beds correctly. Then we had two hours' leave — our first in our white kepis. Most of my roommates went to the brothel quarter, but I was too timid. I had a beer in the American Bar in the main square and looked around the town, where everything looked strange, but I felt disappointed because I had always thought that Africa meant blacks, lions, and virgin forest. Also, nobody was impressed by my new kepi: it was a garrison town, and all the bars were packed with legionnaires.

After completing our training we retraced our journey back to Oran. In those days the Legion wasted no time, because reinforcements were needed in Indochina. On June 15 we sailed on the *Pasteur* from Mers-el-Kebir.

There were seven thousand men on board. As well as the Legion there were French, Moroccan, and Senegalese contingents. Everyone stuck to his own group, the legionnaires mostly playing cards, though I managed to find a Russian chess partner. The voyage took seventeen days, with stops at Port Said and Singapore. Coming after weeks of hard training, it was an easy life, sleeping in hammocks, being left in peace by the NCOs, film shows, and duties restricted to two hours' daily instruction about Indochina, guerrilla warfare, and the behavior of the Vietminh.

The *Pasteur* was unable to sail up the Red River, so American landing craft ferried us to Haiphong, and from there we were moved by truck to an interforces transit camp, where we spent the night in three-tier bunks in barracks roofed with corrugated iron. In the July heat, the atmosphere was suffocating, and it was lucky for us that there was rain. We weren't supposed to leave camp, but while the sentries took shelter most of us took the opportunity to slip off into town. The smells, strange music, pedicabs, and the feverish activity that went on late into the night at last gave me the exotic atmosphere I'd been looking for. I stood on a street corner holding my bowl of Chinese soup, and felt happy.

They had informed me on board the *Pasteur* that I was posted to the Thirteenth Armored Division of the Foreign Legion, and my battalion's rear base was in Hanoi. I was to join the Ninth Company, whose quarters were near the airfield at Bac Mai.

My battalion was bogged down somewhere in the Seven Pagodas area. The Vietminh pressure on Hanoi was not very strong as yet, and Giap had concentrated his forces to the north, in the mountain region around Cao Bang and Lang Son. Operations were mounted on the scale of Mobile Groups (MG), each MG consisting of a number of infantry battalions, artillery, and armored protection, each with its own sector, liable to be shifted as the developing situation dictated to reinforce another MG. The Thirteenth Division was fighting a continual stream of engagements.

I had my baptism of fire four days after reaching Indochina. My company had mounted an ambush after digging in at night near a road junction, and it was we who took the brunt of the attack. I had no responsibilities as yet and was a machine-gun loader, the job they give to rookies when they arrive. My chief, the gunner, a Hungarian called Baradak, was killed and I took his place. I kept it for several months.

This is how it happened. We had dug in and strung out the barbed wire in the usual way, like any other night, and the Vietminh came right at us. Maybe they didn't do it on purpose but were trying to penetrate our line. I was woken by a sentry opening fire. My heart thumped, and I told myself: This is it. I was not afraid (and I never have worried about panicking) because I knew that I was there to fight. I just felt an emptiness in my stomach, like being very hungry. But as soon as our machine gun opened up it was over — I had my job, and there was no time for thinking.

It was rough, but not terrible. The Munich bombing had been a lot noisier. Then the Hungarian said. "Shit, I've been hit. Take over." I asked if I could help, but he refused. A bullet had caught him in the chest. I couldn't see where the exit wound was, but his back was covered with blood. When it was over I asked how he was, and got no answer. He was dead.

I thought the action had lasted half an hour, but when I looked at my watch it showed that only twelve minutes had elapsed since the first shot. At dawn we collected the enemy's weapons, and I saw their bodies, in grotesque positions — real dead men, with contorted features and torn flesh, not at all like the cinema. I cannot describe the way I felt: it was not disgust, but a sense that my existence was over. And in a way it was — I had lost my childhood.

We didn't have many dead that day. Ten to a company was not a lot in Indochina. And now I felt welded to the Legion. The feeling of emptiness subsided, and I was proud of becoming a real legionnaire.

I didn't much like being a machine gunner, because those things are heavy. Lugging a machine gun all day, day after day, plus pack, rations, water, and ammo, through the heat and the paddies, is an exhausting job. Even with a bush hat, the sun gets to you.

The first time I was sure I had killed a man was in September 1951, at the time of Operation Mandarin. With a machine gun you know you're doing damage, but in order to see the results it has to be daytime and the lie of the land must be right. To be sure, you have to have seen the guy standing before he falls.

At three in the afternoon we clashed with a Vietminh company, somewhere between Viet Ninh and Seven Pagodas, in a surprise attack. They were in a village surrounded by bamboo stakes with the points facing outward, and sure to be protected by a minefield. We went in, and when our first scout touched off a mine it was the signal for the Vietminh dug in around the edge of the village to open fire.

We were strung out along the paddy, up to our knees in mud, but although we were dispersed we still made too good a target. I spotted a small dyke between us and the village and made for it fast, followed by the other men. It gave me a solid purchase for the machine gun, which had to give cover to the advancing infantry. We dislodged the Viets and cleaned out the village without meeting any resistance. On the other side were more paddies, and I could clearly make out the last retreating enemy. I got a group of four in my sights, opened fire, and watched two of them fall. It had no effect on me: this was war.

The really rough fighting started at Hoa Binh, a big village on the Black River, west of Hanoi, where we were dispatched in November 1951. The area was infested with Vietminh regulars, and the Saigon High Command had just ordered it to be cleaned out. For Christmas Hoa Binh was surrounded. The Vietminh held all the roads, and the only communications with Hanoi were by river. When they could get through, it was the navy that was keeping us supplied with munitions.

We were commanded by Colonel Vanuxem, a brave man but also clearheaded. In January he realized that we were too heavily outnumbered and decided to pull us back. My company was farthest out, and it was our job to keep the enemy pinned down until the bulk of our force was embarked. When our turn came there were no boats left and we had to wade across the river, then make a two-day cross-country march, continually harassed by the Viets, who luckily overestimated our strength. It was very hard going and we lost a lot of men. I had no trouble because my squad was trailbreaking at the head of the column — a good place to be, because it's never the front men who fall in an ambush.

In September 1952 I took the training course for corporals. I had been a legionnaire for two years and was already a PFC. I did the course in Cochin China, in a village called Arnaudville, built by the Thirteenth Division.

In the Legion, it takes three months to train for corporal, and they make you sweat. You get the same training as a regular NCO, plus discipline. For punishment you might, for instance, be stood in front of a pond, in full combat dress, and have to cross it, carrying all your gear. So far, so good. Then they told you: "Right, kit inspection," and gave you five minutes to have your gear neat and squared off, otherwise it went out the window. And all this sometimes at two in the morning. It seemed pretty mindless treatment, some of it invented by the instructors, most in the tradition of the Legion, but it was not as useless as it seemed. The point was to break the character of the trainee and suppress his critical sense. It gave me some difficulty with self-control, but I held out.

After training I was returned to my battalion, where I was officially appointed squad leader. My first men. I felt no special pride, but I knew that it was a landmark in my life. Before I had been a very introverted young man, with a will of my own, directed only to my own purposes. Now I was no longer alone: I was responsible for a team.

Corporal in the Legion is the most awkward of ranks because it is your job to put into practice everything that comes from higher up. The officers are on the NCOs' backs, but if the NCOs get a roasting it's the corporals who get scorched. I don't know if I was a popular corporal, but the question was irrelevant. A corporal in the Legion is, by tradition, respected — a lord and master. He must be up to his job, or he wouldn't have it.

It isn't even being an example that really counts. A legionnaire works under his own steam. Each man knows what he has to do, and there is no need to tell him where or when. Under pressure, he moves by instinct. The ones who don't are dead men.

Fear ought not to exist. In the Legion you know that when you get the order to advance, you advance. Occasionally I have seen men *show* their fear and lose control of themselves, and it makes matters worse. For instance, I remember one Pole who got wounded in the thigh and started screaming that he was dying. I had the wound dressed, sent him off to Hanoi by ambulance, and four or five days later we heard that he was dead, not because of his injury, but because he let go.

At the other extreme was the Russian. Between Hué and Da Nang we had run smack into the Vietminh 101st Battalion on the plain a few kilometers from the sea. We were outnumbered and taking a bad beating, and the order came to fall back. A mortar shell burst and a piece of shrapnel opened up the Russian from side to side. His guts hung down to his knees. I already had one wounded man on my back, and carrying another was just not possible. The Russian knew it, and he had a solution. I can see him now as he gathered his insides up in his arms and said: "All right, chief, let's go."

"You can walk like that?"

"I'll be okay. Light me a cigarette."

So I lit one, put it in his mouth, and this dead man — as I thought — walked like that for an hour and a half. It surprised me because I didn't know then that a man could put up such resistance by willpower alone: it is very difficult to die if you refuse death. There was a yellowish, foul-smelling sauce trickling down his legs and hundreds of big, metallic-blue flies swarmed after him as he walked, but still he walked. After half an hour he was pale, and his face was beaded with sweat. We covered six kilometers before the medics picked him up and he was shipped off to the hospital in Da Nang. A month later he was back — alive!

The men had a high turnover rate in Indochina, and the Legion suffered considerable losses in killed and wounded. In five years I was hit by shell splinters in the thigh, the groin, and under my armpit, none of them serious injuries. It was like the decorations — I got four, but it meant nothing. One day you do something good and nobody knows, the next you get a medal without knowing why. Most legionnaires could tell similar stories. We were continually in action, and both sides were bound to take casualties.

For the Vietminh we had respect, as we did for any fighting enemy, and I think it was mutual. One day I was on leave in Hanoi and went to eat in a little Vietnamese restaurant. Halfway through the meal I was served a beer I had not ordered. When I asked where it came from the proprietor motioned toward a nearby table where there were three smiling young men with their hair cut very short. I thanked them, and they came over:

"Can we sit with you?"

"Sure."

"You're in the Thirteenth, then?" said one, seeing my badge.

"Yes."

"We're in the Three-o-eighth."

The 308th Division was the one opposing us. They spoke good French, and we talked about one or two operations and had a drink together before saying polite farewells.

I did two spells in succession in Indochina, after signing up again at the end of my two years. I spent my leaves on the spot, but was due some time back "home." In February 1954 I was promoted to sergeant. The course was no easier nor more intelligent than the one for corporals, with the usual constant bullying.

I missed Dien Bien Phu. My battalion was in Hanoi. At the time I did not sense that it was a catastrophe. In our eyes we had nothing to blame ourselves for — we knew that our comrades had done their job. But we discussed the siege, knowing what it was like to be surrounded in the mountains in Viet territory: wait too long, and you no longer have the strength to break out. We also criticized the leadership, because Dien Bien Phu was so utterly indefensible, and de

Castries, because to us he was no legionnaire, just a cavalier who looked pretty good on a horse.

The political consequences of the loss of Dien Bien Phu surprised us. For the Legion the main thing had been to keep a grip on the delta, the center of Annam, and not to invest so much in holding an outlying post isolated in an area the enemy had always controlled. We did not understand why this one defeat should mean dropping everything. Certainly we did not fool ourselves that with the men and resources at our disposal we could win the war of attrition being waged by the Vietminh. The 100,000 men we had in Indochina could not control the forests and mountains which cover four-fifths of the country. But we also felt a sense of frustration because we did not feel militarily beaten.

Then, very fast, came the Geneva Accords of July 1954. At that time the Thirteenth Division was guarding the demarcation line north of Hanoi. We used to play volleyball with the facing Vietminh, who had already taken power. We gave up Hanoi and withdrew to Haiphong, then gave up Haiphong and were transferred to Cap St. Jacques (now Vung Tou) in Cochin China. We hung about there for six months before sailing directly for North Africa, in June 1955. That suited me fine. I was looking forward to spending my six months' leave in the Algerian sun. It was quiet there.

3

Algeria

Algeria was France — an empire, and something more than an empire. We disembarked in time to be caught up straightaway in the July 14 celebrations. We marched in procession, to wild applause, before dispersing into the dance halls where beer flowed, brochettes sizzled, and bands played from Bab-el-Oued to the Champ de Manoeuvres. Nobody seemed to be giving a thought to the National Liberation Front (FLN) partisans and the rebellion, yet the previous year had seen the start of the rising, the famous night of All Saints' Day, November 1, 1954. Already a first army contingent had arrived from France. If you looked closely you could find men in the streets wearing tricolor armbands which would not be removed when the rest of the decorations were taken down. They were members of the defense militia.

I had come back harder, sure of myself and more knowledgeable about other people. After five years in the Legion I spoke good French, not just the language of the barrack room. A good sixty percent of legionnaires are Germans, but to communicate among themselves they speak French. That is the Legion tradition, and traditions in the Legion are ironclad.

The Thirteenth remained off duty for a month, at Camp Zéralda, where we spent most of our time on the beach. Then I took my overdue leave. I rented a room in Algiers, bought a scooter, and got to know several *pied noir* families through girls I'd met on July 14. On weekends we'd go dancing at the casino or La Corniche. On weekdays I spent the morning reading, the afternoon on the beach.

Holiday time ended in November, when I was posted to the Aurès region, the place where the rebellion had started a year before with the murder of two French schoolteachers, man and wife. It was a lousy posting, because at the time we had no helicopters, and every day brought more hard going through the rugged hill country around our base at Khenchela. All winter we searched for the enemy and found no one. It was not till March 14 that we first laid eyes on a group of forty badly armed men.

Our first brush was over in five minutes. The Piper observer planes reported a local band and set the fighters on them to keep them busy till we could get there. It was the first time we had gone into battle by helicopter — just my own section, because there'd been no time to alert the rest. We landed a kilometer away, after seeing how the Corsairs were strafing the *fellagha* hideouts, and when they saw us coming at them from uphill they took flight. We cornered them in a narrow wadi and it was all over in minutes: a brief resistance, and they were wiped out. For weapons they had only hunting rifles and Berettas. We had one man wounded, although we had been outnumbered nearly two to one. After so much time wasted chasing around in circles, it was a welcome success.

Time dragged in the Aurès. Apart from caravans intercepted on the Sahara side, there were practically no civilians, and because we never ran across any FLN regulars we never really had to fight. What clashes we did have were flashes in the pan — the *fellaghas* fired a couple of shots at a range too long to do any good, then they ran. Our losses were negligible: an occasional man killed, maybe two or three wounded, but nothing serious.

In June 1956 we were posted to the Lesser Kabylia to protect a dam which the French were building there. It was much the same setup — one or two shots now and then, but aimed at the dam workers, not at us. All the same, life was more interesting because at least there was country-side, with rivers and forests of cork-oak, and we had a good relationship with the local population. Of course, we searched their villages when the order came, but it always went very smoothly. This was no enemy territory; it was France.

After the Kabylia, I'd had a bellyful. I had been pressing to go on a parachute course for some time, and I took it at Blida in November: six jumps from a Nord-Atlas. I enjoyed it so much that I wished I'd started earlier. The course earned me entrance into the First Foreign Parachute Regiment, the Legion's elite unit, and I was appointed to the first combat company, commanded by Captain Martin. One big contrast with the Thirteenth Armored Division was that in the First Paras we lived with the officers, which made a crucial difference in our relations. Here we rubbed shoulders with our colonel; in the Thirteenth we never saw him. I felt more at home in that atmosphere: still part of the Legion, but with the pride of belonging to a crack regiment. There were various privileges, too: for instance, we now carried out our operations in constant touch with the helicopters, and afterward they ferried us back to Zéralda. No more rotting in the same village for months on end!

Search operations alternated with visits to town, because we were also taking part in what the journalists called the "battle of Algiers," which, for us, meant protective patrols intended to discourage the terrorists. These jobs were a departure from standard military duties: the intelligence officer gave us various addresses, we took two or three jeeps along, and if the door stayed shut we broke it down. When we found a cache of arms or rounded up some suspects, they were handed over to the local troops.

It was not war, and it was never hard. We even had time off to spend Christmas 1957 at Hassi Messaoud. Then we moved to Guelma, which had earned its reputation of being the roughest sector of Algeria. *Fellaghas* swarmed all over the mountains overlooking the town, and they even flew their flag there. They were helped by the nearness of the Tunisian frontier, so we took some months cleaning them out, then lay in wait for them at source. At that time there was only one electrified fence system, the Morice Line, but the National Liberation Army (ALN) kept making the same mistake. After completing their training in the safety of Tunisia, they were obsessed by a desire to cross the line in big units. What they did not know was that wherever they cut the barbed wire it gave the alarm to the nearest post, and we knew exactly where they were. If it happened at eleven o'clock at night, by four in the morning we were ready and waiting to receive them. Supposing they missed the rendezvous, the Piper scouted the area, located them or their traces, and the choppers deposited us all around them.

One day it was a bunch of a thousand who got their foot in the door — on the day before Camerone!* The alert came at eight in the evening, when we were already preparing for the celebration, and we set out in a foul mood. We were meant to be supporting another regiment, which had let the raiders slip through its fingers, and Colonel Jeanpierre positioned us on a hillside to give covering fire. The thousand intruders were below, in a basin-shaped valley, and there

---

* Traditional Foreign Legion holiday to mark the anniversary of the famous battle on April 30, 1863, at Camarón, in Mexico, when sixty-four legionnaires held off two thousand Mexicans for nine hours.

were about seven hundred of us. The other regiment opened fire, and that started it.

We didn't hang about, just formed a line and went in, shouting "Camerone!" The brush was head-high, and we couldn't see a thing as we pressed on behind a barrage of grenades and submachine-gun fire. The only enemies we saw were the dead men we stepped over. A single sweep took us right through the valley. There was no hand-to-hand fighting, and at the end there was no one left. We went back to Guelma, where the goose was overcooked but the beer was still cool.

Camerone was a kind of safety valve, an explosion of collective liberation to vent the surplus of energy screwed down by discipline. Dancing, feasting, drinking, and I mean serious drinking. Tradition has it that Camerone is *naturally* a day of excesses and wild escapades. It can even go so far as pitched battles, as it did at Hué in 1952, when two companies of the Second Infantry Regiment fought a two-hour mortar battle and nobody could stop them. Machine guns were set up on the pavement, and the only thing missing was heavy artillery.

At Zéralda in 1957 our colonel, Jeanpierre, wanted the regiment to stay in barracks on April 30. There was trouble brewing, we were too close to Algiers, and he was playing safe — until a couple of legionnaires got drunk, commandeered a tank, put a shell up the spout, and made for HQ. With the turret aimed point-blank at the officers' mess they instructed Jeanpierre to change his mind before they blew up the mess. They were absolutely out of their heads.

They had their way, and if anybody wonders what happened to them, the answer is: nothing. Jeanpierre did not hold it against them either. It was Camerone, and the colonel had too much sense for that.

It was my officers who made me what I am. Not with useless phrases, but by example alone, they taught me what it meant to be straight and brave, and to take pride in making decisions and carrying responsibility. I respected them all; some of them became my models.

Martin, my company commander during the battle of the frontiers, for example. I was in command of a covering group and stayed by him everywhere, together with the radio operator. Under fire, he would bawl his men out when they didn't take cover, but he himself always stayed on his feet. When I saw leaves getting sliced off the trees right next to us I would tell him to watch out — things were getting dangerous. He just told me not to worry. "It's my job to command."

Lebras took over the first company after Martin left. We had a lot of respect for him, though he was a staff officer. But he didn't like marching, and consequently didn't tire his troops. In combat, no problem — same style as Martin.

Jeanpierre. Every legionnaire in the paras knew him personally. He liked human contact, and called his officers and NCOs by name. We felt real affection for him. He was cheerful, simple, direct, and he knew what mattered, so he could be strict on discipline but not care about external marks of respect; he forbade theft and looting but turned a blind eye to the adoption of an abandoned chicken or donkey. He lived at his men's level and had an eye for every detail, in or out of combat, visiting company commanders without warning, tasting the soup and testing weapons.

Jeanpierre disliked commanding his companies on foot. He used to fly overhead by helicopter, at low altitude, and when the action started he would land immediately behind and tell the unit's commander what he had seen from above.

On May 24, 1958, we were on a sweep near Guelma and flushed out some *fellaghas*. They put up heavy resistance, and we saw Jeanpierre swoop down at ground level in his Alouette II. An enemy bullet perforated his fuel feed pipe, the motor cut out, and the helicopter crashed. Some of the enemy made for the wreck, but we got there first. It was too late. Jeanpierre and his pilot were already dead. When we'd finished, there wasn't much left of the enemy either.

I was fed to the teeth with this phony war. Compared with Indochina, it was a fool's game — a few bullets from time to time, but no real fighting. The Arabs never attacked the military, only civilians. In May 1959 I was already planning to quit the Legion when pulmonary tuberculosis made its appearance. I had been spitting blood and feeling weak, and an X-ray turned up a shadow on my right lung. The doctors sent me to the Maillot hosiptal, and from there I was transferred to Grenoble.

Here I was told that if I did not agree to an operation I could be dead in a few years. That settled it. I had half a lung removed and made a rapid recovery, which would have been even faster if it had not been for a stupid boast. To show what a legionnaire could do, I bet the other patients in my ward that I could complete a three-kilometer march as soon as I came out from under the anesthetic. So after the operation I removed the drainage tubes, stuck plaster on, and set off through a meter of winter snow. When I reached another sanatorium I refused to be returned to my own by ambulance, in order to prove that I had won my bet.

What I hadn't allowed for was the blood seeping inside, once the tubes were removed. When the doctor came to see me at three in the morning I was on the point of blacking out, and my reflexes had gone. I got the roasting I deserved, and Odette convinced me to have the tubes replaced. Three days later we were drinking champagne.

Odette was my future wife, a beautiful dark-haired girl whom I met at a Legion dance, where I fell for her steady eyes and high spirits. We had been going out together whenever my schedule allowed, and we got engaged on my return to Algiers, on February 11, 1960. After my convalescence I had been put on long-term leave, and I already felt as much a *pied noir* as a legionnaire.

My plan was to settle in Algeria. I did not intend to sign on again, and I knew that my leave would be prolonged until my time ran out. I was no longer even bound to live in barracks, just to make a monthly visit to the military hospital for a checkup.

The situation in Algeria was deteriorating fast at that time. In military terms General Challe had the country under control, but it was the politicians who would lose it, as they had in Indochina. In Algiers terrorist attacks on the population, including the bombing of dance halls and cafés, were costing the lives of innocent women and children who had not chosen to fight. Those despicable methods angered me all the more because the previously trusting French population of Algeria had got on the wrong side of the government in Paris, which found its high-level policy at odds with their attachment to their native land.

In the January rebellion of 1960 I was in the university buildings with Odette's brothers, at the side of Pierre Lagaillarde. Facing us was the First Para Regiment, under Dufour. It was he who on the following day disarmed one of his own sections and sent it in to find the "rebel," because he did not want to force Lagaillarde at gunpoint. In fact, Lagaillarde was not arrested till later. He surrendered to the Legion.

Algeria's dilemma was also mine. I still felt as much a legionnaire as ever, as I do today and probably will until the day I die. I had not returned to Germany, and no longer had any contacts there. The news of my mother's death the previous year had drawn a line under my German past, and I considered France my country of adoption, both because of my enlistment and through my family links. The French region where I had chosen to live was the province of Algeria, and I felt just as abandoned by France as did the French people of Algeria.

Through Odette and my in-laws I took part in the daily life of the *pieds noirs*, and in their fears and distress. When Paris threw them over, I felt involved. Whatever de Gaulle's motives, when he had told the European community, "I have understood you," he had been betraying them.

Until then it had all been simple: the Legion was in the service of France. Then all at once I had to choose. How were we to interpret out motto of "Honor and Fidelity"? It spoke for itself. I owed the fidelity to France, not to the policy of its government, and the honor, for me, was that of being with the French. If the French of Algeria were threatened, I owed it to myself to share their fate.

Against that background, and with those feelings, it was inevitable that I should become involved with the OAS. It started in April 1961, at the time of the abortive *putsch* of the "four generals": Salan, Challe, Jouhaud, and Zeller. The First Para Regiment, which had gone over to the insurgents, was dissolved. After Challe's arrest my last company commander, Captain Sergent, brought me into the network. I had to find hideouts for a dozen old comrades who had deserted. At first I stuck to backroom work: leaflets, false papers, arms caches.

In November, however, I received orders to train combat teams for plastic-bomb attacks. I was responsible for the Hussein Dey–Hydra sector. The *pieds noirs* were eager, but talkative and undisciplined, so precautions were necessary. The teams consisted of six men who knew nothing about each other and had no idea how they were connected to the rest of the network.

My first group contained two legionnaires, two members of the Sixth Paras (RPC), and two young and inexperienced civilians. They received their first lesson at Telemly, where our intelligence service had located an Arab tradesman who was collecting for the FLN. At the last minute the boulevard was blocked by riot police roadblocks, and my men would have run the risk of arrest.

I owned a small Vespa 400 car at the time, which I used for doing the shopping. I went by with a long French loaf well in evidence in the rear window, and 500 grams of plastic inside it. There was no difficulty in tamping it down along the doorway; then it was just a matter of placing the detonator and lighting the slow fuse. My guys watched from a distance — it helped in their education.

I was a reluctant exponent of counterterrorism, but the FLN had taken the gloves off, and our orders were to take reprisals against all attacks. All the same, there were some methods I could not stomach, as when I was told to blow up a booby-trapped car at the harbor during the docker's hiring time. At seven o'clock on a late February morning my team was standing by, ready to open fire on an old Simca crammed with explosives. I was to give the order over the walkie-talkie, but when I saw a cluster of Arab workers standing right by the car I called it off. It was too savage.

I was arrested twice. On January 30, 1962, I was passing by the Bar du Commerce, which we used as a contact point, when I saw Momond, the new head of the Delta team, which took on the biggest jobs. He was coming out of the bar with his hands up, in front of some riot police who had machine-pistols sticking into his back. I stopped together with the other passersby, like a casual onlooker, but some plain-clothesmen saw the look we exchanged, and I was picked up.

I was carrying compromising documents, so in the paddy wagon I set about conscientiously eating them. I hadn't finished when we reached the police school at Hussein Dey where the interrogation took place. They put me in a room where there were already a hundred or so suspects lying on camp beds. Immediately I asked for the WC, and finished my meal.

It was just in time. The inspector sent for me, and I was searched: nothing except my papers, the right ones. I was in uniform.

"You're a legionnaire?"

"Yes, First Paras, on extended leave."

"You or your regiment?"

I didn't like his sense of humor, but it was the wrong time to answer him back.

"Your name was found in one of Degueldre's notebooks. How do you explain that?"

"He was one of my buddies at Zéralda. We were in the same unit."

"Get undressed."

They gave me a thorough body search, which did not spare my modesty, but the organ they needed was inaccessible. They had no proof against me. Even so they kept me there for three days, without ill treatment, along with all the others.

The second time, they got it right. On March 5, 1962, at seven in the morning, I parked my car at Hussein Dey, just by the police school. I was worn out at the end of the "blue night" during which there had been forty plastic bombings in Algiers, with ten teams at work, my own starting to run smoothly. I was just about to go into the bistro for a coffee when I was jostled by a young *pied noir*.

"Get out! Get away! The place is going up!"

No time to tell him it should have been done at night, because he was already running. I just had time to get clear before it blew. I went to a nearby bistro, had a leisurely coffee, and as soon as I was back in the car five riot police rushed out of the school and surrounded me, aiming their MAS-36s.

"We saw you! Come out of there!"

They walked me to the detention center, where a lieutenant claimed to have seen me place the bomb. My denial wasn't helped when they searched the car and found a brand-new MAT-49 behind the right-hand door panel. That did it. They kept me at the police school for a few days before transferring me to the Santé prison, in Paris.

A few days later I appeared before the examining magistrate, a very correct old gentleman and a retired colonel. He believed me. A lot of these officers were themselves prone to divided loyalties, and willing to grant us the benefit of the doubt.

We lived like lords in the Santé. The political prisoners' cells were never locked, we got up when we pleased and organized our own assembly each morning in the yard. There were film shows twice weekly, with films provided by the Legion, and you could take educational courses, play volleyball, and even play poker with the warders.

I was still suffering the aftereffects of my TB, and was transferred from the Santé to Fresnes hospital. There I was even more comfortable, because between treatments we were occupying rooms just vacated by the big FLN chiefs.

My trial was set for December 10, 1962, and I was acquitted without charges.

In the meantime my in-laws had left Algeria. At the time I was released they had already settled in Nice, although Odette had stayed near me in Paris throughout my period of detention, and visited me twice a week. I was still a legionnaire on extended leave, but in practice a civilian, drawing my pay and a pension. I took a flat in Nice, regularized our situation by marrying Odette, and tried to adjust to a new life.

I had started to read again. I took correspondence courses, sat at the drawing board, made training visits to factories. Yet family life palled. It's pleasant to have beer in the refrigerator and your feet in slippers while you sit in front of the television. Pleasant for a change. Not for ever.

To keep myself entertained I often went to Legion HQ at Aubagne, near Marseilles, and I used to meet a lot of veterans at the Nice Para Club, where I also trained for a pilot's license. I made some jumps, too. The doctor had recommended fresh air.

The gray period of my life lasted too long — five years. In 1966 my partner Meunier and I opened a small research and development office in Grenoble. I had been working on some inventions: a gyroscopic compass, a hydraulic press, and in particular a new type of hand grenade. But to capitalize on them I had to start a company, and I never did have any head for business. I had intended to patent the grenade in France, but I learned that there was a law by which the Ministry of Defense could oppose the development of that sort of patent for a trifling indemnity. Meunier advised me against risking it, and took it on himself to sell my invention in the United States.

So that was my existence. To the extent that I was absorbed in my work, it satisfied me. I should have been happy, but I was bored to death.

II
BIAFRA

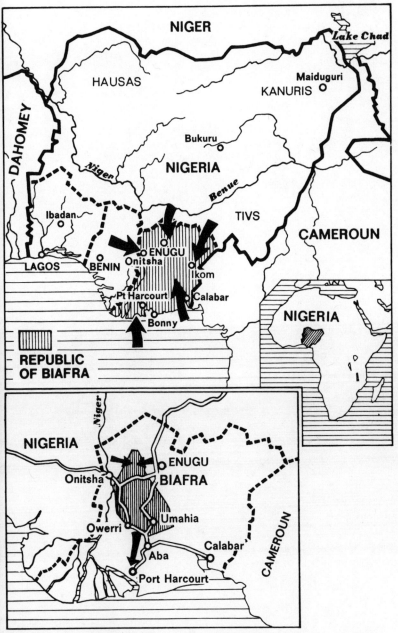

Biafra and Nigeria - showing the main areas of the struggle

4
Biafra

It was in October 1967 that I first heard mention of Biafra.
I had gone to Paris to meet Meunier, and ran into some old
Legion friends, a bit down on their luck after completing
their time or being thrown out of the army after the OAS.
Some were looking for work; others, in search of stronger
sensations, had joined Schramme in the Congo and were
having a hard time. Pinned down and surrounded by the
Congolese in Bukavu, they had been hanging on for weeks,
looking for the chance to break out. We were worried about
them, and every day we would discuss the military situation
there in a little café near the Etoile.

Not to mince words, this was a kind of labor exchange
for the "heavy" brigade. In the little basement room where
the deals were settled you could run into some strange
characters — middle-aged Germans, Chinese, Corsicans, or
Yemenites deep in conversation with hard-looking men with
flat bellies and broad shoulders. In spite of the diversity of
the clientele, they all had a kind of family resemblance:
not so much the long hair and beads, more the shaved neck
and the gray suit worn like a uniform.

The house's reputation was above suspicion. Nobody
would have mentioned holdups, drugs, or prostitution, be-

cause the jobs in question mainly involved African wars and electoral campaigns. The applicants, all serious people, presented proper references. The clients, who were above-board and sometimes official, paid cash down and provided the equipment. I had no intention of selling my own skills and was not looking for that kind of work. But I liked the atmosphere, and the hush-hush side of the proceedings. It was a pleasure to meet old comrades and exchange memories, and natural to find ourselves talking about plans for the future, especially once we'd downed a few beers.

One night I was introduced to two young Africans, sober, soft-spoken men who explained that they were Ibos sent to Europe on behalf of the newly proclaimed republic of Biafra, which had seceded from Nigeria on May 30, 1967. At that time I knew very little about these events; like most other people, I assumed that it was simply a question of tribal warfare breaking out in a former colonial state which had received its independence prematurely.

"Let me start by telling a story," one of the Biafrans began. "A Yoruba, a Hausa, and an Ibo are out walking one day, and feeling thirsty. Suddenly they see a ripe coconut on top of a palm tree. The Yoruba sits beneath the tree and thinks: I'll wait for a gust of wind. The Hausa prays: 'Allah! Allah! make that coconut fall.' The Ibo climbs the tree and picks the coconut."

A silence followed. Obviously he liked to stage-manage his effects. Then he asked if there was a Belgian among us, and big Jeff grunted yes.

"Walloon or Flemish?" the Ibo asked bluntly.

"Walloon, of course."

"You see, you don't like me suggesting that you might be Flemish. If you were, I suppose you wouldn't like my thinking you might be a Walloon. In your country they call that a 'linguistic quarrel.'"

"And in yours?"

"Oh, in ours it's only a tribal war. We are black. But we both suffer from the same problem, even if ours is more recent. To an outsider Nigeria is the richest country in Black Africa, with the biggest population. In fact it's an artificial state set up by the British in 1914 for the colonial exploitation of the Niger basin. They put cat and dog in the same sack — or rather, three peoples with nothing in common inside the same frontiers."

He ticked off the three main ethnic groups of Nigeria: in the north, twenty-eight million Muslim Hausas living under a feudal system which blocked all possibility of evolution; in the west, eighteen million Yorubas, good tradespeople, good workers, but with no great character. And in the east, the Ibos, fourteen million of them if you counted the small neighboring ethnic groups inside the Ibo sphere of influence. "So, if you're going to talk about tribal warfare, you have to be logical — you must talk about all those other tribes, Swedes, Bretons, Basques, Slovaks, Portuguese, Greeks, Swiss, or" — looking straight at Jeff — "Flemings and Walloons."

Jeff said nothing. We went on listening.

"Sorry to give you a lecture, but I think it's necessary in order for you to understand the origins of our fight. Before the English came, in the last century, Yorubas, Hausas, and Ibos all lived in their own places. They were held apart by everything — religion, language, even climate: dry desert to the north, hot and humid weather to the south. The Yorubas are a forest people like ourselves. They traded with the whites through the trading posts on the coast. The Hausas, who had been colonized by their Arab conquerors, had stopped their camels at the edge of the savanna, where the tsetse fly prevented further progress. It is no slander on the Ibos to say that we were a people of the bush, animists, sometimes cannibals, but we already had traditional democratic institutions.

"In those days the only connection among the three peoples was the slave trade. The Hausas were the hunters, the Yorubas were the go-betweens for the European coastal traders, and we were the game. According to the old plantation records I had the opportunity of looking at in Haiti, we were very high quality merchandise, the smartest, strongest cattle available on the world market." He stopped, swallowed the rest of his beer, then asked anxiously whether he was boring us. He wasn't, but it was the man himself who held our attention just as much as what he had to say. He was so different from our previous image of black men that I found myself wondering if he was some sort of exception, the Einstein of his nation. All I knew had been based on the Senegalese in the Haiphong brothels.

"I should have introduced myself at the start," he apologized. "My name is Onyeka Onibogu, I'm twenty-four, and I used to be a medical student at Bordeaux, which is why I speak your language. When our leader, Lieutenant-Colonel Ojukwu, asked us to come home to defend our country, I gave up my studies. At present I'm a traveling diplomat, but I shall be going back to Biafra soon to take my place in the army. And now I'll hand over to my friend, the future Doctor Egbo Okoro. His story is the one that matters."

The other black was shorter and more thickset than his companion, with a less practiced manner. He told us that he, too, had been recalled to Biafra, after studying law in London. He had been born in Kano, in northern Nigeria, and grown up there with his family, and it was they he wanted to talk about:

"My father studied to be a schoolteacher, but he could not find a job in Enugu, where there were plenty of teachers already. My mother's family had a shop in Kano, in the middle of Hausa country, and there was a big Ibo colony there, so they decided to settle in the north. Our quarter was called Sabon-Gari, which means 'Foreigners' Quarter' in

Hausa. The Ibos were there because in the days of the British there had been a big demand for accountants, secretaries, and all sorts of technicians for their businesses, and the Hausas couldn't supply them.

"By the time the British left, the Sabon-Gari ghetto had a hundred thousand inhabitants and was one of the wealthiest quarters of the town. Inside two generations the Ibos had risen to being the civil servants, doctors, engineers, lawyers, while the Hausas were still petrified by their own traditions. That didn't stop them resenting the success of the slave race they once despised, and the more we succeeded the more the resentment turned into hatred."

The next part of his story was palpably hard for him to tell. On September 18, 1966, he was on vacation from London, back with his family in Kano. That day he was visiting some English friends in the middle of town. Around five o'clock he had started home on his bicycle, part of a stream of people on their way home after work.

"Suddenly the people in front of me braked and listened to the sound coming out of Sabon-Gari. At first it was just a murmur, but it turned into a rumble. Some people turned back, others hurried on, thinking about their wives, their children, their parents, and what might be happening to them. As we got closer we could see smoke and hear shots, shouting, terrible screams. A friend of my father's had a shop near the entrance to the quarter. It was on fire. The main street was deserted and full of wreckage — broken furniture, overturned cars, crumpled bicycles. And dead bodies, lying in pools of blood.

"My parents' house was three blocks away. My father had just repainted it yellow, and it was easy to recognize. I stood staring at it. Then I felt myself being grabbed and shaken, and I was hauled into a car. It was my English friends. They'd heard what was happening and had come looking for me. I saw a mob of about a hundred young Hausas flood into sight at the end of the street. They were drunk on looted beer, and armed with broken bottles, old hunting rifles, and machetes. They broke down doors, fired into windows. They dragged out women who'd been hiding in the houses, with their children, who ran behind, trying to catch up. Then they were taken and beaten and trampled underfoot.

"My friends took me to the airport. There were some Ibos there before us, and Hausas too. The Ibos had tried to shelter in the airline offices but the men were dragged out and shot. Some Europeans in transit managed to protect some of the women and children, and my friends took me to a group of whites. The Hausas didn't dare come near, but they prowled around us like wild beasts, and turned the airport upside down looking for more Ibos. I managed to get away at midnight. I hadn't got a ticket, but the pilot took me aboard. That's all."

A silence fell. Not that there were any soft hearts among us, but the Kano butchery was still written on his face, and we could feel his horror.

His friend's voice broke in: "The Sabon-Gari massacre continued for six days, without intervention from the army or the police. The Ibo officers and soldiers were too few in number to do anything. They got rid of their uniforms and joined the survivors who were taking the long road home on foot or by truck. But the pogrom did not only affect Kano. At the same time murder, looting, and arson were committed against the Ibo communities in the northern towns of Kaduna, Gombe, Jos, Sokoto. The death toll was estimated at thirty thousand. From then onward Ibos from all over Nigeria quit their jobs and their homes and began their exodus toward Oriental Province, the Ibo homeland. And the Hausas and Yorubas in our own country, in Enugu or Port Harcourt, packed their bags too. I may as well admit that a Kano-bound train was intercepted by Ibo soldiers and four hundred Hausas paid the penalty for their northern brothers. The Republic of Biafra was declared on May 30, 1967."

Days went by, and I could not get their story out of my mind. I was convinced that they were genuine, and that they were defending a just cause and a persecuted people. I bought books and newspapers and read all I could about their problem, and I was especially struck by one phrase — "the black Jews of Africa." What struck me even more was the indifference of the world. I could not understand how tens of thousands of people could be slaughtered in a few weeks and two million refugees be driven from their homes, with hardly anything said or written about it until one man had the idea of putting a label on the product and calling it Biafra.

One of my old Legion chiefs, Major Faulques, was in Paris, and I happened to know that he had carried out some missions in Biafra. The word was that he was acting for Jacques Foccard, de Gaulle's confidential agent for African affairs. I fixed an appointment, and we met in a bar.

Faulques is one of the few men I admire and respect, and I was glad to be seeing him again. Even out of uniform he looked much the same — lithe, tanned, crop-haired, with a piercing gaze. Without saying so directly, he gave me to understand that he was working for de Gaulle, not as a fighting man but as an adviser helping the Biafran army to organize. He saw the main problem as recruitment, because he wanted nothing to do with trigger-happy mercenaries.

I was very tempted, and I told Faulques that if he thought I could be useful to him he could count on me.

His reply was immediate: "Men like you are always needed, Rolf. Hold yourself in readiness."

My mind was made up. I was bored in France. I believed in the Biafran cause. But before I left I set myself the task of getting some information out of the Nigerians. According to the English newspapers, the federal government had just bought the services of 250 British mercenaries, and I wanted to know how they were to be used. So I got in touch with the Nigerian military attaché in Bonn, Colonel Ikwe, representing myself as a volunteer ready to set out for Biafra but not quite convinced that I was doing the right thing.

At our first meeting Ikwe told me that his government's intention was "to encircle the rebels, then slowly tighten the noose and strangle them." It was a strategy which became obvious later on, but could not be prevented. I discovered during our two other meetings that the leader of the Nigerian mercenaries was a man called Peters, formerly second-in-command to Mike Hoare, the mercenary leader, a tough enough fighting man but also a loudmouth. The recruits were a mixture of former regular NCOs whose main loyalty was the bottle, and riffraff from the London streets. It was a meager harvest, but at least I knew that the federal forces had no real professionals, just opportunists renting out their hides for more than they were worth.

A few weeks later I returned to Paris, where Faulques gave me a plane ticket for Lisbon and the names of my contacts there. He was to remain in France as overall supervisor of the operation. "When you get there," he reminded me, "don't forget you're now a captain. In Africa you can't afford a lower rank."

The Lisbon contacts did their job, and on December 27 I was on board a charter plane bound for Guinea Bissain and loaded with crates of ammunition.

5
First
Impressions

There might be a war on, but inside the long white airport building the officials were waiting. Immigration, customs — we could have been in Switzerland. It was my first contact with the sense of organization, the determination to act like a proper state, which struck me as Biafra's special hallmark and never ceased to surprise visitors, journalists and later historians.

I was met by Major Picot, Faulques's representative in Biafra, an ex-member of the First Paratroop Regiment. I knew him from the days when he commanded the second combat company in Algeria, and I was in the first. Later on we had shared a cell in the Santé prison. It's a good way to get to know somebody. He made a familiar picture in camouflage dress, boots and green beret — a reassuring sight, here in Biafra.

All the same he was pretty gloomy on the way to the base. He'd had trouble getting organized because the federal troops had launched a general offensive and the Biafran general staff had more on their minds than finding jobs for whites. In any case their officers disliked the arrangement, and Picot had to admit that they had a point when they claimed that the men recruited were not only not much good as soldiers but far too big for their boots. The Biafran generals and colonels had been through starchy British staff colleges, and were annoyed by the newcomers' arrogance, bad manners, and poorly concealed contempt for blacks.

Picot himself complained, just as Faulques had, that he'd asked for soldiers and they'd sent him mercenaries. Proper soldiers are hard to get, of course. There were about fifty of these men, mercenaries or soldiers, mostly French, veterans of the Congo and other places, and nearly all of them useless.

I couldn't see much of Biafra through the dark and rain until a group of big white buildings loomed up: we had reached the Shell-BP refinery at Port Harcourt. Before secession it had handled two-thirds of Nigeria's production, and Biafra contained half the producing fields. For Biafra, oil was a blessing and a curse. Twenty million tons a year, the certainty of trebling that figure inside four years — it was enough to make the country the main supplier of oil to Black Africa, and soon one of the world's major exporters, at a good safe distance from the time-bomb of the Middle East.

As if to symbolize that situation, the Shell-BP complex, long since emptied of its British personnel, was now used as a military staff center. When the federal air force had bombed it a week before, they had been killing two birds with one stone. But although the technical installations had been badly damaged, the administrative block and living quarters were intact. Picot took me to his own quarters and we went to the map room.

Biafra: a quadrilateral stuck like a postage stamp on the bottom right-hand corner of the ten-times-larger quadrilateral of Nigeria. Bounded to the north by the savannas of the Hausas, to the west by the River Niger, to the east by the mountains of Cameroon, and to the south by the sea and the marshes of the Niger delta. Population fourteen million. Terrain flat, spongy, and covered with forests cut by a few asphalt roads linking the main towns. The Port Harcourt and Calabar roads meet at Aba; thirty kilometers further on, the road forks northwest to Owerri, northeast to Umuahia, the administrative capital. All this makes a triangle — the golden triangle, center and heartland of the Ibo nation. Farther north the Umuahia road runs on to Enugu, the former capital recently captured by the enemy. The Owerri road continues toward Onitsha, the western gateway on the Niger, by way of the airport at Uli where I landed.

Picot reviewed the situation and made it sound quite ominous. Federal troops were attacking in strength in the north, and they had tremendous superiority both in numbers and equipment. They had the most powerful army in the whole of Black Africa, with land forces of 120,000 men well supported by heavy artillery (particularly Russian 102mm guns) and highly mobile with the help of British-made Ferret and Saladin armored vehicles.

The Nigerian navy was also a tough proposition: it had one heavy frigate mounting 102mm guns, as well as the fast patrol boats which had recently landed a raiding force in the Calabar sector, shooting down one of Biafra's small force of helicopters.

On top of that came the Nigerian air force, consisting of Ilyushin 18 jet bombers and MIG-15 and -17 fighters. They could create panic among the population, and they constituted a permanent threat to strategic installations.

Clearly the federal forces were aiming to impose a blockade. The Biafran breakout attempt toward the west the previous August had run out of steam, and the Ibos had had to abandon the captured town of Benin, which put the Yorubas right on their heels with no river of blood in between.

To counter the Lagos strategy, which was just as Colonel Ikwe had described it to me in Bonn, the Biafran general staff could call upon only one thousand men. True, these could be renewed again and again, thanks to the phenomenal patriotism of the people, but there was no navy, and no air force. Petrol stocks were OK for the moment, but the raid on the refinery made the future look black. As for equipment, there was no way to get it except by air, which meant light armaments only, and daily miracles of maintenance and improvisation from the ordnance services.

"As I see it, we've had it," Picot concluded. "We're wasting our time here."

Coming from Picot, that was serious.

"So what am I supposed to do?"

"I haven't mentioned our centurions yet," Picot grunted. "Right now they're on the Calabar front. You'll find them in the Dunlop plantation. Why don't you look around over there, then tell me what you make of it?"

Next day I drove right across Biafra by jeep, by way of Aba and Umuahia, to reach the Calabar front. There were delays at every ferry, over the Imo, the Cross, and other rivers not named on the map, and I arrived at the Dunlop plantation very late, around midnight.

The white heroes of the Congo were sleeping peacefully, dead drunk, surrounded by bottles. I wasn't impressed. I woke some of them, we talked, and they told me that the fifty of them intended to stop an entire Nigerian division.

"Are you crazy or something?" I asked.

There were pitying looks.

"Listen, Steiner, you are probably a good legionnaire, but you don't know a thing about Africa. We were in the Congo. These niggers know all about us. In Katanga we wiped out four thousand Simbas with a hundred and ten whites. Those monkeys are shit. One look at us and they're gone."

They went back to sleep. About eleven in the morning,

after a whisky breakfast, we visited the front — a quieter part of it — like a bunch of tourists. Instead of splitting up into sections they all stuck together. In their own eyes they were the same supermen commandos they had been in the Congo. Looking over positions, condescending to talk to the natives, strutting in front of the officers . . . it wasn't just crude, it was ridiculous. They were no good for anything. I got sick of them fast. Next day I returned to Umuahia, and when I saw Picot I told him: "Listen, I'm packing my bags and going back to Europe. I'm not going to clown around with those idiots."

"I was expecting that reaction, Rolf." Picot grinned. "But luckily they're not the whole story. You must see the northern front, where there's only the Biafran army."

Five kilometers south of Enugu I saw this famous "front." It was like turning the clock back sixty years: lines of trenches staring across at each other, face to face. Troops rooted to the spot, in spite of the heat, without direction or initiative. A background of charred trees and shell-pocked earth.

I asked to see the commander of this company that was petrifying on the spot, and was taken thirty kilometers to the rear. When I asked the commander for an outline of his men's position he seemed not to understand me at first, then told me he didn't really know. He sent me off to a lieutenant posted this time only six kilometers behind the lines, in the comfort of a disused church. I accepted the beer he offered me, and asked if he was commanding the most advanced sector.

"Yes, sir!" he answered.

I explained that I wanted to see his dispositions, and he reluctantly agreed to come along. After a two-hour search, during which we just missed bumping into the enemy more than once, he finally located his men crouching like rabbits, rifles in hand, in individual holes no more than two feet deep. There they stayed, day and night, like snails in their shells! If they wanted to move from one hole to another they crawled. Even to fetch food they wriggled on their bellies, they were so timid.

I gave the federal positions a close examination through my binoculars. Trenches, dug-in pillboxes. Nothing stirred.

"My God, they're all empty!"

"No, no, no, sir! They're in there for sure!"

Seeing me standing upright, the lieutenant begged me to drop flat before the enemy started shooting.

"How do you know they're in there? Have you sent patrols?"

"Patrols? What for?"

I was too flummoxed to be angry, and besides there was nothing to be said. I wasn't carrying a gun, so I took the lieutenant's automatic rifle, a Russian Kalashnikov. After a few steps I turned and called out: "Just one thing: don't start shooting. I'm going over to have a look."

Not a single Biafran had offered to come with me. I made my reconnaissance solo. Actually there was more risk from behind than ahead. All those scared rabbits had trigger fingers, and there's nothing more dangerous in war than a frightened man. I walked on into the enemy positions, and as I expected they were deserted. Confident that they would not be attacked, the Nigerians had obviously withdrawn at leisure toward Enugu. I entered their trenches and found radio batteries, month-old Lagos newpapers, beer bottles — empty — and wrappings from Red Cross parcels. I even picked up a pack of cigarettes forgotten in the withdrawal. I was in combat uniform, boots, green beret, and it felt good — like old times.

A staff captain and an interpreter had come with me from Umuahia. They told me that the company I had just visited belonged to the Fourteenth Battalion of the East Brigade.

On the way back I looked in on its commander, Major Okoye, a stout man, obviously rather uncomfortable in his handsome red-trimmed uniform, plump hands fidgeting with his swaggerstick. A reservist, so I'd been told. He asked for my impressions, and seemed more startled by my criticisms than by the situation I described. I asked him why he was making the enemy a gift of six hundred meters of ground, and he grunted: "Hmm, you're sure there's nobody left on the other side?"

"Positive. But unless you occupy those positions the people you're worried about are liable to come back."

Major Okoye heaved a heavy sigh which eased his belt below his belly: "All right, if you insist." And he ordered his staff to move the company up into the abandoned positions.

I didn't want Major Okoye to think I was poking my nose into his business, but he was too honest to take offense, and in fact asked me as a favor to look at another sector where the enemy was reported to be attacking with Ferrets. These are light reconnaissance tanks of British make, equipped with Rolls-Royce engines and armed with 13/62 Browning machine guns and a 20mm cannon. They were a real nuisance, ideal for this type of terrain, and the Biafrans were scared stiff of them.

Without meaning to, I walked into the middle of a battle, just in time to see the Biafrans take to their heels. They were retreating in a shambles, for no reason that I could find. Certainly they were under fire, and the enemy mortars and field guns were popping away all around, but that wasn't reason enough. You could hear the Ferrets too, but again there was nothing to set off a stampede. This was war, after all. These men were deserting their posts before being attacked.

The sight of some of them making a run for it in my

direction was too much. I stopped everybody who came near, sat them on the ground and had them wait for some more. That way I collected about forty in five minutes.

The enemy was still making a cautious advance, so I got my deserters to their feet, grabbed a submachine gun, and counterattacked. My men advanced in the classic skirmishing line, three meters apart, and the Nigerians were so unused to the sight that they turned tail and ran. I moved my troops into the enemy's positions, and although they tried another attack they couldn't shift my men and had to fall back.

So it was obviously a matter of leadership; forty men halted on the run had done the job after all. That was the trouble: officers too far to the rear, and noncoms nonexistent.

After the second attack there was a lull, but I was afraid of a third, and ammunition was running low. So I sent my Land Rover to Fourteenth Battalion HQ, the nearest, with instructions to bring a few cases back. An hour and a half later it returned — empty. The driver informed me: "Sir, the major is all for giving you the ammunition, but you forgot to fill in the requisition form."

I saw red. That's the British system then — a piece of paper for everything. At times like this I hardly know myself. I put a burst of fire into the Land Rover. Goodbye Land Rover! "Right," I shouted, "now we've got no more call for ammunition!" So the first vehicle I destroyed was one of ours. . . .

Soon afterward, feeling calmer but still determined, I sent my escorting staff captain back in another jeep, with instructions to warn the major that unless he produced the ammunition straightaway — and without the form — I would be bringing him his very own war.

I had learned a lot during that first visit, and seen a lot. First, the men: they were brave, keen, determined but disorganized. It was early in the war — brand-new battle-dress, with the Biafran insignia of a rising sun on a black background freshly sewn on the right sleeve. The men were well equipped: all of them carried Kalashnikov automatic rifles, which are good weapons. If they were not performing well it was due to errors higher up, and possibly to organizational defects.

I checked with the officers of the Fourteenth Battalion, my hosts, and the company structure was the same as the British, except with double the numbers. The sections, "platoons," sometimes consisted of up to fifty men under the orders of only one officer. For a single officer to command fifty men is impossible without good noncoms — and these they did not have. No subdivision, no groups, nothing. It was bound to produce chaos.

6
I Stay

The air was bracing on the northern front, and there was no need for me to go straight back to Umuahia, as neither Faulques nor Picot had fixed any limits on my reconnaissance mission. Here I could be useful and independent. I started teaching them how to make war.

The Biafrans were absolute beginners, willing but inexperienced. With invasion threatening, they had left their roads wide open, without so much as a trench or a tank trap or even a roadblock. The pillboxes were just sheds which would collapse in a strong wind. The whole job had to be done from scratch, starting with the inventory. On my way I had located three field guns, reliable old Krupp 105mm cannons, camouflaged under dusty netting with hundreds of crates of ammunition stacked up nearby. When I asked why they weren't in action in turned out that nobody knew how to work them!

I showed them how to build good, solid strongpoints using palm trees and sandbags, and how to position and camouflage them. And I taught them to service their guns.

As a practical exercise, I had three defense lines drawn up at two-kilometer intervals, with the help of hundreds of civilian volunteers. The first line was intended to stop the enemy six kilometers in front of a river which could only be crossed at that particular place. The bridge was blown up already, but the bush was too dense to allow movement elsewhere. Three times the Nigerians came, and three times they failed. After that, my people felt comfortable in their bunkers. Nothing could get in: the enemy could blast away as much as they liked but they couldn't touch the men inside.

That was an improvement, but there was still one hitch. The Biafrans were still scared stiff of Ferrets. Just the sight or sound of one and they were on their way. So to prove them wrong I decided to move into one of the front-line bunkers where the enemy was attacking every day. I wanted to explore their mentality. Running away before there was any danger did not make sense, and if their problem was psychological, mine was practical. I have always believed that any man can be a good soldier with the right help.

So I had a strongpoint constructed in a bend in the road out ahead of my first line of defense, commanding the approach used by the Ferrets. It was equipped with a heavy 12.7mm machine gun and protected by pits and chicanes. When I moved in the late afternoon I found three men and a corporal who belonged to the Fourteenth Battalion. This corporal was clearly a relic of the old colonial regime, with sad eyes and a wrinkled face. He stood to attention.

"My name is Wilson, sir. Corporal James Wilson, at your service."

"OK, Wilson. Do you mind if I stay here with you and your men? I want to watch how the enemy works."

The night went by peacefully, apart from about ten minutes of bedlam when one of my men got nervous and blazed away at a hyena or a warthog and both sides joined in at random. Then at five o'clock the enemy artillery opened up again, working at such a regular tempo that it rocked me back to sleep. Later the tempo speeded up, and while

I was shaving a shell fell close enough to shift the mirror I was using. That was dangerous. I might have cut myself. Around nine o'clock the enemy had worked up to a heavy rate of fire, and James confirmed that they were getting ready to attack.

"It lasts for ten minutes, sir. They throw everything they have, then the Ferrets come, with infantry in support."

"And then?"

"Then we get out."

Right. That's what I was here to change. My credibility depended on success today. And this was my moment of commitment. My personal rule had always been not to make war unless I felt morally obliged to, and in principle I hadn't come to Biafra to fight. Now, if we were overrun by the Nigerians, I either violated my status as adviser or got myself killed. No chance. And anyway my conscience informed me that if I hung on it would be a case of legitimate self-defense.

The bombardment had reached a climax, and Corporal Wilson shouted in my ear: "Now comes the hardest part, sir! The Nigerians will attack."

But not just yet. And I am in the habit of making coffee in the morning. I stuffed an empty tin with sawdust, sprinkled it with petrol, then cleaned out another tin for the water. It made a lot of smoke, but it boiled quickly, dissolving the remnants of grease which floated to the top. You notice these small details when it may be your last chance to see them, and the enemy mortars were pounding us with a continual drumroll of fire. The air was thick with dust and smoke as we sat drinking my foul coffee and smoking cigarettes. I felt tense, perhaps the way an actor feels before he walks on stage. My four men were now flat on the floor, and the whole place was shaking — big stuff too: one direct hit with one of those 105mm shells and we'd had it. I was asking James how much longer it might go on when total silence fell.

Looking through the gun slit I could see nothing, not even the sun. While the deathly silence continued, gradually earth and air sorted themselves out and the particles of suspended dust drifted down to form a soft, gray layer over the ground. By now we could see to the end of the road, and we began to hear the sound of engines.

Before I'd had time to identify them as Ferrets, all my positions opened fire in a single convulsion, and without waiting for an order, although the enemy were still out of sight and about five hundred meters away! My own machine gunner came down with the same complaint, and I had to drag him away from the gun by force. I took charge of it personally, and told him to follow my orders and do nothing else. At the same time I sent James out to try and halt the epidemic of gunner's dysentery which had broken out all along our line. I heard a few more bursts, then silence.

Not having a radio with which to coordinate the other bunkers in the line, I took advantage of the hesitation our reaction must have produced in the Nigerian ranks to dispatch two of my men to order those in charge to hold their fire until they heard me open fire. My intention was to let the enemy get to no more than thirty or forty meters away, then to start shooting. I could see three Ferrets through the binoculars, advancing very slowly, with a cluster of men following behind, huddled together like sheep, a hundred, perhaps a hundred and fifty, obviously a company. I flicked the safety off on the 12.7mm and looked around at my men standing at their slits with their automatic rifles.

At two hundred meters the Ferrets came to a halt at the tank traps. It is another of the peculiarities of African wars that everything happens on the roads. Not even tanks dare to venture into the bush. But the infantry kept coming:

they must have been fully confident that the Biafrans were sticking to the rules and had taken to their heels after the barrage.

The Nigerians advanced in dead silence, still bunched together. At eighty meters I could see the leaves on their helmets and olive-green battledress standing out against the blackened bush. Inside the bunker my men were strung tight as bowstrings and were gray with tension. They kept looking outside then toward me, then back outside and again toward me, as if to say: "Shoot! For God's sake shoot before it's too late!" Faces were coming into focus, and we could hear whispers and the snapping of twigs underfoot. That's the time to open fire, when the targets are starting to look like men.

Still they were cautious. No playing around, but a slow advance, crouching low, at the sides of the road. Exactly forty meters away I had located a shattered termites' nest with its dark red debris strewn across the road. That was to be the signal. When the first Nigerian set foot there I pressed the trigger and so did my whole crew.

I didn't pull my punches, any more than they would have, but kept pouring the fire on without trying to see the effect. The solid mass wilted and fell apart in front, and I held my finger down. Those behind scattered and ran for the Ferrets, which were still held up by the tank traps. It took them some time to get there, and I didn't stop firing till the last survivors had disappeared.

The surprise had been complete. Now silence fell again, time to fit a new belt in the machine gun and wait for the enemy reply. It came from the 105mm guns alone. The mortars kept clear. The first shell dropped twenty meters in front of us. Short, but in the right direction. The next might overshoot, but I thought the third or fourth were bound to hit, because now the enemy knew exactly where we were.

Corporal Wilson was speaking for all the men when he said: "Sir, we've won. Now we must get away."

"Why?"

"Because we've had it if we stay."

"That's our job, isn't it? We're soldiers."

The federal infantry were coming on again. This time I opened fire at two hundred meters, and called out for a new belt, opening the breech and holding out my hand for the replacement without looking round. Nothing came. I turned round and saw my loader lying dead, with a bullet through the head. The corporal rolled his body aside without ceremony and took his place. I fired two or three more bursts, then our bunker took a direct hit, right above the machine gun. The explosion only blew us into a corner, and none of us was injured, but the gun was jammed, and I couldn't shift it from under the collapsed roof.

The day before I had left my jeep with all the radio equipment 1500 meters to the rear, ahead of my second line. I told Wilson to get back there on the double and radio Major Okoye at battalion HQ.

"Tell the operator to tell him from me that I want his artillery to open immediate fire on this position."

"On your position, sir?"

"Yes."

"You mean . . . on yourself?"

"Yes. Don't argue, just do what I tell you."

Wilson went off at a trot. He looked worried, but I had no intention of committing suicide. Calling down our own artillery was my best method of getting out in one piece. The Nigerians didn't like explosions any more than the Biafrans. Like all blacks, they would go up against bullets easily, but had no stomach for mines, grenades, and artillery. Since I was going to be bombarded anyway, I would rather be controlling the shells, and they would also keep the federal troops away.

In the meantime there was a lull. The federals must be discussing what to do next; through the binoculars I could see their officers waving their arms and walking up and down. They'd had a hot reception and didn't want another. To remind them that we were still there, we fired a few rounds from the Kalashnikovs, and were echoed by our own machine guns in the front line.

A whimpering noise broke out to my left. It came from one of my men, a very young one, perhaps sixteen years old. He was shaking and writhing, and he started to cry. The cause of his terror turned out to be two groups of men crawling silently along thirty meters away, about twenty of them on either side. That was why their artillery had ceased fire. They weren't coming straight at us but were trying to outflank our position and take us in a pincer movement.

I was crouched beneath the gaping hole the shell had torn in the bunker wall, and my two remaining men were posted in the corners, which were still intact. If they were trying to surround us, they must have realized that we were on our own, or else they would never have taken such a chance. We had to bluff it out. I emptied a magazine of the Kalashnikov, without much effect. Then I spotted a crate of grenades which I had completely forgotten, standing in another corner of our bunker. I hauled it near the doorway and started throwing them. I'd pitched about twelve grenades, blind, before I could risk a glance outside to see the Nigerians in retreat.

There were only two of us in action by now. The boy on my left was badly wounded, with his chest blown open, and I had no time to look after him. This time he had reason to groan. He died in a matter of minutes. At long last there was the whistling sound of a salvo passing overhead — and in the right direction! It landed smack in the middle of the Nigerians, and was followed by several more. When I next looked through the binoculars the infantry were clearing out and the Ferrets were turning back.

The Biafrans kept it up for about twenty minutes, with everything they had, mortars as well as field guns. Each salvo shook the bunker and brought more sand cascading out of burst sandbags through the tree trunks. One more, and finally the roof collapsed. I and my remaining man found ourselves buried to our waists in sandbags and timber, neither of us able to budge, with my rifle jammed somewhere underneath me and the grenades out of reach. It was up to the Biafrans now: it was a question of whether Okoye had thought to send reinforcements or whether Wilson was coming back with volunteers brave enough to get us out in spite of their fear of the enemy Ferrets.

To tell the truth I wasn't counting on them, but it was the Biafrans who came. Timidly, but they came. Maybe they'd been there for some time, and had been waiting for the Nigerians to leave before sticking their noses out. All the same they dug us out of the wrecked strongpoint with their bare hands.

That was my initiation by fire in Black Africa. It was a rough day, but I had made two gains. In terms of my mission I had revived the confidence of the Biafran troops by showing them that Ferrets were not invincible. And for my personal satisfaction I had reminded the Nigerians that a legionnaire is a hard man to shift.

On that day, I decided to stay with the Biafrans, not as a remote adviser but as a fighting technician with a physical and moral commitment. But this trench warfare was no good. I decided to set up my own commando unit.

7

From Company to Brigade

I had been in the Fourteenth Battalion's sector for a week, and had a struck up close relationship with its chief, Major Okoye, whom I nicknamed Coco. He was a good man — cheerful, a bit flabby, fond of beer and cards, and not really cut out for the army. Coco gave me total freedom of movement; he lent me a jeep and kept me supplied with everything I needed.

Apart from the captain's rank awarded by Faulques I had as yet no official position or responsibilities, so one of my main worries was the effect of my presence on the Biafran officers. Apart from Coco himself, there were also unit commanders in the battalion. How were they going to respond to this intruder arriving out of nowhere and bossing them about?

In fact I need not have worried. My arrival was generally welcomed, and I think some of them were quite relieved by my initiatives. Even the general told me one day that if I should need his brigade it was at my disposal. He himself was happy to carry on with his *dolce vita* fifty kilometers farther south, surrounded by girls, booze, and attention. In the course of my career I have often noticed that there is a braid-to-kilometers ratio — the farther from the battle-field, the higher up the hierarchy.

The armchair general commanding the Special Brigade had given me a provisional go-ahead for my idea, which was to form a nucleus of men and give them a Legion-style training. I asked Coco to find me fifty volunteers, and he produced a hundred and eighty, all from fighting units. I also needed NCOs, and one obvious candidate was Corporal Wilson.

The enemy maintained heavy troop concentrations toward Enugu, and one look at the operations map showed that if they could manage to break through the northern front in the direction of Enugu they would cut Biafra in half. The officers responsible for defending this sector were clearly inexperienced, so I felt I must do all I could to fend off the enemy. As I have said, it was the armored Ferrets and Saladins that bothered me most, because of the way they frightened our men. The Saladins, which were bigger than the Ferrets, were combined scout cars and troop carriers, armed with 105mm guns and able to carry a dozen men plus their equipment. Here they were usually used as mobile fire bases, equipped with heavy machine guns or 60mm breech-loading mortars. It was this kind of attack that I was still afraid of.

Then I thought about mines. The Biafrains did not have any, and so far nobody had used them in this war. I had explosive charges buried in the road a hundred meters in advance of the antitank obstacles, and posted a man to set them off at the right moment, but each time the Ferrets stuck their snouts out the man on the spot dropped every-thing and ran. So I remembered the old Ho Chi Minh mines, made of wood and waterproof enough to work after being buried for several days. I had torch batteries, detonators, and all the explosives I wanted. Now I had to find the wood.

My new unit was then stationed in the village school, where the benches had been stored. I put carpenters to work on them and also had the neighboring villages scoured for further stocks, since we would be needing plenty of mines. A prototype was put together from my sketch, and the holes stopped with beeswax. For the demonstration Coco invited the general commanding the East Brigade. I buried the contact device, connecting it by wire to a light bulb at the roadside instead of an explosive charge, and told the skeptical general to drive over it in his Land Rover. The bulb lit up when he did so. Any fool could tell that a real mine would have blown up.

We had a stroke of luck when my commandos returned an hour later with a prisoner taken near Enugu. He was only a kitchen orderly, but he told us that his orders were to prepare cold rations for the following day, a Sunday, because there was an offensive planned for around eleven o'clock. That left me with the one prototype mine available, and only one night to plant it.

When the mine was ready I took a lieutenant and four men, and at ten in the evening we passed through the Biafran forward posts and crawled to a spot about a hundred meters distant from the enemy positions. There was sporadic machine-gunning going on, but the tracer passed safely over our heads, and the flares the Nigerians kept sending up showed us their own forward defenses.

At eleven o'clock I started digging into the hard road surface with a bayonet. It was hard going, because I had to drop flat each time a flare went up. Sometimes there was only a minute to work in between flares, and precious seconds were lost each time my eyes had to readjust after the dazzling light. At two I was running with sweat and making slow progress. It took another two hours before I had dug a trench across the full breadth of the road deep enough to hold a hundred kilos of explosive, several auxiliary detonators, and the mine itself. We finished camouflaging the road surface shortly before dawn, and at five I went back to base and took a bath.

I felt confident that the Nigerians would fall for it. Their first patrols were bound to pass that way, and they always sent their armor first, sticking tight to the road.

I had coffee at six, and at eight I made up my mind that there was no point in going back to the front to watch. The little town of Agbani was five kilometers away, and it had a church and a bar. I would go to Mass, then have a beer with some of my young officers. A hundred kilos of explosive make their own report.

As we drank, everyone was wondering if our mine was going to work, including me. Time crept by, but just when we were starting to worry the big bang came. A roar of joy went up and we went to see the result, which was spectacular. The Ferret which touched off the charge had been blown fifty meters into the bush, leaving a hole in the road as deep as I am tall. And the Nigerians had made a two-kilometer withdrawal (it seems that they never again attacked in that direction). Next day Ojukwu sent for details of the mine, which became the model for a version produced in industrial quantities.

That was my first military action as an officer, on January 12, 1968, and it was the kind of success I needed. Coming out of nowhere, I had managed to make my presence felt inside a fortnight. I had wanted my unit's first operation to make an impact but cost no lives. With that double objective achieved, my boys were beginning to feel confident of their own abilities.

I couldn't stop there, of course, and I spent the next few days preparing for a mission behind enemy lines. On January 23, two days before the raid was due, I received a radio message from Faulques, in French, instructing me to cease all military activity and return at once to Umuahia. There I found my fifty white heroes packed and ready to go, scared stiff of falling into the hands of the Nigerians. They told me that there had been a breakthrough in Calabar and into Ibibio territory at Ikot Ekpene, with ten Nigerian divisions following up. They chattered on like a gaggle of women at a sale until Faulques arrived and shut them up. He had made arrangements to evacuate them, since their safety could no longer be guaranteed. Anybody who wanted to stay could let him know now.

"Me," I said, and I was the only one. The rest called me a mug.

Faulques tried to talk me out of staying, but when he realized that I had no intention of changing my mind he took me to see Ojukwu.

It would be my first meeting with the Biafran leader, and all I knew about him was what the newspapers said — that he came from a wealthy trading family in Newi, that he had studied in England, and that he had some military experience as a member of Nigeria's UN contingent to Katanga in 1964. He received us at the State House, in the center of Umuahia, where we found him waiting alone in a sumptuous drawing room, wearing a loose and colorful African shirt over cotton trousers. Faulques told him that the Europeans were leaving, with the exception of myself, and Ojukwu agreed that the situation was grave.

"We had pinned a great deal of hope on the assistance of the French soldiers. Their experience made them good instructors."

He stopped, and smiled. Ojukwu's calmness was as impressive as his size. He projected a blend of strength and gentleness. He was then only thirty-three years old, which is probably why he had grown the stately beard that aged him enough to help him exert his authority over his elders.

"And now they are leaving," he went on. "Well, that is

their right. And we shall always be grateful for what they have done for us. The agreement was for them to advise, and I personally never wanted them to join in the fighting. Commander Picot fought, on his own initiative, on the Calabar front. You will send him our gratitude. . . ."

Faulques took his leave with a military salue, but Ojukwu asked me to sit down. With tears in his eyes, he thanked me for staying in Biafra, and I do not remember my own answer because I too was moved. Thinking to explain myself and my intentions, I was about to give him an account of my activities when he interrupted.

"I know about the machine-gun post and the mine. You are a real soldier, Captain Steiner, and we are going to need a man like you."

So Ojukwu had already been informed. That made it a good moment to talk about my plan for a commando group, and I rehearsed again what I had worked out in the bunker: attack the enemy rear with a fast-moving efficient unit. And I insisted that it should be independent. I did not mean to take orders from someone who knew nothing about war; I had to be my own boss. He gave me the green light and guaranteed that my unit would be autonomous and separate from the army high command.

"I am appointing you major. You will be accountable only to me, under my direct authority."

Something had happened between us which I still find hard to explain. I found that I respected Ojukwu; he found that he trusted me. I told myself that if Ojukwu had confidence in me I had to do my best not to disappoint him, since my life had equipped me to be of service to this nation.

That gave me an idea. I asked him for Biafran nationality, and he granted it on the spot.

When I got back home to the northern front an enemy advance had split the Fourteenth Battalion's old position and it had fallen back to new lines. My unit was still waiting for me, and I faced the job of sorting out the fighting soldiers from the cooks and drivers among my hundred and eighty volunteers. And I still intended to launch the raid which had been suspended by Faulques's message.

But first I had to settle the officer problem. I had promoted Wilson to sergeant, and I had a few other officers, but these were young and raw. Before I left Umuahia, Ojukwu had told me that Biafra's military academy was about to graduate its first class of officers; he scribbled a short note, and said that I could take my pick.

When I reached the academy I assembled the new crop of eighty second lieutenants and delivered a short speech, informing them that anybody who came with me had a one-in-ten chance of surviving the war, but the certainty of serving his country.

"Those who want to come with me, take one step forward."

Most of the rookies advanced as one man, to be followed rapidly by the shame-faced remainder. I chose ten, on appearances. Nearly all these youngsters were students who had been at universities in Nigeria or Europe at the beginning of the war and had come home to serve their country at its declaration of independence. They all spoke English, some of them French or German, and a few even Chinese or Russian.

Training resumed, and in order to get my men used to combat conditions I sent a section behind enemy lines every day, with orders to approach, observe, but not to start anything.

We mounted our first ambush with a group of twenty men, including the brand-new sergeant, Wilson. At Obe, not far from the frontier, my men had located the HQ of a Nigerian battalion operating out of two buildings separated by five hundred meters of road. Naturally there was heavy traffic on this section, and some good targets.

This time I went along, traveling by night. Early in the morning I located the spot where I wanted to post my men. We mined the road, took our positions, and waited. Setting an ambush has a lot in common with fishing — plenty of small fry before you get the big catch. To stave off boredom we passed the time counting the bicycles, motorbikes, and pedestrians using the road.

It was midmorning by the time a small convoy of three Land Rovers approached from my right. Since we did not know what direction the vehicles would come from, we had laid a classic ambush bringing half our strength to bear on each side, so the men opposite were in reserve. The mine blew, and the first Land Rover overturned into the ditch. We opened fire into the drivers' seats with five machine guns at point-blank range, and the Nigerians had no time to reply. It was all over, with nothing left to do but pick up their weapons.

The second Land Rover had stopped opposite me, and when we ran over to it we found three Ibo women tied up inside. One was dead, another dying and past help, and the third had a bullet through both thighs. By the time I had carried her to the side of the road and cut her bonds the Nigerians were counterattacking with all their available strength, from either side, and in acute danger of hitting each other.

I was stuck by the road looking after the girl, confidently expecting my men to return the enemy fire, but when I called out to them for help with carrying her there was no answer. Mission accomplished, they had already fallen back into the bush. They were still raw. I couldn't blame them for that. The idea of the raid had been to get them combat-fit, with the friendly cooperation of the Nigerians.

Still, I had to save the girl, and I couldn't see how to do it with just a pistol and two grenades. She couldn't walk, and if I tried to I would be spotted, so we moved on all fours, backwards. We finished up in a shallow depression at the bottom of a slight slope, with no obvious way out.

At that point Obu, one of my privates, came back and saw what was happening. As I had taught him, he knelt down, opened fire, and threw his grenades to cover me and the girl. He was a big man in his early twenties, always joking and very sure of himself. Later on he became a sergeant. He wore an amulet as well as a cross round his neck, and I used to tease him about hedging his bets. With his help we got away from the roadside while the enemy still blazed away with rifles, mortars, and what have you. But they didn't dare pursue us into the bush, which was nearly head-high around there.

Layla, the girl we had wounded, was a lieutenant in the Biafran army, captured in her home village near Enugu when she made a reckless visit to see her mother. She had studied at Rouen University, and spoke perfect French. When she recovered she joined my secretariat.

It had been an encouraging start, and I kept up the training, taking the men behind the enemy lines and sometimes sending them out under officers who had proved themselves reliable. A few days after the ambush Major Okoye — Coco, of the Fourteenth Battalion — asked for the loan of what he called my commando company to help reinforce the garrison at Agbani, which his battalion had captured that morning. I congratulated him, and gave him permission to borrow one hundred and twenty men, provided he did not commit them to a battle.

I had to go to Umuahia that day, and did not get back till evening. I was sitting down to dinner when my orderly told me that there were five of my men outside, one of them a lieutenant, all of them wounded. I hurried out to find the young lieutenant, just out of the academy, standing at attention and visibly restraining tears.

"What's happened?"

"Sir, Major Okoye told us to head for the center of Agbani. We went without precautions because the town was already in Biafran hands. On the way we cleaned out a pocket of Nigerian resistance. It was easy. And then . . . then . . ."

And he began to sob quietly. When I pieced their story together, this is what I learned. The Fourteenth Battalion had indeed attacked Agbani in the morning, but without advancing a step. And my men had walked into that hornets' nest with their rifles slung. I'd told them always to follow orders because I would always have a reason, and they assumed that it was the same with Coco. They went on, and were at once cut off, surrounded, and hammered to pieces.

The five wounded men had escaped thanks to Sergeant Wilson, who had stayed outside the town in charge of the unit's mortar battery. When he heard firing he realized what was happening and bombarded the town center, enabling the five to get away. A sixth man arrived next day with a wrist injury. He had been taken prisoner with twenty-seven others who had been tortured and killed. He had been missed because he was covered in blood and had played dead beneath the corpses.

Six survivors. My hundred and twenty men wiped out like flies. Wild with rage, I made for Fourteenth Battalion HQ, to be greeted by the sixty remaining men from my group, the reserve. They had already arrested Coco on their own initiative, and he was shaking with fear.

"Rolf, forgive me. I didn't know. It was my adjutant, Captain X. He is a boaster. He told me that Agbani was taken and I didn't check up. . . ."

I sent for the man and I put him in the hospital. Then I took Coco to the State House and told Ojukwu everything. He backed my actions, and Coco finished up in jail, though I got him out later.

The incident won me great respect in the Biafran army,

but it meant that I had enemies right from the start among some of the colonels and generals. Now I had to build everything up again from nothing. I withdrew my remaining men from the front and transferred them to Madonna 1.

8
The
"Madonnas"

Ojukwu had given me permission to use whatever school I chose as a base for my commando group. Biafra was a Catholic country, covered with religious schools which had been evacuated when war came, so in 1968 Madonna High School, a girls' boarding school, became Madonna 1, headquarters of my Black Legion. It was a vast building, situated at the center of Biafra. Once installed there I set about getting the place repaired, and it was to grow into a self-contained community with its own garages, repair shops, and hospital. In the meantime I had a unit to rebuild.

I had asked for a hundred men, preferably already trained, because Madonna 1 was a rear base and I was anxious to get back to the front as soon as possible. Then I woke up one morning, looked out over what used to be the school yard, and saw two thousand men sitting there waiting — my reinforcements! Three hours later came a dispatch from Ojukwu asking me to use the pick of the two thousand to form a battalion to be known as the Thirty-second Commando Battalion. That meant twelve hundred men: five combat companies, a support company, and the abundance of service personnel typical of armies formed on the British model. I didn't see the use of all that, but I also knew that if things went on at their previous rate — losing a hundred men today, maybe another hundred tomorrow — I'd need all the reserves I could get.

But first I needed a good staff, men who were reliable, efficient, and loyal, able to relieve me of administrative problems. I was lucky enough to recruit several good officers. A former history professor at the University of Nsukka became my quartermaster, responsible for logistical matters. Ojukwu gave me his own chief of security, Major Clement, an ex-chief of police, as my intelligence officer. I was getting the cream of the other army units, and that didn't make me any more popular with various generals who saw me more as an opponent than an ally.

My prize catch was Emeka, who was twenty-three years old and a former pilot in the Nigerian Air Force. As Ojukwu's aide-de-camp he had drawn my attention every time I visited the State House, and it had been his job to find me the administrative staff I needed. I was impressed by his efficiency, discretion, and lively intelligence, and since the Biafrans had no jet planes I considered him available.

Emeka was willing to join me if Ojukwu agreed, but his boss was flabbergasted when I put in my request. When he recovered from the shock he smiled and said: "Ah, you know a good man when you see one." And Emeka quickly became my right-hand man. He was a good organizer who hardly ever needed to be told what to do, with a keen eye for detail and an instinct for putting the right officers in the right jobs. When he came with me to the front he stuck to me like a limpet.

My idea was to train Emeka so that he could take over the unit in the event of my death or injury. He arrived as a lieutenant, but his promotion to captain was already in the pipeline, through Ojukwu. By the end of the war he had risen to lieutenant colonel. As my adjutant he was a lot more valuable in his own right than all the whites I had later.

His bravery and initiative were exceptional. I had other fine black officers in Biafra, but none so thoroughly equipped. Some were excellent under fire, but lacked the education to make good administrators. Emeka was irreplaceable on every level.

My 1,200 recruits had three uninterrupted weeks' training at Madonna 1, instructed by the survivors of the first unit, whose prestige was reinforced by their injuries, and by career second lieutenants, ex–Boy Scouts who thought of training in terms of games and exercise. It might keep up the troops' morale, but it all seemed a bit too easygoing. To replace my "real combat lessons" I would have liked to see my men on the rifle range at least twice a week, but there was no such thing in the Biafran army, because the high command felt that ammunition was too scarce. My view was that it was better to use fifty rounds on the rifle range than to waste a thousand in combat.

Arms, too, were scarce. Despite the patronage of Ojukwu I was still underequipped. I had my Colt .45, like the other officers, and the men used Kalashnikovs, Berettas, Thompsons, etc. Still there weren't enough to go round, and the disparity of calibers made it a real headache to get the right bullets together with the right gun.

One day I was watching my raw recruits in simulated combat with wooden guns, the next Ojukwu had given me five hundred old German carbines and sent me north again, to Abagana, where the enemy was massing. This would be the moment of truth for the Thirty-second Commando Battalion. My five new companies had a quiet journey to the front, to be deployed there along the defensive line left to us by the troops in the sector. I had no armor as yet. My support company had sixteen 81mm and twelve 60mm mortars, with a few thousand shells in reserve. We were ready.

At once we caught the full force of General Mohammed's

First Division advancing on Onitsha. And my virgin battalion held! In ten days of running engagements and violent thrusts, Mohammed could not pass. There were eighteen thousand men in his division, and there was no knowing his losses in dead and wounded. What is certain is that he left three thousand weapons behind him. When he pulled back on March 12, 1968, I took my troops back to Madonna 1. I was sure that he would be in no hurry to return, and I didn't want to molder away in trenches. We had lost two or three hundred men, but we had done our job.

In any case replacements were guaranteed, as I realized back at Madonna 1, where the commandos' prestige had attracted queues of volunteers who arrived barefoot, ragged, without papers and often tired out by a long journey. Their ages ranged from fifteen to forty, and I advised the officers in charge of selection to take the youngest. They learned faster. All of them had the naïve, noble kind of patriotism which in Europe is a thing of the past.

Ojukwu send for me on March 13. During a briefing in the presence of the whole general staff he congratulated me, gave me a bear-hug, and said: "Rolf, I have decided to give you five thousand men, a brigade. It will be the Fourth Commando Brigade."

"Fourth, Excellency? Where are the three others?"

"They don't exist, Rolf." He grinned. "It's simply that four is my lucky number."

I gave back the five hundred old guns which Ojukwu had provided, and next day Effiong, the Biafran chief of staff, came to ask for another thousand. I told him to find his own. The borrowed guns might have come in useful, but his rate of interest was too high, and I considered that my unit had a natural first call on its own captures. I wanted to keep some stocks in reserve, but I made Ojukwu a gift of three hundred rifles for the Umuahia garrison, and received four 105mm field guns in exchange.

In a little more than two months my men and I had been transformed from company to brigade. In the same period we had destroyed or captured thirty-two armored vehicles, when the entire Biafran army had destroyed only three since the start of the war.

It was around then that I received my first white personnel, two of the fifty heroes, who had changed their minds after a few weeks' thinking in Port Harcourt. The first was an Italian named Giorgio Norbiato, a swarthy, tough little man of about thirty, who told me he had served with the Italian marines and in the Congo. I asked why he wanted to fight. Was it for money?

"No, I'm not worried about getting paid."

"What, then?"

"Well, you stayed, didn't you? Why shouldn't I?"

It happened that I had been intending to form a "marine commando." I had placed one of my five battalions, the Eighth, at Port Harcourt, in the marshy delta of the Niger. It was commanded by a Biafran officer, but I made Norbiato responsible for their training.

The second was Taffy Williams, who was British but claimed to be South African, thin-faced, and a graduate of the Congo and Katanga — but a good instructor, brave under fire and authoritative.

Ojukwu and I had never discussed money. He had not offered me a salary and I had never asked for one. Early in May the agent for special affairs told me that he had been instructed to look after my case: "His Excellency wants to pay you what your services are worth." I told him that I had no reason to take pay from the Biafran army. As long as I had food, drink, clothes, transport, and a roof over my head I didn't need anything else.

My men could not be expected to work on these terms, though, and they collected their money from my paymaster in Biafran pounds. But from July onward the Fourth Brigade also had a small amount of foreign currency available, which we spent in Europe on detonators, warheads, and the tools and accessories essential to our home armaments industry. Emeka had worked well, and we had eighteen Madonnas operating all over the country, with cheap manpower provided by the soldiers' families. In co-operation with the ministries for the army and for public works, the brigade had created several factories making small runs of the mines I had designed, as well as more elaborate hardware such as mortars and copies of Russian bazookas. We also turned out armored reinforcements for bunkers and steel plating for converting tractors into tanks.

Enemy armored cars brought in further income. At the beginning of the war Ojukwu, seeing their effect on his troops, had set a price of a thousand pounds for each one taken or destroyed. That gave us thirty-two thousand pounds to spend on stockpiling supplies of yams, the national food, and rearing our hens, pigs, and goats. Later on we added cattle. In the end we were running an almost self-sufficient economy.

I took a special interest in matters of food, comfort, and supply, because no detail is trivial if it helps to maintain morale. But Emeka and I depended on the skills and intelligence of the Ibos. Once a structure was organized and the machinery started it would keep running by itself.

One of my proudest creations was the military hospital, an idea which came to me after the battle of Abagana. My several hundred wounded had been split up among the various hospital centers. A few weeks later I was visited by one of my officers, who complained about being removed from one of these centers and officially reassigned to an infantry regiment. When I investigated I found that the infantry had practically set up its own press gang. Each time one of my wounded commandos was ready to leave he was shunted into some other unit.

According to Emeka I should have felt flattered. He said that they were being taken out of an almost superstitious belief that our success could be transplanted by a kind of sympathetic magic. I could not tolerate our hard-won esprit de corps being bled off, and protested to Effiong, who put a stop to it within a few days. But I was afraid of a relapse, and asked the brigade's medical officer if it was possible to extend the sickbay.

Anthony Aunwa, born in Awgu, had studied medicine in Hamburg and I chose him because he spoke fluent German. He was ready to expand the sickbay to whatever dimensions I chose as long as I found him the right staff, so I had the left wing of Madonna 1 evacuated and the necessary hygienic equipment installed. The quartermaster general in Umuahia supplied beds, mattresses, and sheets, the general staff sent two medical officers, and the Biafrain Red Cross provided the medicaments and operating room. With forty-two nurses from the Ministry of Health we could look after our own wounded from May onward.

The brigade also had its own flag, incorporating the red and green of the Legion as well as the Legion motto, "Honor and Fidelity," a tribute to the courage and integrity of the Biafrans. As for the famous skull-and-crossbones motif of the commandos, every unit had its badge, and I chose this one at the time I was forming the first group. The point was to remind the men that we were there to die, not to play around. It had nothing to do with the pirate flag, or the SS.

I made it my business to personalize my men's equipment as much as possible. When we couldn't get matching uniforms from the army stores we bought a bulk of white cloth from a Greek trader, had it dyed green, and found some master tailors, fifty assistants, and some sewing machines.

That left footwear. We located an old German who had started a small shoe factory near Onitsha in the days of the British. All his capital was invested in it, so he had stayed on when hostilities started. He wanted to move somewhere safer, but didn't have the transport or the petrol. I had his factory moved by my own men, and sent him the moving bill — two thousand pairs of boots.

Tradition also required a personal guard, not for the sake of any personality cult, but because it is customary in crack units to pay that kind of respect to the leader. The best of my men were chosen to form a super-battalion called the Biafran Commando Guard. I owe all my successes to them. Not that I rated my other battalions much lower, but I seldom had cause to use them. Fought in the heart of tropical forest, this was essentially a war of paths and roads. Often the front covered no more than a hundred meters. In a corridor as narrow as that it was impossible to deploy a brigade, so each time I planned an operation of some importance I put my other battalions in support and brought up the Guard.

9
The Marine Commando

Norbiato proved himself the first time he went into action. We set up a raid on the supply convoy for the Nigerian Third Division, which used to sail from Lagos, enter Opobo Bay in secret, and reach the Niger delta by one of its several arms. The convoy was generally made up of small freighters plus an escort of patrol boats which parted company with them at the mouth of the river. For the attack we mounted ordinary machine guns on the bows of three Chris-Crafts commandeered from the Port Harcourt Sailing Club. They were small but fast, with room for four commandos and the pilot.

On the morning of April 4, the three Chris-Crafts were in position, camouflaged beneath the thick vegetation at the river's edge, fifty meters from the navigation channel. Norbiato gave me his own account of what happened.

A heavy tropical storm was followed by a cold night, another rainy day, and another night without a convoy. Waiting became harder as time crept by. Then on the seventh, as the rain poured down in the early morning, two ships crept slowly upriver in line astern, and Norbiato and his men started their engines. One of the Chris-Crafts had a flooded carburetor and refused to start. The other two slid after the enemy, under cover of the heavy downpour.

Norbiato got behind the leader. His second in command took the other, and Norbiato actually boarded his objective, like a true pirate! He and his men jumped on to the ship, relieved to be in action after three days in ambush — and a guard cut two of them down with a burst from a sten gun. Norbiato replied with his Thompson, and the Nigerian fell. The other commando opened fire on the pilot's cabin, and at once the ship veered off course. Norbiato ran forward, pushed the dead pilot into the river, and steered for Port Harcourt.

On the other vessel it was all over without a shot fired. The federal sailors only realized that there was anything happening when they saw their pilot's hands go up. They jumped overboard, and the commandos did nothing to prevent them. Two men for two ships seemed a fair price, but Norbiato was furious to find that the vessel he had captured carried no arms or ammunition, just five Land Rovers, two thousand uniforms, and a load of tinned food. The other ship was the big prize: two thousand cases of 7.62mm ammunition — two million cartridges! — ten tons of Russian 81 and 82mm mortar shells, and a quantity of grenades and other less important hardware.

Still, he had the satisfaction of dismounting the 20mm Oerlikon cannon mounted on board both vessels, as well as knowing that he had gained my confidence.

It was an odd kind of war, in which the Nigerians held one trump card: aerial bombing. The Biafran air force had already been crushed, apart from three or four helicopters and two or three planes which hardly ever left the ground.

I first saw the terrible effects of the federal bombing in the little northern town of Awgu, where I was visiting some of my men in hospital before we opened our own Madonna

1. It was eight o'clock in the morning, and I was still a few kilometers away when the Ilyushins attacked at low altitude. They were aiming at the hospital but were also bombing the nearby market. When I got there I could hear shouts and groans, dogs yapping and hens frantically clucking as they scurried among the dismembered bodies already buzzing with flies. The air carried the sickening smell of shattered flesh. A few children wandered through the desolation, their faces convulsed with tears.

When I saw that marketplace turned into a slaughterhouse I promised myself that I would destroy the aircraft responsible. Our intelligence reported that the Nigerians had based four Ilyushins and two MIGs on the airport at Enugu, the former Biafran capital, which had fallen into enemy hands on September 13, 1967, before my arrival. That was where these planes had come from, and where we had to go. It would take the Russians months to replace any lost aircraft, and at the present rate of a hundred civilian deaths a day by bombing, that would save thousands of lives.

I handpicked fifty men for the operation, under the name of Commando 14, and placed them in waiting at Nara, near the northern front. Each of them received a complete Nigerian uniform which had been removed from a dead enemy and mended and cleaned. I wasn't at all worried that it went against the laws of war to wear enemy uniforms in action: the Nigerians had already stopped observing the rules.

In the meantime I paid a visit to my two battalions in the key sector of Abagana, on the Onitsha front. Onitsha was the one big Biafran town on the eastern bank of the Niger held by federal forces, who had gained a solid foothold there the previous month. They were kept supplied by river, and Mohammed's First Division made periodic efforts to link up with their bridgehead. While we held Abagana there was no way through.

I was on my way there on the morning of April 24, when Daniel, my radio operator, picked up a message from Norbiato's Eighth Marine Commando reporting that the enemy had ascended the Imo River with landing craft the night before, and had succeeded in establishing a bridge-head about thirty-five kilometers east of Port Harcourt. The sector was held by the Biafrain Fifty-second Brigade, which was in a state of panic after its failure to oppose the landing.

This was a vital breach, which had to be stopped. I asked Daniel to get in touch with the commander of the Fifty-second, Colonel Koyolo, a stiff, severe officer, very much in the British mold, whom I knew only from a few handshakes at State House briefings. He got my goat straightaway by informing me that Biafra was done for unless I ordered my marine commando to counterattack at once.

"So you make the blunders and I'm supposed to repair them? I'm not your personal fireman, Colonel Koyolo!"

He tried to adopt a commanding tone: "If you have consulted our officer's manual, Colonel Steiner, you will surely know that the order is to fall back to new positions so as to safeguard our liaison in the event of the line of communication being threatened."

I probably turned as green as my own beret. In that sort of situation I say the first thing that comes into my head. "You're just a parlor soldier, Koyolo! Is that what they teach you at Sandhurst? I've read that training manual. It may be OK on table manners, or how to waltz with a lady, but when it comes to the art of war, forget it! All the English gave you was a superiority complex. . . ."

Koyolo was so dumbstruck that all I could hear was the crackling of the receiver. I told him to go to hell, and broke contact.

I managed to make radio contact with Norbiato, but the noise of battle was so loud in the background that I could hardly hear him. It turned out that he had launched the counterattack of his own accord, and had already pushed the bulk of the enemy force back into the river, but there were two companies still refusing to be shifted from the bank. On top of that, the Fifty-second Brigade was refusing to supply him with ammunition.

"The stupid bastards don't know what they're doing. Send me some more cartridges and I think I can finish the job in half an hour!"

"OK, I'll see to it right now. And I'm sending you the reserve battalion and four field guns."

I headed back to Madonna 1 at full speed to get the reserve battalion on its way, and it left at eleven. I couldn't contact Norbiato again till five o'clock that afternoon when he confirmed that he had received the ammunition and was getting ready to counterattack.

Three hours later, a message from his HQ: Norbiato was reported missing, after being wounded. Without artillery and without the reserve battalion, the fool had gone in full tilt, and had shifted the Nigerians, but he had taken a bullet in the thigh. The men around him had then retreated.

Norbiato's disappearance having been confirmed, Emeka and I set out for Port Harcourt by Land Rover. It turned out that the ammunition had arrived, but not the reserve battalion, which had been held up at Port Harcourt and was still waiting for the Fifty-second Brigade to provide transport. Norbiato was too impetuous to wait — a good captain, but he never gave any thought to the overall picture once he had his head down. I don't mean to criticize. It was a war that called for improvisation and nerve, and he had both.

I collected the remnants of the battalion, but the enemy had no more to fear for the present. They had regained their footing, and had already made four kilometers' progress. There was no question of hitting back before establishing our own position, and in any case there was not the slightest possibility of throwing Biafrans into a night attack. Even in the morning, the most we could do with a decimated battalion, and the certainty of the Nigerians landing reinforcements, was to pin them back against the river.

The overriding priority was to dislodge them from a strategic road junction they had just occupied, which offered an ideal launching platform for an invasion. It had to be recaptured at all costs, and as I sat drinking with the officers of the Fifty-second Brigade in the Port Harcourt HQ I had an idea. When I found Emeka, I told him: "Take some mines and go back to the front. Then pull Norbiato's men back a kilometer and lay the mines in the camp they're occupying now. Leave nobody except the artillery spotters and a radio operator. Then regroup the two battalions and I'll take over when the time comes."

I could rely on a dawn attack by the Nigerians, and my spotters could also fire a few bursts in case the enemy reconnoitered. Meantime I would concentrate everything I had on the camp — the Fifty-second's artillery, plus my four 105mm field pieces and thirty 81mm mortars.

We were ready by four. At seven in the morning the Nigerians started their attack, opening with an artillery barrage from the heavy stuff they'd brought in overnight, which was hard luck on my handful of men in the foxholes, but a necessary sacrifice. Then came the usual procession, led by the Ferrets. When the first of them went up on the first mine, our artillery opened fire on anything that moved in our old positions. They were caught and flattened. As they scattered and ran I took in my regrouped battalion. We were outnumbered by a factor of three or four, but we were able to take advantage of the enemy's confusion to give them a beating they'd remember and to regain all the ground we could.

We did better than I had dared to hope when we took the road junction and threw the enemy back to the river, but it would have been too easy if they had taken to their boats again. Back at Port Harcourt I heard that the Nigerians had opened a second bridgehead overnight, ten kilometers upstream. The ones we had cleaned out had joined up with them. Biafra was starting to crack.

10

The Enugu
Raid

I now became preoccupied with the military situation in Port
Harcourt. We had all our fuel stocks and a lot of material
in that zone, and as things got worse Ojukwu ordered all
armaments factories to be dismantled and machines and
material transferred to the Madonnas. Clearance and removal all took time.

When Port Harcourt fell on May 18, 1968, I had no more
troops engaged in the sector. Although I had no official responsibility for defense, I suggested holding the natural line
of the Imo River and blowing up the bridge on the Aba–Port
Harcourt axis. The line would be easy to defend, and there
was no possibility of the enemy's crossing it by boat to
reach the Aba–Umuahia area which was the heart of Iboland. They would have to outflank it by way of Owerri, a
major detour which removed the advantage of their southern
offensive. Consequently my suggestion would create time to
arrange a counteroffensive, providing we received enough
arms and ammunition.

The events at Port Harcourt had delayed the execution of
my raid on Enugu, which was considered a suicide operation and was frowned upon by the brigade chaplain. I argued
that Jesus himself had in a way committed suicide. Being

God, He could not have failed to foresee the consequences of His actions.

On May 24, 1968, I was finally able to get back to Commando 14 on the northern front. Nara is a small village isolated in the savanna seventy kilometers south of Enugu. The front line, if you could call it a line, ran about fifteen kilometers away. To reach our objective meant a sixty-kilometer march through deserted bush country which neither side had bothered to occupy.

My fifty men had been in clover for the previous month, while I had sweated at Port Harcourt. I arrived to find everything in readiness, even my cook with his field kitchen mounted on a ten-ton Mercedes truck. Twenty-five men were to make the raid, and I gave them their briefing next morning. My intention was to set out that same evening, provided there was rain; I had not been able to send scouts, so I wanted to play safe by using darkness and tropical rain as cover. The men still didn't know what they were doing in Nara. Now I told them that I was after the four Ilyushins and two MIGs at Enugu.

When the chaplain celebrated Mass he blessed each man, embraced him, and wept, much to my own disgust. He might have damaged their morale. In the afternoon the clouds opened and we crammed aboard the truck taking us to the frontier. It set us down, and we started walking through flat bush country where tall grasses and rain cut visibility to fifty meters. The first twenty kilometers were monotonous and gray. Then night fell.

In Africa, on a stormy night you can see nothing at all. The countryside leaves a pattern on your eyeballs after every flash of lightning and you might as well be blind. Your guide is the flop, flop, flop of the boots of the man in front. Walking becomes so mechanical that if he stops you probably cannon into him.

I was walking somewhere in the middle of the column,

followed by Layla, the rescued girl who had become part of my secretariat, who was carrying my knapsack, which contained maps, compass, and binoculars. Around midnight we made our first halt in the ruins of a school, inside enemy territory. Then we went on toward Enugu. I knew that we had to cross a river five kilometers this side of the town, but it was swollen with rain and it took us an hour to find our way across with arms and ammo intact.

Dawn was breaking when we came in sight of Enugu airfield, and as we took cover I could see that we were still several hundred meters short of the target. All around the field the bush had been burned back as a security measure; only an occasional green shoot had sprouted through the scorched earth.

The sun had risen as we crept toward the scant cover provided by the contours of the ground. The control tower was five hundred meters ahead, the planes roughly the same distance to the right, parked at the end of the runway beneath their camouflage awnings. I knew from our intelligence reports that the airport was guarded by four hundred men equipped with Ferrets, and I didn't dare move till nightfall because our position was already so exposed that a man could be spotted at six hundred meters just by getting to his knees.

We were thirsty, but of course we had no water because it would have meant bringing less ammunition. At eight o'clock the mud was warm; at midday it was baked bone-dry and hard, and the sun was trying to do the same for us. Our clothes were torn, through having to crawl along the ground, and we all had scratches full of dirt and sweat, which attracted swarms of flies. Having to keep our heads low meant that we couldn't see each other, but I could hear Layla panting like a puppy dog behind me. . . . Time crawled by. I was lying face down most of the time, but if I squinted upward I could see the vultures flapping their slow circles.

Biafra was the big all-African pilgrimage for vultures that year — always more fresh meat in the larder.

Around three in the afternoon clouds began to appear and the air grew heavier. A storm was brewing, and its interaction with our own tension made the waiting almost unbearable. I kept wanting to stand up and get it over with, but I wanted all the planes, not just one or two. We had to get it right.

We needed that rain. Needed it for our thirst, and for cover. At five it came and we were lapping at puddles like animals. An hour later we were soaked to the skin again and it was hailing. I did not want to take the men straight to the spot where I now intended to attack. There was no point spending the night in position; there was a hillock two kilometers behind us where we could find cover and get a few hours' rest, and we headed for that. We even lit a small fire to dry out our tobacco.

While we smoked I briefed the group. Early that morning we had heard a bugle call, and I had watched the four companies of the guard turn out for assembly. They had raised the colors at seven precisely. My plan was to find a position close to their parade ground and open fire on the Nigerians when they were lined up to salute the flag. It would never reach the top of the mast. I wasn't happy about the resulting slaughter, but there were four hundred of them, plus Ferrets, and our chances were a lot better if we could dispose of them fast.

At 2:30 we set out in single file to within three hundred meters of the control tower, easy to locate against the skyline. Then we made a detour to cross the strip and found ourselves on the other side of a road, behind our objective, and in grass tall enough to hide in. Nothing moved on the airfield as I positioned the men. They were in place at four. This time the wait was easier. We were in the right place, with a clear-cut plan.

Dawn came, with a ray of sunshine illuminating the top of the mast. I made a final check on our positions, chosen so that machine gun enfiladed each of the areas where I had watched the four companies parade the day before. At six the bugle sounded for reveille. At 6:15 a group of mechanics headed for the MIGs, removed the awnings, opened the cockpits and loaded rockets under the wings. I remembered the marketplace at Awgu, and any misgivings faded.

The Ilyushins remained under camouflage. All six planes were bunched together, about three hundred meters away, the MIGs a little apart. I had brought two rocket-launchers, which were to fire on the planes at the same time as the machine guns opened up on the troops. From where we were located there was an angle of thirty degrees at most between our two targets.

At 6:45 the bugle sounded assembly. The federal troops started arriving on parade, all of them impeccably turned out, with the spit and polish you would expect in a British barracks. They wore olive-green uniforms and carried automatic rifles, without magazines. Section by section they lined up, standing to strict attention.

Layla handed me my Thompson.

The bugle sounded.

I heard: "Present arms!" The flag was unfolded and attached.

The bugle sounded again. The colors climbed jerkily up the flagpole.

When it was halfway up I opened fire. Simultaneously all my men opened up on their designated targets. Five machine guns and ten automatic rifles bit into the still figures in front of us and they began to fall. It was like watching a silent film. The sound of our own gunfire drowned any noise from the men dropping in swathes on the parade ground.

I turned my attention to our main objective, the planes, and saw the first rocket overshoot and explode far into the savanna. The second fell short. The third and fourth rockets followed the same pattern, and my heart sank when two more burst with no effect. The seventh — only three left now — and all at once the first Ilyushin came apart like a magic box. Then came the heavy crack of the explosion, the sound of the impact, a second flash of dark red flame, and the whole thing went up. Falling debris set fire to the other crates, and since the Ilyushins were parked so close together they all exploded, all four of them!

Right in front of us it was sheer massacre. Four hundred panic-stricken men running, shouting, screaming, writhing in pain and wriggling like bisected worms. They just didn't know what to do, while my own men kept firing, glued to their weapons. Farther off, the four Ilyushins now made a single giant bonfire, crackling and roaring loud enough to smother even the cries of the dying.

We still had two rockets left, and I shouted: "The MIGs, get the MIGs!"

Fifty meters from the burning Ilyushins the two MIGs were almost intact, although one of them had caught a splinter in the fuselage. The rockets fired and missed — shit, no more rockets. I told Captain Koroko, the group commender, to turn the machine guns on them, hoping for a lucky hit on their rockets, or maybe a fuel tank.

I seemed to have an age to count each following second. The machine guns had switched to their new target, and they kept on and on, a continuous chatter. But the MIGs were a long way off, and I was well aware that the Nigerians were bound to pull themselves together before long. My eyes were pressed to the binoculars, but there was nothing to see . . . and still nothing. . . . I started to despair.

As I was giving the order to fall back, *crrrump!* It happened! I don't know if it was an exploding rocket or the fuel, but first one, then the other, went up. Still the same obsession with huddling close together, just like their infantry. . . .

That was that. The six aircraft were in flames, the shooting had stopped, and in front of us there was a kind of red-flecked, olive-green carpet that groaned and gently stirred. Flies were already swarming in.

Three of my men went to take possession of the enemy flag, while others collected abandoned weapons. It was then that we suffered our first injury, as the Ferrets began to react to a strike which had taken ten minutes at most. A spent bullet had hit one of my men in the shoulder, and I was putting on a temporary dressing when I heard a cry from Layla and found myself knocked to the ground beneath her. There was a brief burst of firing and I felt her body shudder, quite softly.

I pushed Layla away and made for my Thompson. When I turned around I saw a Nigerian soldier standing five meters away, his face and body streaming with his own blood, with a smoking FAL aimed right at me. Before I could pull the trigger, he had already collapsed again. It was the first time I had felt any respect for a Nigerian: this one had used his last bit of strength in trying to kill me.

When I turned to Layla I meant to slap her for playing the old routine of girl-lays-down-life-for-boy, but the shudders had been bullets, three or four of them. I started to open her jacket, but she smiled and said: "No need. It's finished for me." Then she gripped my arm very hard. "Commander, always remember we are fighting to survive. Remember . . ." And she died.

There was no time for mourning. We had to get moving, and quickly. The Ferrets were due on our tails any minute, and there was open ground for eight hundred meters. Although the Nigerians didn't dare advance, their fire was getting more intense. Looking at their casualties, they must have thought we had a battalion in waiting, not a mere twenty-five men. But it did not even occur to them to take over the control tower, which would have given them a clear field of fire, and we reached the thick bush without pursuit, just a few enemy mortars popping away at a target they couldn't see.

The return trip was faster planned. With fifty kilometers to cover in enemy territory and in broad daylight, we commandeered bicycles at the first village we passed through, and a crushing blow to the Nigerians ended up like a country bike ride.

Layla's intervention had saved my life. Elsewhere I had had orderlies or interpreters killed by my side. My continuing survival persuaded many of the more superstitious Biafrans that I was invulnerable, an impression strengthened by the tall stories my men liked to tell. They embroidered their own homegrown epics around a few true incidents.

There was the time at Abagana when I was inspecting a company supporting a counteroffensive against General Mohammed. I noticed a 60mm mortar with its base plate set the wrong way round. We were under fire, the commandos were already attacking, and we had to keep up a brisk fire on the federal positions. I took over from the man using the mortar and put the base plate right. There were forty shells waiting, and I told him to take the pins out and keep me supplied while I bombarded an emplacement of 105mm guns.

In the heat of the action I fired all but one of his shells before moving on to see what was happening ahead. Behind me there was a loud bang, and I thought the enemy was firing with their own mortars. I'd told the mortar's minder to keep the last shell in reserve, but when I turned to look three men lay dead around the burst mortar. The last shell must have been defective. I thought at first that the man must have had his finger over the tube, but it had burst at the bottom as soon as the shell was triggered. If I had fired it, or if the loader had not left it till last, I would have not be around to tell the story.

Some time afterward we were near Ollienba, where my commandos were attacking the headquarters of a Nigerian battalion. My men had the road blocked with trees and elephant traps, as I had taught them, to hold up the enemy Ferrets, but they also held up my car, and I borrowed a messenger's motorcycle to reach the front. As I zigzagged through the obstacles I saw a soldier standing rigid behind the last tree, and I wondered what he was doing standing to attention. Ten meters farther on I could hear him as he yelled: "Stop, stop! Mines!"

I braked hard, and asked if he knew where the mines were.

"Yes sir! Right behind you. You just rode over them."

Just after the fall of Onitsha, some time in April, my reputation crossed the Atlantic. Coming out of a briefing at Twelfth Division HQ, I ran into a journalist, still a rare species at that time. He was curious about finding a white officer in the Biafran army and asked for an interview. I was heading for the front, near Onitsha, so he invited himself along.

We set off in my Land Rover, followed by the general and some staff officers. The Biafrans were still digging trenches, World War I style. As if that wasn't bad enough, I could see from four hundred meters away that the trenches weren't sufficiently deep and that some of them were not covered. I was putting my objections to the general, and getting pretty heated in the process, when the federal troops attacked and he and all his colonels jumped into the ditch, leaving me and the dismayed journalist standing in the middle of the road.

With bullets kicking up dust around us, I told him to take cover.

"Why don't you?" he asked.

"It's different for me. I'm an old soldier. I know the bullets will be spent at this range. If I'm going to be hit, I'll be hit just as easily lying down."

"All right, then; if it's not dangerous I'll stay on my feet."

And just as he was talking a bullet went through the leg of his trousers. Feeling the tug, he looked down and turned pale at the sight of the two holes on either side of the crease. "Look," he said. "Look at my trousers." And he dropped flat.

Again lack of experience. Considering the dispersion of bullets at ground level, he would have done better to climb a tree.

When Robinson returned to the States he wrote the story up and made a big point of my staying upright while the generals dived, and how his trousers suffered when he tried to do the same. I expect he charged them against expenses.

I am not superstitious enough to believe that I was invulnerable, but after coming out unscathed where so many had fallen, I did come to believe in my own luck. Part of it had to do with keeping calm. I am a fatalist. When I'm in danger I tell myself that if the bullet has my name on it I'll be hit, but not otherwise. It isn't that I don't give death a thought; rather I feel that there is no point in letting it affect you, since you can't escape fate. And in the long run, frequent exposure to danger has taken the edge off it. Not that I go looking for the sensation of Russian roulette, or that I enjoy bullets as other people like walking in the rain. But combat does teach you to keep cool and clearheaded.

In fact I suppose that the secret of my luck must be a combination of experience and intuition. The experience has come with time. Although I do have the occasional fit of rage when I forget about personal safety, I have also acquired automatic defensive reflexes — when a shell is falling too close, I know it, and I take an immediate dive.

I also have a lot of faith in my own intuition. I don't know with absolute certainty when there's trouble waiting around the corner, and I can sense whether I should act or stand still. I have taken on enemies whose forces were ten times greater than mine because of an inner conviction that it would work out. And the same kind of irrational knowledge has held me back in positions of superiority.

Bulletproof or not, the legend certainly increased my standing with my men, and I tried to use it to strengthen our esprit de corps. I felt that the "commando spirit" ought not to be confined to military qualities: it should also mean helping each other. Being Ibos, my men didn't need much persuasion, and there was no lack of opportunity. Hundreds of refugees clustered round each Madonna every day, waiting for the soup to be ladled out, because the cooks made extra food for the hungry on their own initiative. That was the sort of "commando spirit" I had in mind.

World opinion constructed an image of the Biafran as a poor, abandoned child, all skin and bone except for the potbelly typical of kwashiorkor, with reproachful eyes staring from a large head covered with reddish hair. Sick and hungry the children may have been, but abandoned, never. No one could believe that who knew anything about the Ibos and their social structures. Among them, a child *cannot* be abandoned, because they do not live for themselves but for their family, for their clan. Theirs is a natural solidarity.

On the other hand, in the great upheavals and movements of population caused by the war some children really did become lost and destitute. This was especially likely to happen among the ethnic minorities — the Ibibios, Efiks, Ijaws, Annangs, etc. These minorities tended to be lower down on the social scale, and often worked as servants among the Ibos. Living on the periphery of Iboland, they watched their own home territory being torn apart by the fighting. Unwanted by either side, scattered and fragmented, many of them went under. Divided families wandered in the bush, avoiding soldiers, often starving to death, particularly the children who had lost their mothers' protection.

Five kilometers from Madonna 1 there was an orphanage run by nuns. The mother superior was always broke, and she had four hundred of these unwanted children, many of them sick. I gave her three nurses on permanent loan and we provided the children's food out of our own.

11

Prisoners
and Spies

The military situation continued to deteriorate. By late May 1968 the northern front was crumbling from the Niger to Cameroon, we had lost Onitsha, and the Nigerian capture of Port Harcourt had cut us off from the sea. That meant that all supplies of food, arms, and ammunition had to come by air. To the west our forces were somehow managing to stand up to the enemy's continual pounding. To the east the Cameroon frontier was closed. To the south neither side could keep any sort of footing in the marshes and virgin forests of the Niger delta.

Our system of defense had not changed. The divisions of the Biafran army tried to protect their various sectors, while my commando brigade remained on call to stop up the holes as they appeared all around our perimeter. But we couldn't be everywhere at once. The future looked grim as the blockade drew tighter around an area the size of Belgium, which the press was already calling "Fortress Biafra," a zone centering on the triangle formed by Umuahia, Aba, and Owerri. The forecast of the Nigerian military attaché in Bonn was coming true: the trap was closing on the Ibos.

I had received my lieutenant colonel's stripes on March 4, and at first I did not wear them. I felt that I didn't need them in order to assert authority. I soon realized that it made contacts with other units a lot easier if I was on the same level as their officers, so when Ojukwu promoted me to full colonel on July 28 I accepted. Even so, it sometimes happened that a general would pull rank on me, and I never made any attempt to correct him — I must have been getting anglicized.

My contacts with General Effiong, the Biafran chief of staff, were always polite but distant. I think he resented my direct access to Ojukwu, when many Ibo colonels had never got near their chief of state. But although the Ojukwu-Steiner connection bypassed him, he kept up appearances, which is the good side of the British style of education. He treated me fairly, helped me to find the right equipment for my men, and even made me a gift of his personal compass when I was preparing for the Enugu raid. In fact, I often went to Effiong when there was something I needed: I knew that he would do his best to obtain it because he was delighted that I had not asked Ojukwu.

On one occasion Effiong made a surprise visit and asked to see the hospital. We toured it, together with about twenty of his officers, and he went from bed to bed distributing handshakes, kind words, and packs of cigarettes. As he moved along the rows of beds he gave the same treatment to a Nigerian soldier who happened to be there. Then I introduced them: "Meet Captain Aluko, commanding the Third Company of the Thirty-seventh Battalion, Third Federal Division."

Effiong goggled at me, and his officers crowded round to stare at this curiosity. They hadn't seen a Nigerian officer, not even a dead one, since the start of the war. Then Effiong took me by the elbow and pulled me aside:

"Listen, Rolf, was it really necessary to bring that man here? Do you think it is right to treat an enemy soldier alongside our own men?"

I told him that no one could make me fight an inhuman war; he sighed and shook his head, but did not take back the pack of cigarettes. He came across three or four other Nigerians on that visit, and this time they got no cigarettes, but Effiong said nothing. He was a gentleman.

This question of prisoners was one of those on which I disagreed with the custom of the general staff. In all African wars the tradition is one of no quarter. No prisoners are taken except when needed. But in my brigade it was my orders which were observed. After every engagement my men collected their dead and wounded as well as the enemy wounded and took them all to the hospital. My hospital. In one of the ordinary military hospitals the Nigerians would have run the risk of being finished off.

I never had any report of my men killing prisoners, wounded or not, once the action was over. In the heat of battle it is different, of course. It is hard to tell just when the fighting is over, and you finish off the wounded, and anything that moves. . . .

Especially in Africa. I know how blacks with no military training behave in combat: in one of two ways, and only two. Either they are paralyzed by an intense, unreasoning fear that sometimes roots them to the spot, sometimes lets them run, or else they are gripped by an equally irrational fit of hysterical euphoria. In that state of mind they massacre everybody who comes their way, civilians included. But I could not hold the prisoners responsible for what crimes they might have committed. A soldier is an instrument. If it hadn't been for the war, they would never have been put in the position of behaving as they did.

With the brigade it was different. It was through the prisoners that we found out what particularly scared the federal troops about my commandos: the officers went first, as they do in the Legion. That was a big surprise for the British-trained Nigerians, and the Biafran regulars didn't understand it either.

Nor have I ever heard it said that prisoners taken by my men were tortured. I would not have tolerated that kind of interrogation, and in any case I couldn't see the point. My attitude was humane. It was also effective. In the come-down that follows the excitement of combat, blacks are not usually brave. A prisoner is afraid; he is likely to talk quite naturally, without being forced, and especially if he is being treated well. Not that he generally has anything useful to say. What could I learn from some Hausa infantryman — since officers were rare in the front line? The number of men in his company? What he had to eat the day before?

Ojukwu felt the same. On one of his spur-of-the-moment visits to Madonna 1 he asked to see two prisoners my men had captured that morning. One of them was a young Yoruba officer. My guards brought him in on a stretcher, and I told him through an interpreter that he was in the presence of Biafra's chief of state. Did he recognize him? The lieutenant nodded. Ojukwu gave him a quizzical look and questioned him in Yoruba, and the lieutenant was calm and pretty talkative. Several times I heard the word "Russian" pronounced in English. He claimed that in his unit there were three Russian advisers to each company.

The second prisoner fell on his knees as soon as he came in and held that position until the interrogation was over. He was a Hausa, and Ojukwu did not speak that language. The interpreter told us: "This nitwit had been marching in our ranks for five minutes, Your Excellency. He was calling out in Hausa: 'Sergeant, sergeant, I need more ammo!' He got the wrong army. Someone noticed him, and seeing how much he liked our company, we brought him along."

Clearly this particular crack soldier was not familiar with

the plans of the Nigerian general staff for their big push. Ojukwu asked: "If I was in your place and you in mine, what would you do with me?"

He hesitated, then announced with a quaver in his voice that he would let his prisoner go. Ojukwu smiled into his beard, and shook his head.

"You're joking, I think. But your life will be spared."

Many superior officers were jealous of the commandos' independence. The Fourth Brigade was Ojukwu's personal unit, and the army leadership had no influence over it, which was why some people with shady schemes of their own tried to neutralize it. They knew very well that any attack on Ojukwu would have had the commandos to deal with.

It all began in April. Colonel Obiagu, Effiong's adjutant on the general staff, often used to visit me, armed with bottles of whiskey, beer, and cigarettes. Obviously he was trying to make friends, and I had nothing against that. Then he started to show his hand, at first with casual remarks: "Don't you think that a combination of your brigade with Colonel Adjuze's Fifty-first and Colonel Ukpana's Fifty-second would make a terrific army? Don't you agree that the four of us should get to know each other better? After all, you have the three best units."

I didn't discourage Obiagu, and from then on I received several visits from him and the other two colonels, who also invited me to see them. On each occasion they were lavish with the whiskey and beer.

Then one day I was astonished to find Obiagu sending me a colonel and two majors with what seemed to be official postings to my brigade. I realized then that what interested Obiagu was not me but my brigade, and that he was trying to elbow me out of my own command by putting in his own nominees. I got rid of the three of them at once — they hadn't stayed for more than an hour at Madonna 1 — then went straight to Obiagu's HQ. Colonel Obiagu was in his office and received me with open arms. It didn't work: I told him that I was annoyed with him for sending me his men and that I was responsible to Ojukwu alone.

"None of you has the right to meddle with appointments to my brigade without consulting him."

He took that badly, and we started arguing. Finally he turned on me: "Do you know that I can have you arrested?"

"You? Just try it!"

Beside myself with fury, I made for the door. Obiagu stood in the way, ordering me back into his office. I shoved him aside and went out, slamming the door behind me. My car was parked in the courtyard outside. When I got in, two MPs ran toward me calling out for me to stop. They had to dive out of the way as I roared off followed by a whole posse of guards, sentries, and MPs waving revolvers. Seeing this, I drew my own pistol. They didn't know it was not loaded, and ran for cover. The gate was closed, and I smashed straight through it and drove back to Madonna 1 jumping all the checkpoints with horn blaring and red light flashing on the roof.

I told the whole story to Emeka, and when Colonel Obiagu turned up within the hour I found that my second-in-command had already stationed five scout cars at strategic points and turned out the guard battalion, without my knowledge. Obiagu arrived with fifty redcaps, the pick of the military police, and as I came out of the mess to greet him I saw this impressive escort confronting the commando guard lined up twenty meters away with their Kalshnikovs unslung.

At the sight of the MPs' apprehensive expressions I burst out laughing.

"Don't worry, colonel," I told Obiagu. "It's not for you, just a training exercise."

Now that I was back in my own base I felt more relaxed.

I took him to my office, and after some more argument I simply walked out and left him.

With nothing definite to go on, and no evidence, I said nothing to Ojukwu, but next day he sent for me. I went in, shook Ojukwu's hand, and sat down. He said: "Rolf, I am told that Colonel Obiagu accuses you of having insulted him to his face in Madonna One."

I then told Ojukwu the whole story — the soft soap, my suspicions and the rest — while Obiagu fiddled nervously with his baton and stared at his cap on the coat-stand. Major Clement, Ojukwu's own security officer before he became my intelligence chief, had been present when the colonel arrived and confirmed that I had insulted no one.

"Good," said Ojukwu. "You can go." I went outside and waited, knowing that he wanted a word in private.

When he came out he told me: "Rolf, I suspected that Obiagu was planning a coup, but I didn't know he was fool enough to try to involve you. But I'm hushing it up. We have more serious business than that to attend to."

Obiagu was put under arrest, and three months later he was given command of a small unit. The other colonels received a warning, and everything went back to normal. The incident illustrated Ojukwu's indulgence, but it also illustrated his subtlety.

12
Seven Minus One

Williams, the white recruit who had argued with me over the question of his pay, returned on July 7, wearing a hang-dog look. He had thought it over — a rare activity for him — and said that he was ready to serve in the Biafran army for nothing.

Next day I reported to Ojukwu that Williams was back, but pointed out that there might be a security problem since he had been in London and might have been in touch with the enemy. Ojukwu left it up to me, so I decided to put Williams in charge of basic training, which was what he was best cut out for.

I met my next white recruit in Umuahia's only nightclub on a hot April evening when I stopped for a drink on my way back to Madonna 1. Apart from a few Irish priests and the German boot and shoe manufacturer there weren't many Europeans left in Biafra, and I hadn't come across the man who introduced himself as Louis Malroony — "but every-body calls me Paddy." It turned out that he had been living in Nigeria for seven years as a Forestry Commission engineer specializing in hydraulics. Before the war he had been sta-tioned in the Abakaliki sector, and his house and belongings were now in enemy hands. He was a powerfully built man in his early fifties.

When Paddy congratulated me on what I was doing for the Ibos, I asked him if he would be prepared to lend me a hand. He was unemployed and did not want to return to Europe, and I could always use a good engineer. I had my answer when he drove up to Madonna 1 the following day. We visited the workshops and I introduced him to my Biafran engineers.

The result was that I put him in charge of my ordnance department, responsible for everything except radio. He never went near the front. That wasn't his job. But out of respect for his position I gave him the rank of captain.

The other whites came little by little. On July 14 two men arrived: John, a quiet raw-boned Rhodesian of about twenty-five, and Ray, a Scotsman who had also fought in the Congo. I could have turned them down, because they hadn't come from Ojukwu.

I took on John because he was an explosives expert. He had been an armorer in Salisbury before he deserted and he really did know his job, as he proved before he died by blowing two bridges for me. One of his specialties was napalm, which he cooked up to his own recipe. The method was simple: into an old oil drum he put ordinary household soap and heated it gently until it was liquid. When the soap was melted he topped the drum with petrol and added gunpowder, in proportions he obviously knew by heart.

To judge by results, it was a good recipe. We also used it to make jumping antitank mines. The big 200-liter containers made an impressive sight when they exploded in midair.

Roy, the Scotsman, was walleyed and sported a Wyatt Earp moustache. He was about thirty-five, but there was something about his streetcorner manner that made it easy to imagine him sitting astride his motorbike in some Glasgow suburb, cycle chain in hand, looking for trouble.

I tried him out at the front in a surprise attack, to test his behavior under fire. The mission was to take a crossroads held by dug-in federal troops with three armored vehicles. He came out of it very well, losing only two men and handling himself like a pro. I kept him.

Later on Roy asked me for a command, and I told him that he must prove himself first. I stationed him at Umuede, as adviser to the guard commander, who was killed soon after. When Roy informed me by radio I told him to take over for the time being, and when it became obvious that he was the man for the job I realized that only a racist would remove him just because he was white.

His later behavior confirmed that he was brave to the point of rashness. He was a chancer, always in the front line, and in two months he was wounded three times — shrapnel splinters in the thigh, a bullet in the hand, and an injured foot when a bazooka shell exploded next to him.

Roy was the best all-around soldier of all the whites I fought with in Biafra. He earned my respect and the responsibilities it brought him.

On August 4 I heard that another white man had arrived from Libreville in the chief of state's plane. During the flight Ojukwu had asked who he was and had been told that his name was Armand and he wanted to join my brigade. I vaguely remembered him from my OAS days when we had passed each other a few times in the corridors of the Santé prison. Three or four days after his arrival I tested him out at the front, and he was wounded at the same time as Roy, also in the hand. It took two of them to change the magazine on the Thompson, and it was a running joke between them for weeks.

Roy informed me that Armand was a good soldier, but

he was different from the Congo bunch. He did not fight for money or for a cause, but for the thrill of living dangerously. At thirty-three he had seen action in Katanga and Angola, and he was equally handy with a Nikon or a Colt, according to circumstance. He got on well with his men, and they preferred him to the other Europeans.

Williams and Paddy were not paid. John and Roy were. It never entered my head to offer money to Paddy — he would have been insulted — but John and Roy were no philanthropists, and they insisted on their salaries. I needed an armorer, and Roy was a good fighting man, so Ojukwu authorized me to pay them a thousand dollars a month out of the funds I had available for buying explosives. Williams had been put off the whole subject by his earlier experience, and Armand never made any conditions for staying.

In case of accident, I guaranteed all of them cover out of the brigade's war chest. It wasn't underwritten by Lloyd's, but they had my word.

Williams, Paddy, John, Ray, Armand, me . . . that made six. One reporter from *France-Soir* wrote: "These are the six mercenaries. They need one more to make a good screen title, and a hundred more to make an army." It was a good line, but nothing more than that, because there never was a white commando unit. The Europeans made up a technical team which I used according to my own needs and their abilities. They had nothing to do with my staff. Emeka was my second-in-command, and if I had been put out of action it would have been Emeka who replaced me.

The arms, munitions, and useful articles which Biafra could not produce had to arrive by air. With the loss of Port Harcourt, Biafra was cut off from the rest of the world, and aircraft could only land by night because the powerful federal ack-ack was so close. The main landing grounds were at Uli and Uturu, before that, too, fell.

The number one airstrip, Uli, was simply a stretch of the main road, widened on either side. For security reasons it was lit up only when an aircraft was approaching. Uli had its own generator, so it could produce something like the normal landing beacons, electric lights mounted on three-meter poles at the edges of the enlarged asphalt surface.

Uturu, which was on loan to the International Red Cross for a while, had no generator, and the strip was lit at fifteen-meter intervals by empty food tins filled with petrol, each one manned by a soldier who put out the fire as soon as the aircraft was down.

Neither field had a control tower, just a radio shack and a small radar scanner mounted on a truck to detect incoming aircraft. The pilots' call signs were changed every day, and they used a secret wavelength for their messages. The plane would make contact, identify itself, then wait for permission to land. In May not more than ten aircraft a night were arriving. From July onward there were sixty or more.

Nine-tenths of the freight was food for the children, and that had nothing to do with me. I had made my own position clear — that you don't win wars with milk. Certainly it was necessary, but it wasn't my business. I had chosen to put out the fire, not tend its victims.

The rest of the freight was the arms and munitions bought on the black market in Europe and South Africa, through Biafra's offices in Lisbon, Rome, and Paris. In our radio contacts with them I always made my brigade's requirements a priority. My sense of our own usefulness was very clear.

At that time the French government was not sending us any arms, and it never did do so officially. If it had the deals would have been handled through the French army, and we would have received their equipment. That way we would not have received, for example, thousands of brand-new German carbines from the Second World War, which could not possibly be traced to France. . . .

In spring the world press began to swarm around, just a few in April, then more and more. To start with it was mainly TV teams, and I could not turn them away because the propaganda was good for Biafra. I made a point of letting them go where they pleased. If they wanted to bury their noses in garbage, it was all right with me: better for them to form their own opinion than for me to make clumsy efforts to influence them and so risk turning them against us. Our cause would speak for itself.

The journalists made a big fuss about me, but I never saw myself as a star. I didn't know what they were writing since I didn't receive any newspapers. As it happened, some reporters drew a phony outline of Rolf Steiner, calling me a "mercenary" because the label was fashionable at that time. I was not ashamed to be in the service of Biafra, but it made me very angry to be tarred with the same brush as the paid killers in the Congo. But nothing real had changed. I still had the same aim of carrying out my mission as well as possible — better than anybody else.

I wasn't fighting for glory, and I never saw myself as a hero. In war there are no heroes. I have no respect for clowns who make a big noise just to attract attention. If a man pushes himself to his own limits, that's enough.

13
The "Agulus"

Six months after my arrival in Biafra my total losses amounted to 8,400 killed, wounded, or missing, almost double the strength of my brigade. An unusually high replacement rate was required. With a permanent available fighting force of five thousand, I kept a number of training camps, each of them housing several hundred men, at full strength. After three or four weeks' training they were ready for service, and I could call upon as many as I needed.

Early in July I wanted to give my men a rest, and they went on leave to seven schools around Agulu, which we effortlessly dubbed Agulu 1, 2, 3, 4, 5, 6, and 7. Agulu was a quiet backwater a long way from the northern front. You could hardly hear the rumble of the artillery pounding Abagana. I kept the men busy with maneuvers and reconnaissance patrols, but in their free time they could dance, sing, or go to film shows. I turned a blind eye to their bringing women into their quarters, being more concerned with their morale than their morals, but I made it clear that whatever they may have been doing the night before they had better be on their toes by morning.

We built up stocks of food in the Agulus, not by capturing them from the enemy but by recovering them from the areas abandoned by the Ibo population with the coming of the federal army. My commandos went deep into enemy-held territory, sometimes as far as Nsukka, to collect these supplies of cassava, oil, dried fish, and so on, and bring them back. Although these were not exactly fighting missions they had their importance in the war because they enabled Biafra to feed its soldiers better. The Nigerians did not know about the existence of these reserves, but in any case they would not have touched them. They were deeply suspicious of food from Ibo sources, thinking that it might be poisoned, and all their supplies came in by truck. Even their meat came from Lagos.

There was a basis of truth to these poison stories. Before the war Biafra had received its supplies of salt from other regions, having none itself, and sometimes the salt had been poisoned. There had also been reports about tinned milk laced with strychnine. All the same, we did have some food which came straight out of the federal stores. It was safe to eat rice, sugar, salt, beans, and other items captured from enemy convoys and intended for their own consumption.

Food, too, is an aspect of morale. No one fights well on an empty stomach. My five battalions produced their own fresh food, and owned five hundred cattle, plus sheep, pigs, and poultry which were tended by men invalided out of active service. The Legion does not abandon a crippled soldier, and neither did I. In Europe they might become subpostmasters, park keepers or gardeners; here I made them herdsmen. They could still be useful, and they were still part of the commando family.

Maybe it was because they were living like fighting cocks that my soldiers became too cocksure. There was a Lieutenant Issoko in the Second Company of my Eighth Battalion who had a reputation as a born comedian. He was always joking or playing tricks, and was famous for his imitations of his friends' and superior officers' voices and mannerisms. One day he was leading a reconnaissance patrol when he ran slap into an enemy patrol which promptly froze with terror and surrendered without firing a shot. Issoko noticed immediately that his five prisoners were all wearing brand-new uniforms. Both sides wore the same uniform; only the insignia were different.

These uniforms were especially tempting because Issoko and his men had worn their own to shreds. So what should be done? Kill them? That was strictly forbidden, and I would find out if they disobeyed. Strip them and bring them back naked? That would be mistreating the enemy, which was also forbidden. It was unthinkable to make a swap and allow them to wear Biafran uniforms, even cast-offs. So they took the clothes and released the men, but Issoko could not resist giving them a note for their sector commander. It read something like this: "We are poor wretches, we have plenty of ammunition but nothing to eat. We are hungry, and if you treat us right we promise to leave you in peace." The note ended: "We like beer too. We will wait for your answer tomorrow morning, on the main road by milestone 45."

The prisoners didn't hang about, and by the time he was back in camp Issoko had put the letter out of his mind — he had meant it as a joke. But milestone 45 was in his sector, and visible when he made his daily trip the next morning to scan the district from the top of a small rise. Five hundred meters away, at the roadside, he spotted a tarpaulin-covered mass which had not been there the day before. At first he thought that it must be a trap, so he cordoned the area off and approached the pile with caution, keeping his eyes peeled for booby traps.

Pinned to the canvas was a brief note, the Nigerian commander's reply. It read: "All right, we agree. Every day there will be food, cigarettes, and beer left here. Good luck, keep it quiet, and remember your promise to leave us in peace."

I happened to be in Agulu 1 around noon when I saw a company march up in single file, every man carrying at least one package on his head, several hundred kilos in all. In the afternoon Emeka handed me a list of the Nigerian supplies — a hundred cartons of cigarettes, corned beef, tea, sugar, ten kilos of bacon, and twenty crates of beer.

"How did they get it?"

"By special arrangement with the enemy, commander."

Then the whole story came out. Issoko thought he had done something heroic, but in fact, from a more serious point of view, it could be seen as treason. It was awkward for me, particularly when I consulted Emeka and he confirmed that Issoko would face a court martial if we went by the book. Meanwhile the lieutenant was still patting himself on the back.

The problem was that the news was bound to travel via the grapevine, and pretty soon everybody would have heard the story, from Owerri to Umuahia. I sent for Issoko's file, and saw that he had been decorated — and wounded — more than once, and that he was described as "intelligent, but tends to put his own interpretation on his orders. . . ." I was sure that he intended no treason, and I was ready to take responsibility for his stupidity rather than see him punished. At the same time I didn't want to encourage anybody else to follow Issoko's example.

I thought for a while, then told Emeka: "Right, here's what we'll do. I don't really want any trouble with the Nigerians here, because we're supposed to be resting. So we'll leave this sector in peace for the time being, and you can tell Issoko that from today onward he can make it his job to collect anything they're fools enough to leave."

The system worked for ten days until Ojukwu got to hear

that we were smoking Nigerian cigarettes and drinking beer from Lagos. He laughed when I explained Issoko's deal, then added: "Call it a day, Rolf. The joke is over. Please stop it right now."

So we stopped. Some of the higher Biafran officers had seen their chance to take a crack at me, and I heard from Ojukwu himself that my enemies had got him out of bed at two in the morning with the news that I was in collusion with the enemy and they could prove it.

In addition to the Fourth Commando Brigade and its associated Madonnas and Agulus, Ojukwu trusted me enough to give me one "top secret" responsibility: to prepare guerrilla zones for the day when we might need them. This work was independent of the brigade, and none of my staff except my intelligence officer knew about it.

From February onward it had become clear that Biafra could not hold out militarily and the conventional war would sooner or later be decided in favor of the enemy. Ojukwu knew that he could no longer rely on any outside help. The only substantial aid had come from France, and at that time France had just withdrawn its support. What was needed was to create a guerrilla infrastructure throughout the territory, so that units which had been beaten in battle could break up and take to the bush. (Ojukwu was to drop this scheme after my departure in late 1968. The military situation had stabilized then, and he had high hopes of renewed and massive French support. But that is another story.)

Since March, Ojukwu had been sending picked men to each region with orders to lay the groundwork for local resistance and to hide stocks of food and arms. For my part I had begun to set up guerrilla bases in enemy-occupied areas. Ideally I would have preferred to be waging a guerrilla war already against the federal lines of communication, but my men and I could only be in so many places at once, and we were stretched to the limit.

All the same I had managed to bury a three-month supply of ammunition, enough for a brigade, at Madonna 14. It was not to be touched except in case of a general collapse, when my men were to disperse into the guerrilla zones at top speed. And among these zones there was one which offered special advantages: the uninhabited mountain area this side of the Cameroon frontier, in the north of Calabar. It was there that we planned to make our last stand if things went really badly.

I had selected Calabar for several reasons. The town itself was an important harbor in the extreme southeast of the country, and it had its own airport. The hinterland was covered with virgin forest. Calabar, which had fallen to the enemy almost without a fight on October 20, 1967, would have made an impregnable stronghold, protected on one side by the sea, on the other by thick jungle inhabited only by pygmies and wild animals. On top of that it was right next to Cameroon, whose main ethnic group, the Bamileke, were old allies of the Ibos. Instead of requiring an expensive and vulnerable airlift, we could have obtained all our food and arms officially, across an easily supervised frontier.

All that was left was to recapture Calabar, and it would not have been a difficult operation, because the Nigerians had left a slender garrison. They were not anticipating an attack from the west, and although I would have had to cross two hundred kilometers of jungle there were only two companies to deal with. I knew this because I had sent a scouting expedition made up of commandos born in Calabar.

On May 20, just after the fall of Port Harcourt, I submitted my plan to Ojukwu. I already believed that the enemy was planning to seize Aba, although as it happened they made a try for Owerri first. Eventually it was inevitable, given the balance of force, that we would lose Aba, and I urged Ojukwu not to defend the town and use his reserves, but to let me mount an expedition against Calabar. He liked the idea, but kept telling me: "Wait a bit, Rolf. Not now, not yet. . . ."

14
The Beginning of the End

The enemy had been occupying Onitsha since March 24. The eighteen thousand men of the Federal First Division held the town and its approaches. They were cut off from their bases by the Niger, but were supplied by boats which could shelter from our mortars under the bridge. On July 5, while my unit was on stand-down at Agulu, two Nigerian divisions launched a heavy attack on Onitsha from the north, aimed at breaking out own circle round the town. The attack succeeded, and the two enemy forces joined at Abagana. At four in the morning I received a call for help from General Amadi, commanding the Thirty-fourth Brigade. I refused, seeing that the game was already over.

Ojukwu asked me if I could make a personal reconnaissance of the bridge, to find out if it could be reached by river.

"Do you really think it's a good idea, Excellency?"

"Yes, Rolf. Frederick Forsyth has noticed that the water under the bridge gets much shallower in the dry season. He believes that the commandos could reach it by night with one company by walking along the exposed part of the riverbed."

That made sense, so I decided to take a look.

At that time Forsyth was an unknown young journalist who had managed to win Ojukwu's confidence. He was living in Umuahia and was consequently a privileged observer. Forsyth was clever and discreet; he kept his distance from visiting colleagues. He went wherever Ojukwu went and was familiar with all of Biafra's political and military problems.

I drove as close as possible to the enemy lines and went another few hundred meters on foot to a viewpoint which enabled me to see the pillboxes the Nigerians had built at the entrance to the bridge. The binoculars also showed that there was no exposed riverbank; it was steep at that point, because that was where the current flowed fastest. I sent a soldier into the water to make sure, and it was three or four meters deep. No chance of wading along. It was on the other bank of the Niger that the falling water level had left a broad expanse of sand and gravel.

I reported to Ojukwu that the operation could not be carried through as Forsyth suggested, and he accepted my judgment. But he did not abandon the idea of taking Onitsha by other means, and shortly afterward General Amadi asked me for reinforcements to attack the Onitsha bridgehead by land. The short-term aim was not to retake the town but to dislodge the enemy battalion guarding the bridge. Ojukwu felt that if we could hold that position the Nigerians would have trouble keeping their division supplied.

I told him: "Excellency, I only have two companies available. If you want, I'm ready to include them with the Twelfth Division contingent, but I'd like to command them myself."

Ojukwu conferred with Amadi on the telephone and said I could go ahead. The mission was simple: I had an infantry battalion to my right, another to my left, and I held the center with my two companies. After a heavy preliminary bombardment, my men advanced as planned at eight in the morning and succeeded in storming the enemy lines. It cost us fifty men, a big price, but the federal troops had been dislodged from their bunkers at the entrance to the bridge.

But just as we were overrunning the Nigerians in the central sector, the men in the right-hand battalion began to waver and run, and they were quickly followed by the battalion to our left. I had no authority over either, and no means of contact, so I held my position but stopped the attack because I wasn't crazy enough to try to take the bridge alone. The Nigerians still had a battalion between the bridge and the town, and my two companies were not strong enough to dislodge them or to hold off a counterattack. I waited for Amadi to regroup his battalions and move them back to reinforce my flanks.

Two long hours passed before one of my own captains came stumbling up to me from the rear, breathless and in tears. I had never seen a captain break down so completely. Finally he managed to get a sentence out: "They are all dead, all dead, commander!"

"Who are you talking about?"

"All dead! Colonel Chigbu has killed them."

After patient cross-questioning I eventually got the full story. When the two battalions had broken, the colonel had tried to regroup his retreating men, working himself into a red rage as he did so. It was in that state that he had come across the advanced rear base where I had left my vehicles and drivers, and where my cooks were preparing food for the fighting men at the front. Chigbu stopped and started firing at them like a madman.

I drove straight to the scene, to find fourteen men lying dead. The survivors now emerged from cover and confirmed the story. As we were talking, the colonel himself arrived with an escort and came swaggering up with his hand outstretched. I was already close to boiling point, and asked if it was true that he had killed my men.

"Yes, and I would have done even better if the rest hadn't run away."

"Why?"

"Because they are cowards, deserters."

"But they're my men."

"I know that. But why did they leave the front?"

"Because they were cooking for the men who didn't leave, you damned bastard!"

With that I drew my Colt and took two shots at his epaulets, aiming to shoot them off. I hit the first, but I suppose I was shaking with anger, and my second shot nicked him in the shoulder, I forget which one. His eyes popped and he ran off howling like a dog. None of his bodyguard had moved a muscle.

An hour later Ojukwu sent for me. He was very frosty when I arrived at the State House.

"Is what I hear true, Rolf? That you tried to kill Colonel Chigbu?"

"I don't know about trying to kill him, Excellency, but I wouldn't give a damn if he was dead."

"Really? You think you can kill my officers just like that? You think we haven't had enough killed by the federal forces?"

Ojukwu wasn't happy, but neither was I. I explained the whole business, and he ordered me to return to Madonna 1 and hold myself in readiness. That night I received a second summons to the State House, and this time Ojukwu shook my hand.

"I'm sorry, Rolf, I was misinformed. If somebody had killed men of mine in circumstances like that I think I might have had the same reaction."

A week later I received a clumsily written letter from Colonel Chigbu. It must have been the right shoulder I hit.

"Sir, can you ever forgive me an action that I cannot forgive myself? It was a dreadful misunderstanding and Our

Lord Jesus Christ will punish me for it one day. Please accept my eternal regrets, which will never cease pursuing me."

Behind Chigbu's chastened tone it seemed to me that I glimpsed the shadow of Ojukwu. I never again lent my men to another commander without the express order of the chief of state.

He had to give that order several times. That's war. . . . On August 3, on the eve of his departure for Addis Ababa, Ojukwu told me: "Rolf, the situation in Owerri is critical. The federal troops are only nine kilometers away, and the town could easily fall in two or three days. If that happens during the negotiations I'll be put in a very delicate position. I want you to send your commandos to reinforce the regular army."

I promised to send them, and gave him my word that Owerri would not fall while he was away, though I couldn't help hoping that he would be back soon.

I intended detaching seven companies, but at that time my brigade was holding a thirty-kilometer section of the northern front, so I could not withdraw all my units at once. They had to be replaced by the infantry, and that took time. I sent one company on the same day I saw Ojukwu, and the other six followed next day.

When I reached Owerri I found the town completely evacuated, and a general air of panic. General Wakama's Eleventh Division was responsible for the area, but most of his men were youngsters with no real military training and no combat experience. Obviously I couldn't expect much from that quarter.

The threat to Owerri came from the Nigerian Third Division, and I decided on an immediate operation to loosen their grip. Ojukwu had given me a free hand to use Wakama's division, and I told him to post three of his battalions along the main road occupied by the Nigerians, with instructions to attack at daybreak. That would hold down the bulk of the enemy force while my seven companies attacked them from the rear at three different points.

My commandos moved into position at night, and at six-thirty they expected Wakama's raw recruits to engage the enemy. Nothing happened. Seven o'clock came, then eight o'clock, and at eight-thirty we gave up on them and decided to put in our own attack. It was unplanned, but it would be a bad blow to my men's morale if I took them out without a fight.

Our objective was the village they were using as their main supply base. When we attacked there were about three hundred Nigerian soldiers sitting in the shade eating their breakfast. The front was twenty kilometers away, and they felt perfectly safe. Within five minutes we had the place cleared: one look at the commandos and the federal troops took flight, leaving a trail of toast and marmalade and bacon and eggs.

Ten minutes later we received a bonus when a motor-cycle messenger arrived from their headquarters. Everything had happened so fast that he had no idea that the village had changed hands, and when one of my men flagged him down he took him for a Nigerian. The intercepted message was an important one, concerning a planned enemy offensive against Aba. We reset the trap, and along came a truckload of ammunition. One of my corporals took it back through the bush to our own command post in Owerri.

The raid had been a walkover. We had destroyed their advanced rear base with practically no resistance, captured a mass of files and papers, and cut the federal lines of communication. So a missed chance had been turned to our advantage. On the other hand, if the three Biafran battalions had attacked as planned we could have cracked the enemy front in a day and pushed them back fifty kilometers. I was very annoyed that Wakama had not done his job, and back in Owerri I asked to see the officer commanding the battalion that was supposed to have started the offensive. His name was Lieutenant Colonel Magiyagbe, and he was wary enough to bring his general along.

"Tell me, colonel, how is it that you didn't show yourself when you had strict orders to attack at six-thirty?"

"Well, sir, I wasn't disobeying because my medical officer was ill."

I didn't get it. So he took out his Sandhurst officers' manual and showed me where it said, in black and white, that every active battalion was to be accompanied by a medical officer. So I took a swing at him. I was very much on edge at the time. I was worried about the military situation, and my health was suffering. Anyway, Magiyagbe went off very aggrieved, and although General Amadi didn't say a word I certainly had not made myself a friend.

Next day we were able to measure the effect of our action: the Nigerians had been pushed back fourteen kilometers in spite of the infantry's failure. I used this additional territory to reorganize our defenses into successive lines — for the Eleventh Division. As for my commandos: their role was over.

Ojukwu was pleased to find the situation better than he had hoped on his return from Addis Ababa. He himself had not been so fortunate: certain of Russian and British support, Lagos was refusing any concessions and insisting on total surrender by the "rebels."

At our own level, although the enemy had fallen back in front of Owerri the Nigerians had not stopped the hunt for a breakthrough elsewhere. They had found a gap in our defenses farther south, and were now threatening the sector between Owerri and Aba, previously a very populous region where, instead of a single main road, there was a network of paths and tracks. Seeing that they could no longer hope to reach Owerri directly, they had decided to do it by infiltration.

The Biafrans had never guessed that this terrain could be used by the enemy, and had left it unguarded. That kind of bush country, with its palm trees, giant termitaries, and marshes, was unsuitable for the Nigerian army's light armor. On top of that, their infantry, which was officered by Yorubas but largely manned by Hausas more at home in the broad spaces of their own savannas, detested having to operate in a land of tall grass and jungle where they could not see farther than ten meters.

Those Yoruba officers must have had their work cut out to persuade their men to penetrate that unfamiliar territory. Their success, in fact, put the whole of Biafra in danger. It opened a third front, enabled the enemy to threaten us from two directions once they reached the Aba–Owerri road, and offered them a direct route to Umuahia by way of a disused minor road. As soon as Ojukwu was informed he asked me to reinforce the infantry once again.

The sector seemed quiet when I got there. It was one of the odd facts about this war that before or after a heavy clash the campaign took on a holiday look. I sent three companies and kept four, not wanting to be fully committed without a clear notion of the enemy's intentions. My first elements quickly made contact with the federal forces, who at once halted their advance. But by evening I knew that they had time to seize an important center of communication, the village of Umniede. I ordered the guard to recapture it.

I knew that it was going to be a hard job, because the enemy leadership was backed by Russian advisers, but we attacked in the early morning and the village was in our hands by noon. Although we had incurred heavy losses, that action enabled us to enlarge Aba's defensive perimeter to the northwest.

Next day the enemy, seeing that there was no access through Umniede, discovered another approach farther south by putting a pontoon bridge across the Imo River. That southwest front was like an air cushion — compress it at one point, and it bulged somewhere else. Now the federal forces were cutting the Port Harcourt–Aba road behind our own positions, and threatening to cut off the Biafran force guarding the east bank of the river. The enemy knew that our troops were there, but the Biafrans didn't know yet that the Nigerians had got in above them. A real shambles!

So while I was still supposed to be containing the Umniede front, itself as porous as a sponge, Ojukwu ordered me to hurry south to stop this new intrusion. I went down to examine the situation and, to say the very least, it was confused. There was a general free-for-all. No one knew who was fighting whom, and the advancing Nigerians popped off in all directions: unlike ourselves, they had no need to conserve ammunition. Fortunately they were making no attempt to forge ahead too fast. They fought in the English style, allowing the commissariat time to catch up.

Even so, their offensive was gaining ground, and the situation looked urgent enough to make me send north for eight additional companies out of my total of twenty-four. They went straight into battle. My opposite number, Adekunle, felt sure that he had a breakthrough this time. After failing to find an opening through Owerri and Umniede, it now looked like plain sailing to Aba. I reported to Ojukwu at once. What made things even more critical was that we were almost out of ammunition.

Ojukwu had no confidence in the infantry and thought it incapable of replacing my commandos. The fact is that it was not reacting at all. Its units usually occupied quiet sectors a long way from the front, so three-quarters of its strength was unusable. It was a question of leadership.

Ojukwu gave up worrying about his generals' hurt feelings and put me in charge of Aba's defenses, placing the eighteen thousand men in the sector under my sole command.

My first step was to move my HQ to Aba. I left Emeka to run operations around Umniede, where our troops and theirs were still playing hide-and-seek, and I engaged my nine best companies in the defense of Aba. At the same time I concentrated the infantry closer to where the action was, and used it to construct strongpoints to reinforce our lines of defense. That left very few troops in Aba itself, and not one commando. In town there was just the army chief's empty HQ (he left ten days earlier, when things had started to look dangerous) and my command post. I had installed myself right in the middle, in the residence of the Justice minister, who graciously put it at my disposal now that he himself felt uncomfortable there.

When my men entered Aba on August 15, a good half of the population had already evacuated the town in a panic. I decided to try to create a more cheerful atmosphere by having the nine companies march through Aba with the brigade band playing before going on to the front. Later I heard that de Gaulle had been very displeased with me when he saw my band on TV playing the "Marseillaise" in the streets of the besieged town. He felt that it was a clumsy attempt to commit France. I don't know whether his own initiatives were any less clumsy than mine. At least my own actions were performed without an axe to grind.

For two or three days our own thrusts put a brake on the enemy advance. South of Aba the Nigerians had already reached the main road axis and were occupying a two-kilometer stretch. With their backs to the Imo River they were trying to consolidate this advantage by rebuilding the bridge we had destroyed, so as to be able to bring their supplies direct from Port Harcourt.

There was no concealing our own shortcomings in that

area. Certainly we were receiving more fuel, material, and ammunition than before, but we consumed it so fast that deliveries could barely keep up, especially since we always had to make allowances for mistakes. At that time the supply of Czech weapons via Tanzania was petering out under pressure from the Russians. Our principal supply source was the Ivory Coast, which was a front for France by way of Gabon. Unfortunately there were a lot of hitches: DC4s arrived every night from Abidjan loaded with cases, but most of them contained 82mm mortar shells, which were no good to us with our 81mm mortars.

Biafra had based its independence plans on its rich oil resources; now it was importing its fuel. But not all of it. Since the loss of Port Harcourt the Biafrans had controlled only one oil well, near Ahoada, and they had created a home industry to distil its production. They built their own stills, soldering spiral steel tubing onto old oil drums and connecting it to empty drums. Fires were lit under the full drums, and the oil vapor passed along the tubing, which was wrapped in rags kept constantly water-cooled. This operation was repeated two or three times, except for diesel.

They were an incredible nation. Ibo ingenuity and courage were remarkable in everything they did, and they did nearly everything for themselves. The press was too busy spotlighting the exploits of white "mercenaries" to point out Biafra's self-sufficiency. The Ibos formed a genuine society: not just lawyers and diplomats, but also civil servants, workers, and technicians. And no beggars. A country to be proud of.

15
The Battle
of Aba

General Gowon was determined to capture Aba at all costs. The town had crucial importance for the Lagos government: in capturing it the federal army would demoralize the Biafrans by trimming one corner of the "golden triangle" of Iboland. At the same time the way to Umuahia and Owerri would be wide open. With that one stitch cut, the whole of Biafra would unravel. That explains why the Nigerian chief of state took so much care with the southern offensive, which he entrusted to an ambitious, temperamental character, Colonel Adekunle, nicknamed the "Black Scorpion." Gowon simultaneously used and distrusted him.

Adekunle was twenty-eight years old, fast on his feet, clever, and a good strategist. He would have made a worthy opponent if we had been fighting on equal terms. As an Ibo he had all the resentment and bravery of the turncoat with a need to justify himself. He was popular with his men but unpopular with the journalists, having drawn himself to their attention by executing one of his own men for killing a prisoner, in front of an American TV crew.

For three weeks we were face to face at the gates of Aba. A lot of men were to die in that battle, which was a constant ebb and flow of attack and retreat. We would lose ten kilometers one day to regain them the next, but on the whole the three-steps-forward-two-steps-back routine tended to work in Adekunle's favor. On the morning of August 25 the federal troops found themselves ten kilometers away.

As I drove out to the front all the civilians were coming the other way, mingling with retreating soldiers. It was dark by the time I returned to Aba for a council of war with my officers. We wanted to counterattack but we were out of ammunition, with less than a day's reserve left. Every night we had to meet and unload the incoming plane and send its cargo where it would do most good. The previous night we had received nothing but 105mm shells, which were no use to the infantry. My calculations showed that for every rifle needed at the front there were only three rounds left. No chance of getting any more. Now what?

The situation produced one of the best of all the dirty tricks I played on the Nigerians. I got the idea from a visit to the front line a few days before, at Umniede, when I had been inspecting one of my companies which was dug in under fire. I was stretched out next to a machine gunner who wasn't giving an inch, and feeling pleased with his performance. All of a sudden he was folding his bipod and telling me: "We've got to get away, commander!"

"Why? What's the matter?"

"Didn't you see? Whites!"

I scanned the palm trees in front of us with my binoculars, and caught a glimpse of two white faces. Seeing that I wasn't moving, my machine gunner opened fire again, but he had been cool before and now he was nervous. I asked him some questions afterward, and talked to some other commandos, but there was no getting around the traditional prestige of the white man. It was a sort of neocolonial witchcraft. My people had stayed because I had stayed, but their confidence was seriously undermined.

In that case, I thought, if an intelligent Ibo loses his

nerve because there's a white soldier facing him, then the average Hausa must certainly have the same reaction. For some reason, there were a good many albinos in Biafra. I gave orders to collect every albino in the division; although I didn't yet know how to use them, I wanted them available. I grouped them into one unit about the size of an under-manned company and held them in reserve.

And on August 26, with Aba in danger and no ammuni-tion to defend it, I played this final card. Instead of mount-ing a classic dawn attack with my surviving commandos, I brought up my albinos, after a preliminary artillery bom-bardment to use my 105mm guns and draw the enemy's attention. Then the time came for the albinos to show them-selves. One look, and the federal troops loosed off a wild fusillade and turned tail. We went after them, and at the end of the day we halted thirty-four kilometers from Aba, all because of a half-strength company of imitation white men.

On the subject of the presence of Russian and British mercenaries (or advisers) in the Nigerian camp (there is the same distinction as between a craftsman and a laborer in civilian life): I never captured one alive. England had twenty-five hundred military "helpers" in Nigeria in 1968. Not more than three hundred were attached to the enemy forces, and we had files with their photographs, service records, and notes. They were not organized into self-contained groups but worked as advisers to the federal officers.

In the Umniede and Aba sectors it was not the British we faced but the Russians — three to each company. I got this information from the Yoruba lieutenant questioned by Ojukwu, and it was confirmed by other sources. In any case we had concrete proof: one Russian was killed near Umniede in a Saladin. On him we found letters in Cyrillic characters, identity papers, and an old copy of *Pravda*. He was half burned, his body hanging out of the turret. In his wallet we also found photos of him with a woman and children, presumably his family.

It is hard to say whether the Russians had a different job from that of the British advisers. What I do know is that at Umniede they were often seen reconnoitering from armored scout cars a few hours before an attack, and that their attacks were totally different from the conventional offensives usually launched by the Nigerians. My officers noticed it straightaway. It is true that the Russians, like the Germans, are no beginners in tank warfare. Maybe they had a few Stalingrad veterans left for export. . . .

In spite of all our efforts it was getting harder and harder to contain the enemy attacks. We were getting pulverized on all fronts, with the Nigerians pushing forward everywhere at once, not just at Aba but also at Umniede and Owerri. They kept on coming, and I couldn't stop a lava flow with a team of firemen. According to our intelligence they had thrown three brigades at Aba alone.

After August 16 all my reserves were committed and were taking terrible losses in every sector. That left me with a single battalion around Madonna 1, which I was reluctant to touch. New recruits in our camps had their training period cut to two weeks. I would have liked to be able to keep pace with my losses, but it was impossible with so few replacements left.

My headquarters were still at Aba, which was being bombed by Nigerian planes every day. There were few visitors, and a rising desertion rate among the infantry. Discipline started to suffer in the general confusion, and the high command took stern measures to maintain it. I became personally involved in one sad episode which began on September 2, while I was driving back to Aba from a briefing with Ojukwu.

On the way I met three commandos walking together with

their rifles and kit. They said they were on their way to Owerri. There was something familiar about the sergeant's beaming face, and I asked him about himself. He turned out to be Obu, the man who had come back for me after the ambush when I had found Layla in the back of a Nigerian staff car. In other circumstances I would have been glad to see him, but no one was being sent on leave and I told Emeka to bring them back with us.

Next day a message arrived asking me to hand the three deserters over to the military police. They were to be taken to Umuahia and executed. The order was signed by Effiong. I knew that there had been similar executions a few days before, and there was no denying that they had been caught leaving the front when the fighting was at its heaviest. But I felt that they had been acting out of ignorance, not fear, and refused to hand them over.

Two hours later came another message from Effiong: if I wouldn't let them go I was to have them shot myself. And he sent a photocopy of the verdict, which came from a military tribunal. There was no possibility of asking Ojukwu to make an exception of them.

The three were being held in a garage, and I ordered the doors to be left open and the sentinels to be removed. I couldn't very well warn them to run for it, but I hoped they would have the sense to catch on and return to their unit, where it would be easier to fix something up. But at two in the morning they were still there. I was forced to go in and tell them that they were to be executed next morning, and there was nothing I could do about it.

They heard, but they did not believe. I even sent Father Nweze, our Catholic chaplain, to warn them, but although he stayed all night they would not take their chance and leave. They just laughed. I was their leader, I would not let them die. Finally I went in again to tell them that I'd done all I could, and that now I was putting them back under guard. Perhaps that convinced them. At any rate they made their confessions.

The execution was timed for eight in the morning. I was left with one last course of action — to sacrifice one man, so as to be able to say: "Look, the other two saw him die, that's a good enough lesson." I came into the yard at 7:55, just as the execution squad filled in. It was made up of commandos who had drawn lots overnight. Then Sergeant Obu was brought in. He stopped and saluted when he reached me. He refused a blindfold, took his place against the wall, and listened to the quick orders and the rattle of rifle bolts. He was still looking at me when the shots rang out.

He went first because he held the highest rank and it would have been unjust to kill a private and spare his superior. The look on the faces of my watching commandos told me that the lesson had been learned, and when the second man was marched in I waited till the last second and then stopped the execution.

I sent the two survivors back to the front. Obu had to lie there in his own blood. He was the example. He had to be seen.

One privileged witness to all these scenes was Julia, a German who had made herself a permanent guest at Aba. She had turned up at Madonna 1 in February claiming to be a journalist and carrying a suitcase full of medicine. She took no persuading to tell her story. In Germany she had been engaged to an Ibo studying at the tropical medicine hospital in Hamburg. He had left the country after completing his studies, and Julia had heard nothing more. But then the civil war broke out and she became involved with writing articles, collecting money, and circulating petitions on behalf of Biafra. She had even started a committee to support Biafra. Eventually she had found her way into the country, but was confronted with one of the brutal realities of African life — her fiancé had more than one wife already.

Julia was small and wiry, an intense intellectual of the type who readily link their emotional lives with the defense of great international causes. If she'd been twenty years older it would have been Schweitzer at Lambaréné; twenty years younger, militant Maoism at Vincennes. As it was, at thirty-seven, and whatever her motives, she was one of a growing number of people in Germany who had been shocked by the fate of the Ibos into realizing that humanitarian aid was not enough. Biafra's children could only be saved by saving Biafra itself. I used to lend her transportation and an escort when she asked for them, and she spent her time among hotels, hospitals, and camps, paying several visits to Madonna 1 and spending some time with my commandos on active service. When she met Williams, at the end of August, it was love at first sight. After that she was never far away from him.

Everything was going from bad to worse. Nigerian firepower kept growing, and although I had stepped up my emergency interventions the Biafran infantry was crumbling. Our situation in Aba was practically hopeless. Early in the afternoon of September 4, seeing that my commandos were still blockading the road at Milestone 19, the federal troops decided that if they could not go through us they would go around us. Without using their tanks, they slipped through along various bush trails, and the infantry units guarding the southern outskirts of Aba were taken by surprise. As usual they panicked, and the breach was open.

I was in my HQ in the middle of town with no guards, no staff, not even the cooks. Everybody was committed. The Nigerians started up with mortars, but were too cautious to advance farther. Around four o'clock Adekunle laid down an artillery barrage. In view of our lack of response, it seemed to me that they were bound to catch on that there was nobody to respond, so I decided to shift my HQ back to a prepared base on the northern edge of town.

As I set out to supervise the move, taking Julia with me, a young lieutenant saluted me and asked me for a decision about four Ibo deserters who had been sent back by the enemy and were now prisoners in the garage. This was a very much more serious case than Obu's: they had tried to change sides. I asked what his instructions were in case we had to leave.

"To kill them on the spot, but I need your consent."

"Nothing to do with me. See the military police."

"There's no one left, commander."

Time was pressing, and I didn't take long to decide.

"Right, if those are your orders, now's the time. Go ahead!"

I got into my car, and Julia sat next to me. Before I had started the engine we saw the four Ibos brought out, half naked, in chains, and with battered faces. The soldiers pushed them into the individual holes which had been dug for antiaircraft protection and opened fire, point-blank, under our eyes.

Julia looked at me with an expression of horror mingled with admiration. She didn't say a word. She who used to criticize me so often never said anything to me about that scene. I did not regret the decision I had had to make, but I have tried to forget it.

When I got back I phoned Ojukwu. It had occurred to me that there was one more thing we could try.

"Excellency, the enemy is now a kilometer away from my HQ. Tomorrow morning Aba will fall. I suggest pulling my commandos out from Milestone Nineteen and back into the suburbs. That way we could hold up the federal forces for a few days more."

"OK, Rolf, talk to the army chief."

So I called him. "All right, if you like, but inform the divisional commander."

I couldn't contact the divisional commander at his own HQ, so I drove off to look for him and eventually found him with a couple of girls, getting drunk, not at Aba but farther to the rear, where it was safe. He told me the idea was impossible. If one of his battalions took over at Milestone 19, the enemy would just blow it away like feathers in a gale. He might be right, I thought, but we had to try something. He just dug his heels in. So that's the end of Aba, I told myself, and went off to evacuate my HQ.

On September 5, at seven in the morning, the Nigerian army entered Aba, now an empty town. Meanwhile, on their side, my commandos had pushed several kilometers farther south and were now at Milestone 22, meeting no resistance because the enemy were too busy capturing Aba behind their backs. They had to be warned before they went straight through to Port Harcourt, but the lines were down and the radio link cut, and I had no way of telling them that their retreat was likely to lead to disaster.

I jumped into the Mini-moke and set off into town, where I could hear the rattle of gunfire all round me as the infantry continued to cling on. But I still had half of Aba in front of me, and the federal troops would have control of the road any minute. I drove like a maniac, swerving around the shell holes and the corpses, till on the outskirts of town I almost crashed into another car coming the opposite way at the same speed. By a stroke of luck, it was being driven by one of my captains on his way to ask for orders.

"Aba is under attack," I told him. "Don't fall back directly on the town, but take the road round the Protestant church, behind the water tower. You'll find me near the river north of town. I've had bunkers built there."

With the captain on his way back, I turned back to cross

the town. I was surprised to find the center still full of soldiers, who seemed to have regrouped so as to retreat in good order. They had stopped firing, and watched me go past with no apparent surprise. A bit farther on a group of foot-sloggers opened fire on me. It was bound to happen. Naturally they weren't shooting straight, and when they recognized me they shouted that the Nigerians were inside the town. No, I told them, I'd just come from there. Then the troops I'd passed in the street started setting up machine guns and firing in our direction, and I was forced to concede that I had driven right through the Nigerians.

The battle of Aba was over. I returned to Madonna 1 with only fifty men still standing out of the nine companies which had set out on August 15. On September 6 Ojukwu ordered me to reform my units. As usual we had handed over the fortified positions to the infantry. It took me two weeks to withdraw my men from the Umniede and Owerri fronts, but together with the wounded discharged from hospital and the new recruits graduating from the Madonnas I was just about ready for action again by September 20.

16
The Calm before the Storm

I haven't yet mentioned Felix, my adopted son, who came to me after the Aqwa massacre. The background was this. When my commandos recaptured Umniede the federal troops had to look for another way to Aba. Up to then the region's lack of roads had kept it clear of the war, and so the civilians had stayed quietly in their villages. The Nigerians fell on them like vultures.

I was informed of a massacre at Aqwa, the main center, and the general staff asked me to make the "vandals" pay. The map showed Aqwa in the midst of the bush twelve kilometers from our present location, but it was impossible to withdraw even a single company from the forces who then had their hands full at Umniede.

Soon after that I had word from Ojukwu: "Rolf, you must get help to Aqwa." So I took a section and went there myself. The place was a mortuary — five hundred and twenty-two civilians hacked to death with machetes, pregnant women eviscerated, men's genitals hacked off, mutilations . . . the standard procedure, in fact, and none the less horrible for that. And there was nothing I could do except give instructions for a body count.

Three days afterward the federal army got through the

forest and opened the Aba front. Then came those three weeks of cut and thrust with a constantly shifting front line. In the middle of one offensive news reached me that in an attempt to pierce through our left flank the enemy had wiped out four or five villages. This had to stop. I sent two companies straightaway.

The first village was another Aqwa, except that among the dead women and children was a three-year-old boy, miraculously unhurt, sitting and gazing about him with no visible response. The commandos took him with them, dressed only in a waist-length short and the customary talisman tied around his neck. They brought him to Aba, where the siege was only just beginning, so I was able to find a nurse to look after him and sent my men out looking for clothes for him.

With the town almost empty, they had no trouble finding spare children's clothing, and one man came back with a child's cot painted blue. I had it put next to my own bed. They also brought food, and I noticed that although the boy made no response to anything, he ate and ate without stopping. It was all he knew. There was no laughter, but no tears either. In fact, the Biafran children never seemed to cry, as anybody who went there will confirm. Why, I don't know.

Around eight o'clock that night he got sleepy, resting his head on his arms on the low table. My orderly took him to bed, and when I went to bed at two that morning he was sleeping with his thumb stuck in his mouth. I slept late, as I was very tired, and at seven I was still in bed when I felt something stirring next to me. I turned over and found him burrowing up against me like a little animal. He wasn't used to air-conditioning, and he had crept out of his own bed into mine in search of warmth. Sensing that I was looking at him, he half-opened his eyes, looked up, and went trustingly back to sleep. That was when I fell for him.

From then on I decided to take care of him. When I got up I couldn't get hold of the nurse, so I showered and dressed him myself, and took his hand to show him round my HQ. He was clearly a bit less than three years old, and I decided not to hand him over to an orphanage, where he would be lost among so many refugees. I took my earliest opportunity to inform Ojukwu that I had a small problem.

"What is it this time, Rolf? You've been fighting another of my generals?"

"No, it's simpler than that. I've found a little kid who has lost his parents, and I like him. Will you let me adopt him?"

"Ah, that's better! Yes, all right, if that's what you want."

So the minister of the interior took care of the formalities. There was no way to discover his real name, so because he had been lucky to live I called him Felix, and he was baptized Felix Ojukwu Emeka Steiner. Ojukwu was his god-father. I had a little boy, and I felt lucky too.

The Nigerians seemed satisfied with their victory at Aba. They, too, must have needed a breathing space. Before they fell, my men had inflicted heavy losses, and one heard that all hospitals in the middle west were overflowing with patients. Nevertheless it was an inept decision to halt their offensive when its momentum had looked likely to open all Biafra to invasion. The Biafran general staff used the truce to reinforce our new lines of defense with artillery, and the enemy let it happen. Don't forget, though, that their objective was not a military collapse, which would have exposed the victors to all the daily problems which face an army of occupation. What they wanted was a straightforward surrender resulting from slow strangulation by their blockade.

In the lull I asked Ojukwu for permission to spend a fortnight on leave in Libreville. Since my arrival on December 27, 1967, I had not set foot outside Biafran territory and I was suffering from overwork, lack of sleep, and nervous tension. Ojukwu agreed, but on September 24, the day before I was due to leave, Uli airport was evacuated. The enemy had come to life again and had reached a point twenty kilometers from the landing strip. I had to go to Uturu, the Red Cross airport.

Biafra's contacts with the outside world were not maintained according to any fixed schedule. You had to wait, sometimes for a long time. I had my little boy with me, and we watched the air traffic — two planes from the French Red Cross. The second carried ten tons of powdered milk, which the International Red Cross refused to unload because the consignment had not been cleared with them. Those were the days when the cold war between the French Red Cross and the International Red Cross Committee was at its height, one tending to support Biafra, and the other having tacitly colluded with the Nigerians on more than one occasion. When the pilot found out that I was in the area he came and asked for help. It was simple: I just ordered my own men to unload the plane.

The International Red Cross Committee's representative in Biafra happened to be at the airport at the time. Carl Jaegger was a starchy forty-year-old Swiss, always equipped with jacket and tie, thin gold-rimmed glasses, and a plump respectability that was out of place in Biafra. I swore at him, of course, and the quarrel must have lasted for the next hour. His style put my back up, and mine must have had the same effect on him. The sparks flew every time we met.

In Libreville I rediscovered the sea. It was not the deep Mediterranean blue I had learned to love in Algeria, but through it I was restored to wide horizons, calm, and solitude. And there was the sky, too. At the airport I hired a small private plane, although I hadn't flown one since 1964. I strapped Felix in behind me and we went for a spin over the virgin forest. When I made a few nose dives on clearings, for amusement's sake, the copilot was worried by the vibration.

"This isn't a military plane," he said through gritted teeth. "These machines only have a hundred-and-twenty-horse-power engine!"

But I heard a noise behind me, turned round, and saw Felix shaking with laughter. It was the first time I'd seen him laugh.

From that day on he began to loosen up. When we went out to sea in a rubber dinghy with an outboard motor Felix stood up at the bow like a commanding officer, took all the waves in the face, and was fascinated by everything he saw. When the spray really enveloped him he would shoot a glance at me to find out whether or not to be afraid . . . and he smiled.

We used to go bathing near the Hotel des Cocotiers, and when the water was up to my neck Felix, who was knee-high to a grasshopper, would run down the beach into the water to join me. He couldn't swim, but he came! When the water came up to his mouth he paddled like a puppy and kept on coming! He trusted me.

At Libreville I met several Frenchmen who weren't there on holiday. First there was Colonel Durieux, the French military attaché. As orchestrator of the little clandestine world which revolved around Biafra, it was he who supervised the air-freighting of supplies. Being also — by pure chance, no doubt — the official representative of the French Red Cross, he was better placed than anyone to know how the cargoes were to be distributed. . . .

Another important figure was the mysterious Philippe (that was all the name he had), a discreet, distinguished gentleman who controlled the local network of the Service de Documentation Extérieure et de Contre-Espionnage (SDECE), the French intelligence department. His men sometimes came to Biafra for talks with Ojukwu. Naturally I knew them and approved of their activities in so far as they served the interests of our cause. But I wasn't allowed behind the scenes, although I knew that to them I represented a reliable point of leverage. When the arms from Abidjan had started landing from July onward, the crates had been addressed to me personally. Without actually taking offense over this, Ojukwu had asked me to have the labels altered; I already had a tendency to see my commandos served first, and he did not want to be totally dependent on my goodwill for his army's equipment.

I had a few serious talks with Philippe, in the course of which it was decided to set up a permanent radio link between us. During my absence, Ojukwu had resolved to raise my brigade to divisional status and make me wholly responsible for the Calabar operation. I therefore had to supervise all the logistical problems — control of the airport, arms drops, the provisioning of the expedition — which an operation of that scale involves.

My return to Biafra was to be marked by an intensification of my running battle with the International Red Cross. Shortly afterward the papers reported that an IRC plane had crashed near Port Harcourt with forty Nigerian soldiers on board. Lindt, the secretary-general, claimed that his organization had been forced to carry them, but the press protested bitterly. Then, on October 20, the IRC representative in Biafra had the nerve to complain about my evacuating one of my bodyguard to Libreville after his leg was blown off in a raid. He claimed that it was a political action to remove any of the surrounded Biafrans.

I was exaremely annoyed by all these incidents. The IRC had forty Volvo jeeps, painted white with Red Cross markings, parked on a lot. I told Ojukwu I had plans for them: "Excellency, the International Red Cross is working for the

Nigerians. We have proof. Give me the authority to requisition those vehicles."

"It can't be done, Rolf — not officially. But if you're so
keen, I'll look the other way. . . ."

I sent for Emeka.

"You know the Volvos with those Red Cross Swedes in
charge? Well, I need them!"

He gave me a sardonic grin. "Is that an order,
commander?"

"Not exactly, but Ojukwu says he'll turn a blind eye, and
you can be sure I'll do the same."

A few days later there were eight new vehicles in the
commando pool, freshly painted and perfectly camouflaged.
The painters had used the red cross as a guidemark for the
crossbones in our emblem.

The real, more serious war persisted, and I continued to
lay the groundwork for the Calabar mission. But there had
been trouble between me and General Ifionu for some time,
and this began to undermine my relationship with Ojukwu.

Ifionu was a severe character with a VIP's belly, one of
the few Biafran soldiers to have seen service as an officer
before 1960. Unlike most of his colleagues he held himself
aloof and never raised his voice. With his bulbous eyes,
heavy jowls and grayish, baggy skin, he resembled a snooty
bulldog, and this elder-statesman appearance gave him a
certain amount of pull with Ojukwu. But he didn't like me
much, and was jealous of the trust placed in me by his
leader.

In order to deceive the enemy, my division kept on the
move in its own sector to make the Nigerians think we were
up to something there. But Ifionu, who wasn't in on the
Calabar plan (Ojukwu and I had mentioned it to no one),
thought that we really were finally going to launch the big
push on Onitsha which he himself was unable to bring off,

and which he'd been trying to drag me into for some time. By getting me to attack in his place he would be pulling the chestnuts out of the fire and taking the credit in the event of a victory; in case of a defeat, though, I would carry the can.

I saw his game but couldn't fully counter it. In order for our decoy operation to be credible it had to be aimed somewhere fairly important. South of Onitsha there was a hilltop which was one of the key positions in the enemy defenses, and Ifionu convinced Ojukwu that my men should mount an attack. I was reluctant and out of my sixteen available battalions I committed only one, which I put under Armand's command. For corroboration I sent a weak brigade across the Niger "in support."

Armand took a beating, which was only to be expected. Ifionu was unhappy because I had only committed a single battalion to his operation, and it seemed to him a tiny investment in his vast project. He tried to force Ojukwu to involve me in a larger-scale offensive, and got his permission to have me attack Onitsha from the north. But the more I thought about the Calabar operation the more suicidal the Onitsha mission appeared. Onitsha was defended by Nigeria's best division, well dug in. The suggested direction of attack was over open ground. It would be a shooting gallery with my men for targets. I said no.

Ojukwu insisted. Again I refused, and to prove I meant it I withdrew the brigade I had sent to the middle west. After the bloodshed at Aba I could not take the responsibility for starting the slaughter again, with no chance of success. I felt disappointed and aggrieved, and it was at that moment that I thought for the first time about handing in my resignation.

17
The Fall

There were other pressures to get out of Biafra, and the most serious of these was the change in the attitude of the French toward me. In 1967 the situation seemed clear-cut: France was Biafra's ally, and it was Faulques and Picot, working for Foccard, who had sponsored my arrival. After Faulques's departure France stopped direct aid. Subsequently the new element introduced into the war by the creation and effectiveness of my commandos induced some more or less official representatives of the French government to contact me directly.

The first time, in June, I had a visit from an anonymous messenger. I gave him a clear account of my own point of view, stressing the fact that in January we had been dropped because people in high places had given us up for lost, and yet here we were five months later, not just alive but kicking. So if the flow of aid resumed we would have every chance of strengthening our positions and forcing the enemy to concede our independence. He promised me an early resumption of arms deliveries, and he kept his word. The first French planeload of arms landed at Uli from Gabon on July 13, and military aid kept coming regularly.

In October, during my stay in Libreville, Philippe had

pledged himself to supply me with arms directly, telling me that my division would receive everything necessary to maintain it as a crack unit. All I had to do was send him a list of my requirements. That was very satisfactory, and I was particularly happy about the prospect of receiving up-to-date equipment, because I was working on the Calabar plan at the time.

All the same I was not unaware that other emissaries from Paris were already hard at work trying to replace my position with Ojukwu. I couldn't see why. I had no responsibility for any of our military reverses, and in fact it was the heroism of my commandos which had enabled us to contain the enemy's crushing numerical superiority. But I had caused displeasure in the Elysée, perhaps because my band played the "Marseillaise" that time in Aba, and I sensed the wind changing.

As soon as I returned from Gabon I started to receive crates of ammunition, and crates of champagne, too, daily. This came from Paris by way of Libreville. I didn't understand why, since I never drink champagne, and in any case it seemed far too crude a gesture not to have strings attached.

I soon found out what they were. With the tenth case of champagne a top French civil servant arrived on Philippe's behalf at the Newi command post where I was now installed. He tried to play it casual: "My dear Steiner, now that you and our own services are working hand in hand I can let you know about one of our problems. It's like this: Ojukwu is refusing to transfer part of the nationalized Shell-BP concessions to SAFREP [Société Anonyme du Recherche et Exploitation du Pétrole, the French oil company]."

I didn't see how I could further the French interests in Biafra's oil, and I told him so.

"Make no mistake, you can help. They say you have a lot of influence with Ojukwu."

"I see. In other words, because you've been supplying me with crates of champagne and promising heavy machine guns, I'm supposed to go to Ojukwu and insist on his granting what he's just refused?"

"Your frankness is a little heavy-handed, but basically yes, that is what we expect from you. In a more diplomatic style, of course. . . ."

"Listen, I realize that to pay for our arms Biafra has to give you oil sooner or later. I expect that's why they're called concessions. But it's like this: I am a soldier, and haggling isn't my job."

That seemed to annoy him: "Look, Steiner, you and I are not children. It is another way of serving France, my dear chap, and you have already served her well!"

"Maybe so, but that isn't reason enough to persuade me to try to convince Ojukwu to go back on his decision. A few liters of fizz for a few million tons of oil may be a good deal for you, but not for me."

"You want more?"

"Nothing — and no more talking either. I don't wear a French uniform now. I'm a Biafran. If Ojukwu refused your proposal it was because it wasn't in the best interests of his country, which is also mine. So I can't help you. I'm not the man you need."

"So it seems," he said tersely.

After he left I expected the supply of champagne to dry up, but French diplomacy is tenacious and it didn't stop. Perhaps they just decided to use up the allocation.

I wondered about the meaning of Philippe's approach. SAFREP already owned a tiny share of Biafra's petroleum concessions, dwarfed by the holdings of the British represented by Shell-BP. I knew that Ojukwu has made a secret offer to de Gaulle to pay for French aid by ceding some important zones of exploitation after the war. The principle of the deal was accepted, so if Ojukwu was refusing the

French proposal it was either because the French were being too greedy or because he had received better offers from the Americans. They were keenly interested in African oil, situated so conveniently far from the crisis area of the Middle East. So they didn't want to interfere, not only because they did not want to embarrass their ally, England, but also because it would have been rash to back a side in danger of losing when they could afford to back both at once. And that is what happened. Their representatives occasionally turned up in Umuahia, as I suppose they did in Lagos. Biafra's income came in part from American companies, and so did Nigeria's. We had no illusions about that.

In the range of our alliances, China played a small part (as usual lining up opposite the Soviet Union, which supported Nigeria); Tanzania, Gabon, and the Ivory Coast were mere transit points; Haiti a symbol, and Portugal and South Africa compromising friends. France was our main hope. If French aid, which was vital to our cause, was contingent on my being sacrificed, I was ready to pay the price.

I didn't have long to wait before steps were taken to remind me that I was becoming an undesirable. "They" had made use of me, and now that I no longer suited I was to be replaced. The candidate appeared on October 31. He was around fifty, military-looking, with a white shirt, khaki trousers, and something of a Mussolini strut. He wore a plastic canteen filled with whiskey at his belt, he was dead drunk, and he called himself Colonel Reps.

I received him in the mess at Newi, together with Armand and a few high-ranking Biafran officers. It was embarrassing for Biafran colonels to see a French colonel in that condition, but there was nothing I could do about it, and in any case there was no other way in which he could have brought off his spectacular entrance: "Steiner, you're a cunt, de Gaulle is a cunt, Ojukwu is a cunt, and you don't know how to fight!"

If he had said that in private, all right, we still might have worked something out, but in front of the Biafran officers I was paralyzed.

"With the morons you've got," he went on, "it isn't guns you need but bows and arrows. And if I, Reps, were in your place I'd take ten thousand savages, spears and all, and we'd be in Lagos like that!" Grunting and wheezing he reached for his briefcase and took out a letter of introduction addressed to the Biafran chief of state, written on notepaper with the heading of the President of the Republic and signed by General de Gaulle. I took him to a room on the first floor to continue the conversation by ourselves, but things didn't go any better.

"Listen, Steiner, don't be a dope. You know very well that you're here because France sent you. Right, you've had your little game, you've cut your caper for the press, and you've made your bid. You think you're clever? A cunt, you are. A coward! What the hell are you doing here? You're on your backside, and there's fighting at the front! Why don't you pick up a gun?"

"Because it's not my role now."

"Oh, it's not your role? And you're supposed to be a legionnaire?"

I could barely prevent myself from taking a swing at him.

"All right, that's enough for now. If this is all you have to tell me I want you out of my HQ."

"Oh, sorry," he said, "there's another thing. If you don't give me your division and settle it with Ojukwu, it's simple — no more aid!"

"Tell that to His Excellency, he's my chief. And now get out."

Later on I often wondered where Colonel Reps came from. He hadn't been sent by Foccard, because his people were in Libreville and I knew them. Yet the letter really was signed by de Gaulle. I never did find out exactly whom he was working for, but it was common knowledge that the French intelligence services in Africa were split into at least two factions which were always sniping at each other.

As soon as he was out of Newi I sent for my secretary and dictated my letter of resignation. The official pretext was my falling out with Ifionu, but the true reason was my gut feeling that, rightly or wrongly, I had lost the confidence of the French secret services, and it was best for me to leave before de Gaulle turned off the tap.

When Ojukwu received my letter at the State House he sent for me. He was his usual calm self, but rather cool, as he told me: "Rolf, I cannot accept. Of course you're a European, as people keep reminding me at the moment. But I who am black must remain with my people. And do not forget that we are both Biafrans."

"Excellency, what did Reps mean by saying that if it came to the point he could stop the aid?"

"I am not to be blackmailed so easily," Ojukwu said.

So I withdrew my resignation. It was November 1. We never mentioned Ifionu.

I went back to Newi and never saw Reps again. Next day at Uli, no plane came. The following day, again no plane. No champagne, no munitions. After four days with no messenger from Libreville I had to yield to the facts: he had not been bluffing.

I felt dog-tired, worn down by a combination of the incompetence and playboy attitudes of many of the Biafran officers, the neocolonial pressures from the French, and a kind of moral and physical erosion. Another thing preyed on my mind: some Frenchmen I really respected, Faulques and Picot, had devoted themselves body and soul to Biafra before dropping out of the game and never coming back. Could I succeed where they had failed? The war was dragging on, more people were dying, and where was it getting us?

On November 6 there was to be a meeting of divisional commanders at the State House under the chairmanship of the chief of state. Once more we were supposed to debate the advisability of an attack on Onitsha. I made up my mind that I would submit my resignation again, with all the generals present, and this time Ojukwu would be unable to refuse.

Things were accelerated by an incident involving some new white recruits. I did not know any of them, and put them on trial with my commandos. Two of them were French, one Belgian, and one Irish; all were young and under the impression that they were still in the Congo. Every night they went to Uli to scrounge petrol from the planes. The airport commander, Ojukwu's own uncle, warned them that they were abusing their uniforms and that they had no right to go onto the airstrip. The little bastards couldn't think of a better solution than drawing their revolvers and making the commander undress and crawl naked along the airstrip.

Next day at breakfast, as soon as I heard what had happened, I had them all confined to barracks. They hadn't killed anybody, but they had humiliated the commander, and to anyone who knows the Ibo temperament that is worse still.

Ojukwu sent a message to me demanding their punishment. I told him that I was for expelling them, and he replied: "All right, they will be expelled." He was furious about the treatment of his uncle and summoned the guilty parties to the State House on the day we were due to discuss the Onitsha question.

Ojukwu's office was a huge room on the first floor, furnished with a conference table in black marble surrounded by upholstered leather chairs. I arrived in driving rain at three in the afternoon of November 6, parked my car, and saluted the generals waiting outside. The door of the audi-

ence chamber on the ground floor was open, and I had time
to see my four white recruits waiting inside.

Effiong and Ifionu were already there, and the other
generals joined us. Ojukwu came in, visibly tense and tired.
We got up, and he shook hands all around as usual. He was
about to speak when I said: "Excuse me, Your Excellency —"

"Yes, Rolf?"

"I want to renew my resignation for personal reasons."

Ojukwu paused, then in a sad, gentle voice he said:
"Colonel Steiner, you have been with us for a long time. You
have done a tremendous job. Your moral qualities and
military experience have been of immense service to the
nation. . . ." He stopped, and looked at me with unusual
intensity. "I am certain that as a Biafran patriot you wish
to be of further service. I regret your decision but I cannot
oppose your wishes. I accept your resignation."

There was a long astonished silence. The air conditioner
droned on. The rain pattered against the window panes. I
felt very moved, and so did Ojukwu, I believe. I thought I
saw Ifionu smile. Then I stood up, gave a soldier's salute,
and walked out.

I was bitter and on edge. Deep down I would have liked him
to refuse my resignation, but I realized what was at stake.
At least things were clear now: my good standing with
SDECE had been due to my influence on Ojukwu; now I
was refusing to make use of that influence, or perhaps I
was losing it because of Ifionu, so SDECE and the other
secret outfits whose job was to observe and use me were
throwing me overboard without a lifebelt. There was no
point in trying to fix the blame somewhere. If the arms
shipments were to start again, I had to go.

All these thoughts were passing through my mind as I
left the room and went downstairs past the audience chamber. Seeing my four recruits still waiting there I decided to
talk to them. There was an armed guard by the open door,

and any visitor, black or white, who went into the chamber was supposed to be searched. It was standard practice. But not me. Yet now this guard barred my way and started patting my pockets. He's new, I thought, he doesn't know me. I removed his hands. He gave me an arrogant stare and this time thrust his hands into my pockets. I gave him a hefty shove; he reached for my throat and I hit him.

Some more guards now appeared and I was seized, pinioned, and pushed into a side room. They didn't dare to hit me, but it felt as if a world was coming apart. Baffled, I waited for the bad dream to end and for Ojukwu to come and put everything right. My head was seething with the decision to leave, humiliation and shame. . . .

From the alcove where I was being held, surrounded by guards, I heard Ojukwu come down. He did not come to me but entered the audience chamber, where I heard him address the waiting recruits in a harsh voice quite unlike his usual controlled tone. "I've had enough of you!" he shouted. "You can bugger off!" And there was a sound of something breaking. I heard later that it was a Chinese vase.

When I asked to return to Newi a guard captain told me: "Sorry, sir, our orders are to take you straight to the airport. You are to fly out tonight."

"Whose orders?"

"Military security, sir."

I wanted to collect my belongings. And there was Felix.

"Sorry, sir, we can't let you."

I was stunned. It could only be a misunderstanding. I could not and still cannot believe that Ojukwu himself had ordered my expulsion. At nightfall we left for Uli. I was allowed to drive my car, but with an MP captain sitting next to me. The other whites followed in a Land Rover, and there was an escort in front and behind. It looked normal enough, and the civilians were waving as usual as we drove by, but my heart was sinking and my mouth tasted of ashes.

At Uli the airstrip was deserted. Once again there had been no plane that day. The escort left after passing on instructions to the airport police. They were not to let us leave, and we were to be put on the first plane for Libreville. They were reinforced soon afterward by an MP company.

We were shut in the waiting room in silence, with only the flies for company. They lumped me together with the deportees, who were wondering why I was with them, and I myself was left with a number of questions. Why was Ojukwu abandoning me? Something had happened behind my back which I was unable to understand. Reason of state it might be, but once my resignation had been tendered and accepted, what had I done that justified my expulsion? What was I guilty of? The scuffle with the guard was too trivial. There had been worse actions on my part. The behavior of the whites? Not my responsibility. Obviously several things had combined — Ifionu, Reps, the aid question — and my new men's behavior had been the last straw.

We spent the night there and the following day, forbidden to leave or even to make a phone call. In the evening two Red Cross planes, after unloading their tins of milk, refused to take us. I tried to keep my dignity. Did Ojukwu know what was going on? I wasn't sure, and I wanted to find out, but the captain in charge repeated that he was forbidden to let me make a phone call. His men kept pointing their Thompsons at us. Some policemen arrived and removed my badges, the Biafran one, the commando insignia. It was a nightmare.

It wasn't usual to leave the chief of state freely and find oneself under arrest a few moments later. Had they been carrying out Ojukwu's orders correctly? Was he being deceived? Had he been misinformed about me? Against all appearances I still trusted him. I tried several times to make the guards take me to Ojukwu's uncle, so that he could pass on a message, but the airport commander was still hopping mad about his maltreatment by the four whites and he refused to see me. Perhaps he thought that I was responsible for what had happened and that Ojukwu was punishing me for the same reason. The vicious circle was complete.

On the third day the monotony was broken in the morning by federal MIGs bombing the airport. In the afternoon I had some welcome visitors, a stunned Emeka, accompanied by my own staff. Coco, Major Coco of the Fourteenth, was there too, uneasy and unhappy, and old Wilson. Their presence brought back the ten extraordinary months we had survived together, and other images came in their wake — Obu, Layla, Norbiato, all those people dead, my friends . . . My staff were dumbfounded; they could no more understand the reasons for my disgrace than I could. I had the impression that if I had ordered them to march on the State House right then they would have done it.

I asked for news about my son, and told Emeka to put him in the care of the bishop of Umuahia, together with the nurse.

Even today it is hard to recall what passed through my mind during those painful hours. I refused to accept the evidence of my senses, and found myself in such a dazed, numbed condition that instead of fighting back I let everything go. My life was coming apart and losing its meaning. I was so disgusted, so disillusioned, that I stopped caring what happened to me.

In combat I am clearheaded and decisive, but injustice disarms me. Later on I was to suffer a lot more physical pain, but I do not believe I have ever felt so torn apart as I did in those hours in which I found myself alone and betrayed. I only had one thought — to get out as soon as possible.

But there was one other thing I couldn't help noticing. During the three nights at Uli airport, I had not seen a single planeload of arms flown in. They were still being held up in Libreville. That proved that there really was a link between the acceptance of my resignation, the stoppage of arms shipments, and my diplomatic repudiation. I understood Ojukwu's dilemma. I should have taken Reps seriously.

In the continued absence of shipments from Libreville, on the evening of the third day the airfield commander requisitioned a Biafran aircraft with an Ibo crew. But they refused to take us, claiming that once we were on board we would be looking for revenge and might overpower them and hijack the plane to Lagos. To reassure them, I myself made the suggestion that we should be handcuffed, and it was done. We boarded the plane like criminals being deported.

An hour later, Libreville restored my honor and my liberty.

III
THE SUDAN

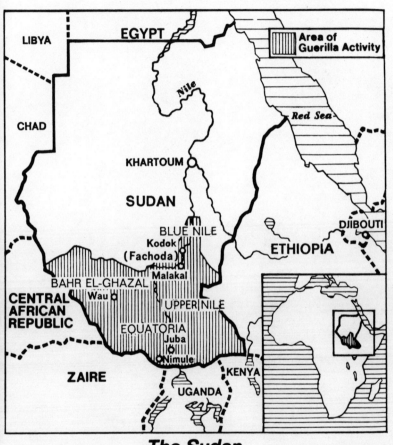

The Sudan

18

Between
Two Wars

I had hoped to drop out of sight in Europe. Instead I found that wherever I went — Rome, Frankfurt, Lisbon, Zurich — I had been preceded by tall stories, mainly in the yellow press, which had turned me into a "personality." I had enjoyed being popular in Biafra, where I felt I'd done something to deserve it, but my new reputation was baseless and artificial, and I didn't like it at all. But I quickly realized that it brought me one advantage. As an unknown my prospects had been limited; this temporary fame gave me the opportunity to organize my future. Quite unintentionally, I had reached a level of independence which gave me the chance of realizing my dreams while remaining true to my principles.

For the moment I could take my time looking around for something useful and interesting to do. I had recovered from the mental beating inflicted by my departure from Biafra, and I had become too involved with the Ibos to cut myself off overnight. In Lisbon I got in touch with the head of the Biafran missions in Europe, Dr. Mojekwu, who rather shamefacedly passed on the chief of state's regrets for the brutality of my expulsion and told me that the men responsible had been punished. He unofficially confirmed my ideas about the background to Ojukwu's decision, but asked me to continue to help Biafra by working for the cause in Europe, where various Catholic movements were busy collecting money. The centers of Biafran activity were Lisbon, Geneva, and Rome, so I did a lot of traveling.

Three weeks previously, on the day after my arrival in Libreville, I had been surprised to find Roy, my star white Biafran recruit, following in my footsteps. With his usual bounce he explained that now that I had left Biafra he was no longer interested in remaining, and that he had asked Ojukwu's aide-de-camp for permission to rejoin me. I had a soldier's affection for the Scots hothead, in spite of his gangster qualities, and so I thanked him for his gesture of solidarity. He tested my gratitude straightaway by asking for a loan.

Roy suggested a trip to South Africa, but Pretoria refused me a visa at the last minute. The north of Africa might accuse us of working for European neocolonialism, but the south saw us as potential agents of revolutionary Marxism! So we went to Rhodesia instead. We were tourists, of course, but the local Special Branch didn't know that, and we were followed wherever we went. I stuck it out for a while, then told Roy that I was flying to Zurich.

"Hey, that's great," he told me. "I've got business there — it's where I bank my money. Mind if I come with you?"

On our first night in Zurich I took him out on the town, and found myself paying for his drinks and even for the nightclub hostess he decided to sleep with. But before retiring with her he kept up a stream of anecdotes about his heroic past — gold smuggling in the Congo, looting the banks in Stanleyville, massacres here and there. . . . He had one story about when he and his friends located a gold storage depot near the Congo-Sudan border and wiped out a score of Congolese guards so as to leave no traces. This was a thug's life, not a soldier's, and I felt disgusted. To clear the air I jokingly asked him: "Roy, we're friends now, aren't we? Tell me, if the Nigerians had offered you a million dollars to kill me in Biafra, would you have done it?"

He was in no state to think twice. "Even for ten thousand," he rapped back. I didn't take him seriously and went off to bed, leaving him with his girl.

While I was in Zurich I was approached by all sorts of people, ranging from sensation-seekers to scroungers — and even politicians. One or two mercenary leaders looked me up, expecting to find a brother in arms.

Some offers of work came in too. The first came from a group of associates of Modibo Keita, formerly prime minister of Mali, who was being held prisoner in some out-of-the-way place in the Sahara after one of the upwards of a hundred coups which have happened in Africa since 1960. It wouldn't be very difficult to free him in a commando raid, and they suggested operating out of a base in Conakry, in Guinea. I could name my own price. I refused because I didn't know enough about Modibo Keita to judge whether or not I would be furthering the cause of Africa.

The second offer came from Tshombe's secretary, a beautiful platinum blond German of about twenty-six, who was living in Munich. When the Katangan leader's plane was hijacked over the Balearics on June 30, 1967, she had been sharing his Madrid apartment. He had left two million dollars in cash and she was willing to spend all of it on getting him released. She didn't care how. That was how she put it to me, having read the papers and concluding that I would want to talk money. I turned her down, for the same reason as before, and found out later on that she had made the same offer to a couple of Congo veterans who had conned her out of half a million dollars and skipped to South America.

Some of the other propositions were too far-fetched or too small-scale to be worth mentioning, but they all cast me as a sort of Third World strong-arm man, a Skorzeny of the tropics, or a knight of the African bush looking for just causes. I had to make the best of my new image. After all, in 1964 who would have come looking for Staff Sergeant Steiner, Rolf, who had left the Legion by the back door, to offer him millions of francs for the rescue of Y or Z?

In the meantime there was an odd episode which started with a phone call from a Nigerian colonel. He had a particular request to make and wanted me to meet him at his hotel in two days' time.

I accepted out of curiosity, and when I arrived he introduced me to three of his fellow countrymen — according to him, members of the government. I had taken no special precautions before going to meet them — they could not risk abducting me, any more than I could make any attempt on them. That is the rule of coexistence in Switzerland, where so many opposing factions live side by side.

Their proposition was simple: "Do you remember Captain Norbiato?"

"I remember him very well. You killed him."

"You're wrong. He is alive; he was only wounded."

And they were ready to free him if I would help. They told me that my commandos were still loyal to me personally, that I had been badly treated by Ojukwu, and that if my commandos turned against him the "rebellion" would be finished. They were banking on my holding a grudge. All I saw was a chance of getting Norbiato out. But first I wanted proof that he really was still alive, and they agreed to provide it. We met again a week later, and they produced a note dated January 1: "Rolf, I'm in good health. Help me to get out of here. Giorgio."

It was definitely Norbiato's handwriting; I had to seem to be playing their game: "Okay, but your idea of using the commandos won't work. I can't be sure of having all the officers behind me now. But what I can do, if you agree, is to give you my personal evaluation of what must be done to win the war quickly."

They were interested, but suspicious, and they asked for guarantees. I suggested giving them the information in two installments — the first straight off, the second when Norbiato was out — but I made a bad mistake by deliberately understating the manning level of Biafra's operational units. What I should have realized was that there was no chance of giving damaging information, because the Nigerians would know the facts already through their own spy networks. But when this occurred to me it was already too late to correct myself. On the eighth I received a telex: "Meet January 11 for second installment. All well. Package will be delivered." The eleventh came and went, then the twelfth, and I phoned the colonel, to be told that he was in Lagos.

Not having any great reason to trust me in the first place, the Nigerians had realized that I was trying to con them. Norbiato was probably killed.

Weeks went by, and at last the ideal cause felt its way toward me in the shape of two big, timid men totally unlike the hustlers I usually met. They wanted to tell me about southern Sudan, and did not ask for anything because they thought they could not afford me. Their country was poor and unknown, and there wasn't a drop of oil beneath the ground. Through an accident of history and the calculations of the old colonial powers, their people, who were black and Catholic, had found themselves shut inside the same frontiers as the Arabs of Khartoum and were suffering under their crushing domination. Their Church had abandoned them, the world ignored them, and with no funds to keep them going their hopes had run very low.

They themselves had been keenly following every twist and turn of the Biafran war for independence, which they saw as an example to follow and a model to imitate. My name had cropped up in their scrutiny, and they felt that they needed someone like me.

I was very tempted, but after my experience in Biafra I did not want to commit myself without a thorough briefing on the situation in the Sudan. In Rome I met some Catholic missionaries who had been forcibly repatriated six years earlier. They knew the country well, but suggested that the man who could bring me up to date was a Father Gypkens, in Frankfurt.

I went to see him in the house in a Frankfurt suburb where he occupied a single room furnished with a wooden bed and a big desk crowded with files and papers. On the walls an ebony crucifix and a Bantu mask recalled his missionary past in Africa. Now he was aging and soft-spoken, but his harmless manner concealed a fighting spirit. It was he who three years before had received the first reports from some Italian missionaries on the crimes committed by the Sudanese Muslims against the black Christians and animists of the southern provinces. In the space of a few years about five hundred thousand had been massacred while the world looked the other way. Their information had shocked him into realizing that his faith could only be defended by total commitment.

In 1966 Gypkens had set up the *Forderungsgesellschaft Afrika* — the FGA — and bravely committed it to the side of Biafra. He was quite ready to take risks, and among the supplies he had dispatched to Ojukwu were a planeload of inflatable boats for navigating the Niger, medicines, several tons of copper tubing, machine tools and diving gear, not to mention powdered milk.

"For two years now we have had sizeable sums of money available," he explained. "But we don't know how best to

use them for the Sudanese because we haven't found anybody to go there and report on what's going on."

The missionaries had been expelled in 1962, and the few
journalists who had visited the country since then had not
been far enough into the interior for the FGA's purposes.
The information sent by the southern Sudanese themselves
had been scrappy and often inaccurate, so not only did the
FGA have no idea how to go about delivering and distributing aid, it didn't even know what was really needed. And
meanwhile its budget was growing by about a million marks
a year.

I told Gypkens that if all he wanted was somebody to
look, listen, and learn, I was his man. He accepted grate-
fully, and I fully expected him to pick up the phone and
book me onto the next flight for Kampala. Since there could
be no question of obtaining a visa from Khartoum, I would
have to enter the Sudan in secret, across the border with
Uganda. But Father Gypkens explained that the FGA did
not organize their operations themselves, but used a sort
of general manager who looked after the purchase, ship-
ment, and distribution of all the aid they sent.

It made sense to use a businessman's know-how instead
of relying on the hit-or-miss amateurism of so many other
charity organizations, but when Gypkens handed me a letter
of introduction to his manager I was startled to read the
name Gregor Klemann on the envelope. I had come across
the name before. He had been a rag and bone man; then
he had moved into scrap metal, after that into property, and
at thirty-five he had carved himself a comfortable place in
the business world.

The Biafran war had enabled him to enter an even more
lucrative field of activity — relief work. There he had had a
chance to show his paces, organizing, buying, transporting,
and distributing, and he had done remarkably well. On
Biafra alone his commission on the aid collected for starv-

ing children after the press campaigns in Europe had made him a millionaire.

I knew that Klemann had done two or three stretches in prison, but Gypkens did not, and I decided against telling him. I didn't want to kick up the kind of scandal that might harm the Biafran cause.

I told my two timid visitors that I would be paying their country a visit, and they promised to inform the man in charge of their resistance movement, whom they called General Taffeng. A few days before leaving I asked Klemann to get me some staff maps of the Sudan, which were only obtainable in London, a radio transmitter, and a rifle — not a military weapon but a Winchester, to be used for hunting and, if need be, for self-defense.

Roy insisted on coming with me, since he was broke and in need of excitement. I agreed to put him on the FGA payroll but there was a last-minute hitch, because under his real name Roy was forbidden to enter any African country. He had been one of the mercenaries surrounded at Bukavu in 1967, and they had all had to promise never to set foot in Africa again before they were released. I had no time to wait for him, and asked Klemann to try to get him a fresh passport so that he could join me later.

19
First Visit to
the South
Sudan

The Ugandan general staff organized a special reception in my honor. Standing on a green lawn by the shore of Lake Victoria, surrounded by his own officers and a few representatives of the southern Sudanese resistance, was a giant of a man. He came toward me, gave me a thump on the back, and roared. "General Idi Amin, glad to meet you, Colonel Steiner!"

The former heavyweight champion of the Ninth Rifles had not lost his punch. At that time he was commander-in-chief of the Ugandan army, a post bestowed on him by President Milton Obote in gratitude for his help in overthrowing the president's predecessor. His future seemed assured and already the men and women around him were treating him with a mixture of fear and admiration.

"The general is a great friend of our cause," one of the southern Sudanese quietly said. Amin overheard him, and came up to us.

"Ah, Colonel Steiner, you are a great soldier too! You commanded the biggest black army a white man has ever led. I tell you, not even the British! Now, do you know why I love my brothers in the south Sudan? It is because I belong to the Kakwa tribe myself. I was born there and my family is still living there. We are of the same people. There can never be a frontier between us and them."

I found out how right he was when, instead of having to creep past frontier posts and risk my neck in the wilds, I was landed by a small hired plane on a grass airstrip where a reception committee was waiting. I had entered the Sudan without knowing it. In fact, although movement was not easy, it was not the government soldiers who caused difficulties. Over an area of 55,000 square kilometers — about the same size as France — ninety percent of the country was "off limits" to the Arabs, who controlled only a few checkpoints along the main lines of communication. If they ventured into the bush, they never came out.

There was no Arab administration, and even the frontier posts were now held by the Anyanyas, so that away from the roads there was something like total security, and even on the roads the guerrillas could feel reasonably safe, with the Arab checkpoints well over a day's march apart. I had better clear up the common confusions by explaining that Anyanya is not the name of a tribe or of the southern Sudanese people as a whole. In the language of the equatorial tribes it is the name of a lightning poison secreted by one of the local snakes. The freedom fighters of the eastern Nile area had taken this formidable name, just as the young warriors of the Congo had called themselves after the lion — Simba. Gradually the name Anyanya came to be applied to the members of the Liberation Front.

It was hard to tell who were soldiers and who civilians among the fifty men in my escort. Very few wore uniforms, most were barefooted, and their arms were an assortment of rusty German carbines, antique Brandt machine guns, hunting rifles, and old Kalashnikovs taken from the routed Simba groups who escaped from the Congo in 1964. Those who were too poor or too clumsy for firearms carried bows and spears.

We were passing through rolling country crisscrossed by trails cut through very thick vegetation. At a height of around eight hundred to a thousand meters above sea level the temperature was quite bearable. It was June, the start of the rainy season, and razor-sharp grass grew in profusion to a height of up to two meters. The route plan took me through a number of villages so as to show me the conditions of life for the refugees here. No one knew the real numbers of the population of the south Sudan, but four million seemed to be the best guess. The state of war prevailing for the past ten years had shattered their traditional way of life, and hundreds of thousands of people had left their homes for the frontier region, where they lived a wretched life in widely separated camps.

We reached the seat of the provisional government after a three-day march. It was here that I was to be introduced to General Taffeng. I knew that he had been one of the few "natives" to be promoted to second lieutenant by the British just before they left in 1955. On January 1, 1956, the day the Arabs took power, Taffeng had been arrested and held in jail in Khartoum for two years without any reason being given. After his release he took to the bush and started training black guerrillas. The Arabs took him for a rebel — very well, a rebel he would become, the father, in fact, of the revolutionary movement.

The "capital" was a refugee camp of several thousand people, situated near a river and sheltered by enormous trees. The whole population turned out for our meeting, grouped into concentric circles with women, children, and the aged on the outside, and ministers, officers, and VIPs making up the inner ring. Taffeng was not a politician in the Western sense but a charismatic leader and a venerated symbol. He was tall and thin, like all Nilotics, and looked younger than his sixty-five years. The energy of his gaze won his fellow countrymen over before he opened his mouth.

After exchanging the usual compliments with General Taffeng, I spent two days at his camp before leaving again with the minister of the interior and his staff to continue my tour of the villages. These were usually small in size, because the bush could not support larger concentrations. The walls of the round huts were of woven grass and branches, the roofs of thatch. The inhabitants fed themselves by making clearings too small to be spotted from the air and planting cassava. Each village kept back part of the crop for the Anyanyas who defended them.

Every thirty or forty kilometers there was a village where you could pick up supplies and spend the night. A section of the escort went three hours ahead to pitch camp, and officials ate and slept along with the rest. The food was boiled cassava with bits of fish or game.

I would have liked to evaluate the Anyanyas' military capabilities, but it wasn't possible. They didn't even bother to post sentries overnight, because it would be unthinkable for any Arab soldier to venture so far onto their own ground. The real enemies here were the insects, particularly the mosquitoes. Without a mosquito net the only way to escape them was to sleep by the fire, where a kind of wood was burned which produced a thick, pleasant smoke that drove them off.

The Anyanyas were champion marchers. They never seemed to tire, and I was hard pressed to keep up. Later, on my second visit, I walked them off their feet, but I admit that on my first visit I suffered a little through blisters until my feet got used to my boots again. In any case I had very little inclination to feel sorry for myself as long as we went on moving through such enchanted country, with animals so plentiful that it was often like strolling through a huge open-air zoo. After Biafra I also noticed a significant absence: there were no throngs of feasting vultures.

The ants were another story. Here they had a species with

the habit of invading human dwellings in their millions and covering the occupants with a living skin. Once in place they all start biting at once. The Anyanyas showed me how to prevent their invasions by scattering ashes all around the camp. These ants dislike fire, and even cold ashes are enough to deter them.

I was on a fact-finding mission, so I applied myself to observation. I saw how the population lived. A delegate of the Red Cross would have been dead within a week in that bush. There was nothing there, not even the most ordinary objects which seem to have invaded the entire planet — not a plastic bucket, a box of matches, a nylon shirt nor even a bottle of Coca Cola. Nine-tenths of the people went naked. They lived like animals, and the women didn't even have pots to cook in. Instead, the men hammered bits of sheet metal into usable shapes.

The sanitary situation was a disaster. There were no doctors, and on the whole of the trip I met only one nurse, who was called "Doctor" because he had once worked in the hospital at Juba. He showed me his bag. All it contained were a few dirty syringes and empty tubes of ointment. At every stop we were surrounded by children suffering from all the chronic illnesses of malnutrition, none of them sad or cheerful, just indifferent. Deprived of medical care, the people had reverted — if it had ever been abandoned — to the remedies of the local witch doctors, based on roots and herbs, some of them effective but most of them harmful.

At the root of the situation lay the refusal of the Anyanyas to be dominated by the Arabs. This was a historic conflict, since the north is populated by Arabized Muslims, the south by animist Nilotics. Peoples of the sands and those of the forests: here were the basic elements of the Ibo-Hausa opposition which, under different names, has always divided the peoples artificially united into states by colonial powers ignorant of the natural frontier where bush meets savanna.

This conflict of races and customs had been complicated in the course of time by religious antagonism between the Islamic north and the more and more Christianized south, but here the resemblance to the Biafran war ends. In the country of the Ibos the missionaries had been followed by trade, culture, and wealth — the whole range, in fact, of Western civilization. In the Sudan the incurable poverty of the soil had prevented any such development, and I soon discovered that the human material here was on a level well below what I had come to expect in Biafra.

Previously they had lived in a subsistence culture in villages built close to the lines of communication. Their houses had been burned by the Arabs, and if they did not run they were killed, so they had left, taking nothing with them. But the losses had been spiritual as well as material. Before the Arab aggression seventeen percent of the southern Sudanese had been Catholics, the rest animists, with a very few Protestants and Muslims. The Catholic population, although very small, had constituted the core of all the social structures and practically the sole force for progress. General Taffeng himself was a Catholic. So the exodus of the priests, black as well as white, decreed by the Sudanese government in 1962 had come as a crushing blow. Yet the people had retained the Catholic faith and ritual, even without priests, and the number of Christians had actually increased.

My mission lasted six weeks. We traveled about forty kilometers a day, with three weekends' rest, and I acquired some idea of what the southern Sudanese needed. From information provided by tribal chiefs the number of refugees surviving in the bush of Equatoria Province could be estimated at around three hundred thousand, and of those who had crossed the frontier, at around two hundred thousand. They were homeless, sick, and starving. In my report to the FGA I intended to indicate how the necessary food should be distributed, but first it had to be delivered, so before leaving I began the construction of a landing strip on a flat, well-sheltered spot not too far from the frontier. When I left, hundreds of southern Sudanese were working to clear the bush with their bare hands. Tools were something else they lacked. I had never seen a people so destitute.

I was not there as a military observer, and had not spoken to anybody competent to provide information on that subject, but I could not help noticing that the Anyanyas were almost weaponless and no good at using the arms they did have. To complete this account, I should add that I did not realize then that the southern Sudanese had internal rivalries of their own. They gave me the impression of being a united people with a single leader, General Taffeng, as had been the people of Biafra. Later I was to find that although he was respected, there were deep-seated and historic differences among the tribes. I noticed nothing, and nobody saw fit to inform me.

Back in Kampala I found a telegram from Germany, signed by Klemann, informing me that Roy was in Nairobi and would be arriving any time. He had been supplied with a brand-new British passport. I had to leave for Cologne, but I sent Roy into the Sudan to supervise the completion of the airstrip and to start organizing teams to distribute food and medicine to the villages.

In the plane back to Europe I rehearsed my report. In my opinion the errors committed in Biafra could be avoided. First, the southern Sudanese had to have doctors, nurses, and welfare workers. The best medicines in the world were no good without someone to explain how to use them. Also there was no point in spending vast sums on airlifting food from Europe or America when it was possible and far more practical to buy their traditional food on the Ugandan market.

Feeding them need not be hard or expensive. For instance, these people had previously owned small cattle herds, while now they had none. This was savanna country and, except in the tsetse fly areas, why not buy cattle in Uganda and share them out among the new villages? Their milk would feed the children, who were incapable of absorbing powdered milk because they tended to lack the necessary enzymes to digest it.

I was suggesting setting up a buying office to organize supplies from Uganda. It would buy goods wholesale, ship them across the frontier by truck, and distribute them to the tribal chiefs. Among the southern Sudanese this is not a hereditary office: the chief is elected, and goes on being elected only as long as he proves reliable. For a ton of food to benefit the entire group it only needed to be given to the chief for allocation.

In Kampala President Milton Obote disapproved of my plans, fearing that an organization of that kind operating from his own territory would harm his relations with Khartoum. Idi Amin was for helping the Anyanya struggle but didn't much care about truckloads of blankets! Still, he was sharp enough to spot that my plans could well lead to diversified forms of aid more in tune with his own aims. At that time, although not all-powerful, he was strong enough to order his army to turn a blind eye to my harmless smuggling service.

My main aim was to make sure that the FGA's aid went where it counted most. Taffeng had other ideas, though, and tried to work on my feelings a few days before my departure. "Medicines and food are all very well," he told me, "but we are much more interested in you than in anything else your government might send — apart from arms, that is. . . ."

He wanted me to make a commitment, but I was tired of fighting and besides I still wanted to serve Biafra. All the same, I promised General Taffeng that the FGA would start backing relief work for his people.

The first hitch came as soon as I arrived back: Klemann had been asked by some of his associates to stop using me because I had objected to airlifting supplies from the port of Mombasa to the south Sudan. I had found that the job could be done more economically by rail, which meant a loss for those sharks who usually supplied their own planes, at a price. I gave Gypkens the comparative figures and he naturally went for the cheaper solution.

Three or four days later Gregor Klemann phoned to tell me that Roy had alleged in a message from the Sudan that I had exceeded my mission by meddling in military matters. I was supposed to have offered arms to Taffeng, who had given me command of his army. This was ridiculous, and I reminded Klemann that neither Taffeng nor I had that kind of cash available, and we weren't likely to get credit from people like himself.

I hung up on him, but I was perplexed, not about Klemann's activities, but Roy's. Then I started to fit some facts together — his insistence on following me, his remark in the Zurich nightclub, that second passport which came so easily. Now I came to think of it, perhaps he had already been working for British intelligence in Biafra. I ought to have suspected him a lot sooner and seen that his fascination with danger led him in search of stronger and stronger sensations — the cruelty, double-dealing, and treachery which, far more than the love of money, make up the real mercenary.

In the following weeks I had a flood of invitations from all sorts of organizations to speak about the situation in the south Sudan, and I did a lot of public speaking, sometimes with monks, even bishops, in the audience. I always emphasized the call for the missionaries to return and to remain loyal to the religion they themselves had taught. Failing that, the departed black priests at least should return, in spite of Vatican opposition. Doctors and nurses, too: like the priests, they would be working under difficulties, and their safety could not be guaranteed, but that was their job and they had chosen it.

I added that the southern Sudanese also needed political help, which would mean circulating documents on the true state of the region, as well as financial help to buy arms. My principles had not changed: to combat the effects of war, it had to be actively discouraged. These people were being attacked; they must defend themselves. I developed the same themes in my report, and awaited a reply from Father Gypkens, but he refused to see me and had me informed that the FGA was unable to follow up my suggestions.

My reaction was violent. It was scandalous to have aroused so many hopes only to dash them again, and unthinkable to repudiate so much distress. Father Gypkens was an old man with bad advisers, and I could not change his mind; instead I redoubled my activities in Cologne, Frankfurt, and Bonn, campaigning for help wherever I could find a sympathetc hearing. Yet at the end of September 1969 I had to accept that the FGA categorically refused my program.

I had given my word to General Taffeng on behalf of the FGA. I decided to keep it on behalf of myself, and to put myself at the disposal of the South Sudan Liberation Front for the space of a year. Not wanting to arrive empty-handed, I got in touch with a Biafra-Sudan action committee which had already helped the Ibos a lot and whose founders were ready to mobilize public opinion about the troubles in south Sudan. When I got in touch with their head office I was surprised to find an old acquaintance — Julia, now an influential member of the committee, and a hard and dedicated worker. Their financial resources were limited, but thanks to Julia and her associates I was able to collect a ton of medical supplies, a generating set, tools, a hydraulic pump, a chicken incubator, and a hundred kilos of tomato seed and dispatch them to Kampala, where the archbishop agreed to store them till I came to collect.

I had no preconceived ideas about the kind of help I would provide to the southern Sudanese, except that I intended to improve their condition. My immediate plan was to start an experimental farm and organize a system of distribution for the food produced or imported, so to begin with, I had to retrain myself as an agronomist. Before drawing up a list of requirements I did a lot of serious reading to prepare myself for this next phase of my life, which I saw as a new kind of battle. That meant learning the techniques which would make my work effective, so I studied gardening, agriculture and in particular poultry farming, tropical diseases, natural fertilizers, the role of vitamins, animal hygiene and feeding. I reviewed everything which could be produced on a farm in that climate. One of the objectives was to augment the daily protein ration, one of the main dietary deficiencies. There was also the question of getting hold of the necessary piping to go with the water pump. There was plenty of water, but it would have to be taken where it was needed. My aptitude for mechanics was helpful here. Of the fifty-odd books I took with me, fifteen were concerned with cultivation, with soil analysis, irrigation, grafting, fertilizer use, pest control.

By the end of October I was ready to leave again for Kampala. It looked as if it would be an absorbing experiment, this attempt to make the population self-supporting. I saw it as a civilian role, but of course I also expected to have a few small military questions to settle. I was not naïve enough to believe that my conversion to the ploughshare could be absolute.

20
Living among
the Anyanyas

Some Anyanya representatives were waiting for me when I flew into Kampala and they took me to their headquarters where Taffeng was waiting. He thanked me for keeping my word, and seemed pleased that I had come back. He also had some more news about Roy. My Scots "colleague" had been telling Taffeng that I was an impostor, that I had never been a soldier, and that although I had fooled Ojukwu by claiming to be a colonel I wasn't even capable of commanding a platoon. He had also offered, on behalf of the British, to set up a military camp in the Sudan and to provide arms and ammunition for the Anyanyas. Coming from a country which was a known supporter of Khartoum, the offer had seemed so suspicious to Taffeng that he had reserved his reply.

I had to lay my hands on Roy to find out what he was up to, and although I couldn't find out where he was living he saved me a lot of trouble by walking in while I was talking to some southern Sudanese officials a couple of days later. He must have thought that I was right out of the game, because the blood drained from his face and he stood in the doorway unable to move.

Not seeing any reason to involve our hosts in our troubles,

I spoke in French: "Look, Roy, I can tell when there's something wrong, and I want to know what kind of dirty tricks you've been playing. I do know you've been working on something completely different from the job I gave you. You force me to poke my nose into your business."

He had lost his usual grin. In the mood I was in, he knew that I would stop at nothing, so he started to talk. His story was that he was working for Blunden, who was in Kampala with instructions to get rid of the Ugandan president because the British didn't like his policies. The training camp for the Anyanyas in the Sudan had been Blunden's idea: it would give him a free hand to train a unit for a coup against Obote under cover of helping the southern Sudanese. I had been the thin end of their wedge, and I didn't like it.

"Right. You're going to take me to your boss."

At the Apollo Hotel the desk clerk told us that Mr. Blunden had left for Addis Ababa the previous day but was expected back in a few days' time.

I had one strong hold over Roy — he was a prohibited visitor in Africa — so we made a deal. The hotel staff must have seen him around with Blunden. They would swallow his story when we returned next day to say that he had received a phone call instructing him to look for some papers that Blunden had left behind. They would let Roy into Blunden's room, and he would remove all the documents we found there. If things worked out he could be on the plane to London by tomorrow evening.

Everything went as planned, and I went back to Anyanya HQ with the secret dossier under my arm. As we sifted the papers the first thing that caught our eyes was a receipt for one hundred thousand pounds sterling, signed Bataringaya, who was Obote's own minister of the interior. We also found the radio code used by Steve Blunden for his transmissions to London, and the code for his exchanges with Roy, enabling us to decipher a stack of carbon copies which left us in no doubt about the nature of the operation he had in mind. These messages had been sent from the British embassy in Uganda.

When I asked Roy about the receipt he denied all knowledge of it, but said that Blunden claimed to have the Ugandan minister of the interior in his pocket, bought and paid for. We went through the rest of the dossier, then I had it sent back to the Apollo Hotel, with my card and my thanks. All I had learned agreed with what Taffeng had told me. I asked Roy to write down all he knew about the plot, and when he had finished his deposition I asked a final question. Who did they have in mind to replace Obote — Bataringaya?

"No. Idi Amin."

I was certain that Amin wasn't in on the coup, not because it was beyond his ambitions but because the southern Sudanese representative in Kampala, Serafino Swaka, his own brother-in-law, had confided that the ebullient general did not yet feel ready to assume supreme responsibility.

"You're wrong," I told Roy. "Idi Amin wouldn't have gone for it."

"Maybe. But he would have been obliged to take over because as army commander he would have had to establish order."

"And is that the only reason you thought of him?"

"No. Blunden told me that the British knew Idi Amin well and he was their first choice because he was the stupidest and the easiest to manipulate."

Events were later to prove who was the most stupid.

I had Roy driven to the airport and the following day I sent his confession to Idi Amin, with a request to pass it on to Obote.

After this interlude I returned to the Sudan by truck,

taking with me the material which had been forwarded by the archbishop of Kampala. On the previous trip I had found an ideal location for my first experimental farm, close to a river, with more than a meter's depth of black soil never before cultivated. My hope was to locate similar spots for the time when a second generation of production centers was hived off from the first, which I called Fort Amory. It was a day's march from the frontier.

My intentions were civilian, but my military subconscious was unwilling to let itself be taken by surprise, so I had my camp protected by strongpoints and an advance warning system. For this I was able to rely on the Anyanyas. General Taffeng had provided eight hundred of them for my protection. I began to build the farm on November 1, 1969. Counting the civilian population, the volunteers sent by various chiefs, and my own Anyanyas, I had a work force of above five thousand. They made short work of clearing the land.

The idea was to make a modest start. Our first objective was to rear chicks in the incubator and dispatch them in batches of five hundred to each village, so that the inhabitants could rear their own from then on.

The first twenty chicks to emerge from the incubator became my friends. When I called them they would come and perch on my head and shoulders. Perhaps I made a more presentable mother than the machine which hatched them. . . .

After three months the first generation of Fort Amory chickens was ready. Our losses amounted no more than ten percent. On February 1 my people set out on foot into the surrounding villages, with bamboo cages, each holding twenty plump pullets, on their heads. The tribal chiefs had been warned, and I had advised them to make sure that their original stock stayed out of the pot. My working capital eventually stabilized at four thousand chicks. When they reached twelve weeks I had them distributed to the villages. In nine months I produced just over fifty thousand.

In the first quarter I concentrated exclusively on the farm. By daybreak I was in the garden where I had made my first tomato sowing. The African sun is too strong for new plants, and they had to be sheltered by day beneath a kind of straw awning. It was a simple but delicate task which forcibly reminded the workers of their power over the products of the soil and made them pleased with the results obtained. I had left a demonstration patch which withered in spite of frequent watering, while the others became green and healthy.

With the first crop we had too many tomatoes and had to sell some of them on the Kampala market! The money went toward buying three bikes, some kitchen utensils, and a sewing machine for the collective.

Dozens of sick people arrived at Fort Amory every day and slept on the ground outside my hut. Those who could not walk came on other men's backs, or by stretcher. We had to put them somewhere, and that gave me the idea of building a hospital. I had not lost all hope of doctors becoming available someday, and they might as well find reasonable working conditions when they did come.

My men cleared a broad area which was to contain a number of small separate buildings. There was no problem about roofing these with straw, but the walls had to be solid and the forest had nothing to offer but wood and grass. After a lot of searching we discovered deposits of clay mud, and I made a test brick by hand, let it dry, and put it in the fire. When it came out with the right consistency and color, we were able to go ahead. Following the instructions in the book, I made a mold using wood from the medicine crates. I had brought a book on the use of clay, as I had foreseen a possible need for pots, tiles, guttering, and various other receptacles in commercial quantities.

I called on childhood memories of Bavarian peasants making charcoal, and to bake the bricks I built the same kind of fire, digging a hole in the ground, and putting in a layer of bricks, a layer of wood, another layer of bricks and so on, before covering the lot with earth. It burned underground for three or four days, the wood smoldered away, and usable bricks emerged. To make more brick ovens I had teams of men scouring the forest for dry wood, others cutting it to the right length, others finding the clay and molding the bricks.

Poultry, tomatoes, and brick-making now took up most of my daily life, but my biggest problem was the sick, who presented a comprehensive range of the illnesses native to these latitudes. I had given myself a rapid course in nursing, but it didn't always help. Malaria I could manage: I had a microscope, and I could take a blood sample and compare it with the color pictures in the textbooks. The virus was easy to identify. Venereal diseases were not difficult either for a former legionnaire. As long as it was just a question of giving streptomycin injections or handing out aspirin and Paludrine, I could handle it. When I could not identify the trouble I sent the patient to an American gynecologist, Dr. Jackson, who ran a hospital twenty kilometers across the Ugandan border.

I had ten marks in my pocket when I reached Kampala, but I had no living expenses at all, and in order to be closer to the southern Sudanese I deliberately cut my needs to a minimum. If you wanted to help these people you had to live, sleep, and eat like them, even if it meant going hungry. My one luxury was electricity. We ran a pump off the generator, and after filtering the river water was pure. I also had a small radio transmitter, an American GRC 9. I had brought only essential clothes — jeans and sandals — and I never wore a uniform throughout my stay. My food came from the people, who gave me cassava, flour, and salt, to which I added the meat I brought back from hunting trips.

That bucolic existence was not unpleasant. All the same, the war was not far off. Early in January I was informed that a mass grave had just been discovered in a village near Juba, about forty kilometers from the farm. A big pit had been dug, the bodies of the murdered civilians thrown in and covered with earth, and trucks had been driven back and forth to level it all out. When I went to make an inspection I found the village burned to the ground and a total of four hundred and thirty-two bodies when the pit was cleared. It wasn't the first time I had seen the enemy's handiwork. A week after my arrival they had attacked a hamlet eighty kilometers north of Fort Amory, near the main road, where the Anyanyas were thin on the ground. My men had been alerted and had found five civilians nailed up alive on trees and left to die by the men from Khartoum.

Fort Amory and its farms now stretched over an area of ten square kilometers. By February there were nearly ten thousand people living off the land where previously there had been virgin forest. They were quite different from the Biafrans, and lacked the education, method, and imagination of the Ibos, although they did possess other qualities.

I was no commander, and I had no aide, but I struck up a friendship with Taffeng's minister of the interior, Eliaba Surur, who had had a bungalow built out of our bricks on the other side of the village. We consulted each other on all the important questions that cropped up, and I relied on him as I had done on Emeka. He was about forty, shrewd and quiet spoken, educated by the missionaries in Juba, then spotted by the British while working as a schoolteacher and appointed a provincial chief in the days of the colonial administration. He had been in the ranks of the South Sudan Liberation Front ever since independence, and was in charge of planning and education as well as the interior, because qualified men were rare.

Himself a father of three, Surur was very preoccupied by the need to educate the children who swarmed around. This was another void left by the missionaries, and at first we considered filling it by recruiting southern Sudanese students in Nairobi or Kampala, even in London and Rome. But we realized that it made no sense to decapitate tomorrow's elite, and that if they were to be used, it should be as officers. Instead we combed Fort Amory and the principal villages for all the young men who could read and write, and Surur worked out a necessarily accelerated teacher training course. Soon every camp had its own teacher, sometimes as young as seventeen. It wasn't perfect, but it was better than nothing.

The big problem for the southern Sudanese was the feuding among different clans inside their own ranks. A few months after my arrival two thousand Anyanyas of two northern tribes had fought each other for three days, and hundreds of men were killed. My own men became restless and informed me that the time had come to make war on the Morus. Why the Morus? Because my men were Baris. What did the Morus and the Baris have against each other? They were old enemies.

This was elementary but logical. Nevertheless I wanted to know more and I consulted Eliaba Surur. He told me that the Baris had belonged to a great people of central Africa which had kept its own special protein stock — the Morus. Over the centuries they had eaten almost the entire tribe. I decided to try to make a settlement.

Naturally none of the Baris wanted to come with me on that kind of mission, and in any case their presence would be liable to get us massacred on sight. As a white man, though, I was accepted and respected by all the tribes. The devaluation of the white man in Africa which had begun in the Congo had not yet spread to the Sudan.

My Bari Anyanyas escorted me for two days up to the mountains which marked off the territory of the Morus, and I covered the last few kilometers on my own. I didn't know just where to find them, so it was the Morus who saw me first. They held me at gunpoint for half an hour till a young English-speaking officer arrived. Word spreads fast in Africa: he knew who I was when I introduced myself.

The Moru leader was a fierce-looking lieutenant colonel of thirty. We had a lengthy discussion in which I under-lined the stupidity of killing each other off when all the Anyanyas had the common aim of liberating their people. These crazy rivalries were playing the Arab game, I insisted, and I must have convinced him because he agreed to make peace. I immediately wrote a message to my waiting escort in the foothills, and when my men arrived the commander of my guard shook hands with the lieutenant colonel. That is how the Morus and Baris were reconciled.

Once Fort Amory was a going concern I wanted to get to know the south Sudan. I needed to gauge the dimensions of the conflict and to understand the protagonists, friend and foe.

First I visited the Kukus, a tribe of the Bari clan which inhabits the west bank of the Nile. I hoped to be able to advise them on making better use of their region's natural resources. Water is plentiful in Equatoria Province, and huge fish can be caught in streams three meters wide, as well as in the Nile, which is also peopled by thousands of hippos that come out of the water every evening. The alluvial banks should therefore have been producing meat or crops, and if properly managed, both. Of course the river people fished and hunted on their own account but it had never occurred to them to increase their catch to sell or give to others. I saw things on a bigger scale. I wanted dried fish and meat as reserves for our army and as produce to sell on the Congo markets.

Mila, the Kuku chief, fell in with my plans and we succeeded in increasing our food reserves considerably. Yet the wise old man was not satisfied, and he finally got round to telling me why:

"The Anyanyas, sir. They take our poultry, and our girls. . . ."

Bows and arrows were useless against the Anyanyas' guns, and something had to be done. They were supposed to be guerrillas, not bandits. For the moment there was so little pressure from the Arabs here that they could throw their weight around in the villages. Mila told me that some of them were even taking charge of the part of the crop meant for their fellow-soldiers, so that some had too much food and others too little. Instead of living with the people, the Anyanyas were living on their backs.

My first move was to take twenty rifles from my own escort and hand them over to the Kukus. I gave Mila a chit appointing him military chief of his region, and made him a gift of my Winchester to seal his authority. Next I came to a decision which runs counter to Mao Tse-tung's famous saying that a guerrilla must be in the people as a fish is in water. Here in this primitive country where a nobody with a rifle felt more important than the greatest tribal chief, it was impossible. I therefore set up buffer zones around the inhabited regions, which were forbidden to the military. An Anyanya who entered without permission could be arrested, and in case of any resistance I armed the villages for self-defense by disarming as many soldiers as necessary.

With equilibrium reestablished, things went back to normal and there were a lot fewer clashes than before. All the chiefs of Equatoria Province spontaneously adopted the same system, so the different elements among the people could now concentrate on resisting the common enemy. They became unified by neutralizing each other.

21
Tribalism and the Israelis

Unifying the tribes had become my principal concern. Without it neither war nor peace could be made. I felt no popular unanimity here, as I had among the Ibos. Certainly they had their hatred of the Arabs in common, but that cement crumbled as soon as the old demons of tribal warfare stirred.

Without even telling me, Taffeng had given me an official title: commander of the regular army of Anyedi, which was the historic name chosen to designate the future Republic of the South Sudan. I had not come to make war, but I accepted in order to be able to help with matters of military organization. Holding authority in the army would enable me to consolidate national unity, but I lacked the cadres to provide a good infrastructure: the officers already serving had their own habits, some of them pretty untidy, and I couldn't sweep them away overnight. However, I soon adapted to the situation and they quickly accepted my authority. As I already knew from past experience, Africans are generous with their loyalty to the people they respect.

Once the Anyanyas were operating under a single command it was my intention to create small five-man groups in all sectors; for more important operations I would keep in reserve strike companies to be stationed near strategic points. Naturally all units would be a mixture of different tribes. This seemed a sensible as well as a cautious plan. The army obviously needed strengthening before it could be sent into action. To harass the enemy too soon would only lead to reinforcements being sent. For the moment there could be no question of making commandos out of these men, but merely of inculcating a minimum of discipline. Later on, when the Anyedi Liberation Front had forty thousand seasoned men available, I or my successor could launch them simultaneously against the enemy rear, and so liberate the greater part of the south Sudan. In order to protect our own preparations I ordered the main roads to be mined but I stayed on the defensive.

Thanks to my own explorations I now knew the enemy strength as well as the opposing general. About eight thousand men: Yei, their command post in Equatoria, was held by two battalions; Juba, their commander in chief's HQ, had a garrison of about thirty-five hundred men, counting a few black Muslim or renegade families. I knew the exact location of their combat positions, which could be observed with binoculars from a hilltop a kilometer away from the road.

All in all the enemy establishment was fairly thin, limited to posts located along road axes and sometimes fifty kilometers apart. In each there was a company, or at most a battalion, quartered in abandoned missions or guesthouses. They all lived in perfect peace, most of them not even defended by trenches, foxholes, or so much as a string of barbed wire. That made them so very vulnerable that I couldn't watch them lounging about without thinking that the day we started our own Vietnam they would be blown away.

So it was straightforward on their side. On our side, though, apart from the tribal feuds and lack of discipline in the Anyanya ranks, I soon realized that Taffeng was involved in a silent but ruthless struggle for power with one of his own lieutenants. He was the true charismatic leader, but his rival, Joseph Lagu, had the Israeli arms on his side.

Lagu was a man of about thirty, one of those timid, taciturn people whose ambition is expressed by too much arrogance toward subordinates and too much obsequiousness toward anyone they stand to gain from. Educated in Khartoum, he had been promoted to second lieutenant in 1963 and sent south at the outbreak of the rebellion, when he had gone over to Taffeng. In 1967 the Israeli ambassador in Kampala had asked for a young officer to be sent to Tel Aviv to plead his country's case and he had stayed for eight months.

Their interest in the south Sudan was anything but humanitarian. By stirring up trouble in the area they wanted to pin down a fraction of the Arab potential: it meant that many less soldiers to bother them in Sinai. Lagu was easily led. Once back in his own country he became an agent of the Israelis, and when they started parachuting arms in September 1969 it was to Lagu's camp, not Taffeng's. For some time Taffeng knew nothing about this mess, and I took it upon myself to inform him.

Lagu's response to Taffeng's summons was that he was too busy to travel, but Taffeng might come to see him if he wanted. The situation was turning sour, so I arranged a meeting of all the Anyanya leaders in Kampala under the supervision of General Idi Amin, with the purpose of reaching an agreement on the leadership of the Liberation Front. So that I should not seem to be interfering in their affairs, I stayed away.

On his return, a downhearted Taffeng told me that Lagu was arguing that it was time for younger men to take over. The tribal chiefs were hesitant, but the younger ones were for him because they were eager to fight and he had the

weapons. Not wanting to widen the divisions in the movement, I advised the general to agree. One title more or less
would change nothing essential: when the time came, it
would be Taffeng the Anyanyas obeyed.

So Lagu became the nominal leader and handed out all
the gifts from Israel. His HQ became known as the company
stores. Some came my way, and my men were equipped
with arms captured from the Arabs during the Six Day
War — 120mm mortars, British repeating rifles, Russian
grenades and mines in plenty, and Brand light machine
guns in industrial quantities.

Personally I had no contact with the Israeli advisers who
came in from Kampala and spent five to six weeks at a time
at Lagu's command post at Owing-Kibul. There were four
of them, led by a Colonel John, and they included a doctor,
a radio specialist, and an infantry instructor. We had no
wish to meet because they claimed that I was working for
the West Germans and wanted Lagu to get rid of me. Lagu
was clever enough to see that the Israelis were pursuing
their own interests, while Taffeng, he, and I were working
for the southern Sudanese. Then, too, he needed me. The
Israelis had never sent him any guerrilla warfare instructors;
what they supplied were experts in conventional warfare of
the kind appropriate to their own country and their own
modern armaments, but totally unfitted for fighting in
Africa.

Although my most pugnacious Anyanyas were straining
at the leash, I reckoned that we were not yet ready. On their
side the Arabs were not looking for trouble. The Khartoum
government was short of cash and no longer as optimistic
about a military reconquest as it had been a few years
before. Bombing was safe enough, though, and their raids
were haphazard, conducted against any target — a hut, a
village, a herd. The aircraft they used were twin-engined

Antonovs or small British-made Provost training jets, dropping Russian 50-kilo bombs. All we had for protection were 35mm ack-ack cannon. The Israelis never provided any artillery, and besides it was impossible to move heavy material through the forest.

More demoralizing for the civilian population were the first Arab heliported operations, when five big Russian choppers would land a hundred paras near an isolated village at dawn. They massacred everything that moved and left again without waiting for our counterattacks. All we could do was to bury the dead and tend the wounded, and since we never did get hold of a doctor this job fell to me. One day they bombed a school and I had a twelve-year-old girl brought to me with her arm almost off. I did my best for her, and at least stopped gangrene setting in. Later, during my trial, I was blamed for looking after her. The Khartoum judges resented their soldiers' work being sabotaged.

The only military operation which can be credited to my account was forced upon me, as I shall explain. And it so happened that it was witnessed by the same journalist, David Robinson, who was with me when he got a bullet through his pants outside Onitsha. Journalists were rare in the south Sudan, but Robinson was stubborn, and found me during one of my few visits to Kampala. He asked me how to get into the Sudan, and I told him to consult Lagu.

"That's what I did last month, but he said there was nothing he could do unless I got permission from the Israeli embassy in Kampala. It seemed a bit strange. Still, I went, and they refused."

Robinson had persisted, and his search had taken him to Tel Aviv, where Golda Meir sent him to the war ministry, which passed him on to various other services. The final office told him to go back to Kampala, where in fact nothing had been arranged. I promised to take him into the Sudan myself.

By then I had shifted my HQ thirty kilometers beyond Fort Amory to an abandoned plantation by the road I was having built. Eight kilometers away was the village of Kajo-Kaji, occupied by an Arab company. They knew that there were Anyanyas in their sector but took good care not to come out looking. Our spies informed us that they had a few light machine guns and two 60mm mortars, so attacking them would have been easy enough, but pointless.

The Arabs themselves broke this balance, in the following circumstances. Reverting to my old habits, I had gathered four companies around my HQ under my direct command and put them through intensive training. On July 7, 1970, I was forced to send some of these men into action when I heard that the Arabs were holding about two hundred southern Sudanese women prisoners in the Kajo-Kaji sector. This was intolerable, and I decided to combine their rescue with a training mission by sending a young lieutenant to work his way around the village and free the women.

It should have been a simple map-and-compass march, but what I did not know was that the Arabs had a forward post several hundred meters out. Since it was four in the morning and raining heavily, and the position was not marked on their map, one of my sections walked smack into it. The sentries shone searchlights around, and my men fell flat. Now the young Kampala student in charge of them was stuck: if his map was wrong he might be only just outside Kajo-Kaji, and he had no way of knowing whether the sentries had gone back to sleep or given the alarm.

The sun rose, and still the young student (his name was William Allau) could not make up his mind. He had strung his men out in a line, but with no idea of attacking, while retreat was getting more impossible by the minute as the light improved. At nine o'clock a woman left the post to fetch water, and walked straight toward the Anyanyas, who were concealed in two-foot-high grass. They were forced to grab her and hold her in case she reported their presence, but of course the sentries came looking for her. This time Allau's men opened fire and so exposed their presence. If they had been more experienced they would have retreated; as it was, the Arabs sent some men to attack them from the rear, and only then did they try to retreat, blazing away with all their weapons and firing on the post with a bazooka. The huts caught fire and the whole post burned down. About thirty men were killed. I was told later in Khartoum that it was the biggest victory the Anyanyas had ever won!

On our own side we had lost five men, two dead and three missing, including William Allau. We waited for several days before deciding that they must have been liquidated, the usual fate of black prisoners, made even more likely by the beating the government forces had taken.

I was sorry about Allau, who was a promising young man. On the other hand the incident had shown that the Anyanyas were nearly ready: they had put up a good fight and withdrawn efficiently and with relatively few casualties.

Because of racial tensions between the communities, there were no light-skinned people left in the villages of the south Sudan. They were either gone or dead. Yet one night I was informed by one of my adjutants that an Arab civilian making his way from Juba toward the frontier had fallen into the hands of an Anyanya patrol and was being held prisoner in Fort Amory. He was to be hanged in the market-place at dawn next day.

In theory it had nothing to do with me, but I could not allow such a mistake to be made. I went straight to see Eliaba Surur and asked him to send for Lieutenant Colonel

James, the sector commander. I wanted to tell him that since I was there because Arabs were killing blacks I couldn't be expected to accept their execution of an Arab without even knowing whether he was guilty. If the man was hanged I would take up arms against the Anyanyas; otherwise I wanted him released and sent to me.

At seven o'clock two guards brought the Arab to me, still rubbing his bruised wrists which had just been untied. He was scared stiff, and threw himself at my feet to ask for protection. I discovered that his name was Mohammed and that he was an Egyptian national, thirty-two years old, and had been working in Juba as a tailor for the past twelve years. Since Juba was one of the few places where an Arab was safe, I asked why he had left, and he told me that he had been in trouble with the police after having a bit too much to drink and making insulting remarks about Nasser and Numeiry. If he had stayed he could have been beaten to death, or he might have rotted in jail for years. When he got the opportunity to escape he had decided to take the chance of freedom, hoping to set up in business in Uganda.

James told me that it was his fellow Anyanya officers who had demanded the death penalty, so I got them together for a talk, and the outcome was that I took Mohammed under my own protection. I promised him an escort to Uganda if he still wanted to go, but told him that there was plenty of work here if he stayed. For a start, my men needed uniforms. When he chose to stay, the minister of the interior found him a sewing machine and I installed him in the village of Morta, with a promise to keep him fed until he started making money, and to pay him two chickens for every pair of trousers he turned out for my men.

Mohammed didn't take long to get on his feet. He was unpopular at first because of his race, but when his story got around the villagers were proud that he was ready to trust them, and the deputy chief even allowed him one of his daughters in marriage on credit, which was very unusual. After that, each time I asked after Mohammed I was told that he was doing fine. He had a wife and a job, he went fishing . . . he was integrated!

I had spent a whole year in the south Sudan, and had kept my contract with myself. My impression was fair: the Anyanyas now had an infrastructure which was not perfect but which worked. Out of groups of armed bands I had made soldiers. The whole territory was now divided up into military zones and covered by radio. Thirty thousand men made up a regular army and ten thousand were involved in guerrilla operations. They had learned Vietnam-style techniques of communication, information, and sabotage, and each village had its own defense system which could be used just as well against an Arab offensive as against robbers, who had become rare. Lagu could now think in terms of larger-scale actions in the near future, such as attacks on vital objectives in the north — bridges on the Nile, dams, or railway lines. It was even becoming feasible to carry the subversive war to Khartoum.

So when I balanced the accounts for my visit I had good cause to feel satisfied: I had set the machinery going, and the organization would remain. All the same, although you can improve the soil and make it produce tomatoes, poultry, tobacco, or bricks, men's nature is not so easily altered, and here I was slightly disappointed. Tribal feuds, lack of discipline, and a general absence of drive and urgency did not encourage me to stay on. I did not feel drawn to dig deep into my reserves for these people as I had in Biafra. And I also did not want to commit myself fully in this war because I had realized that there was no military solution. We could keep harassing the enemy and dissuade him from attacking, but once out of the bush we would have had to fight a conventional war for which we did not have the means.

A year after my arrival I said my farewells to everybody and decided not to return. The Sudan had been an interlude, and my place was elsewhere. On October 4, 1970, I boarded an army car sent by Idi Amin and went back to Kampala, intending to go straight on to Europe.

22
Hijacked
to Khartoum

A top Ugandan minister was waiting for me in a luxury office in the Parliament Building built by the British for the comfort of their successors.

"Colonel Steiner," he said, "we have not forgotten the service you did us by warning us of the plot organized against us by the British secret services. Would you like to help us once again?"

"If I can."

"I won't beat about the bush with you, colonel, since you have already demonstrated your loyalty. It involves General Amin."

"What has he done?"

"He is trying to overthrow the government."

"And what do you want me to do?"

"To speak out against him. He has the army, unfortunately, but it will be less loyal to him if the officers see that soldiers of your standing do not hesitate to stand up to him."

"Let's be precise. You want me to incriminate him. How?"

"Well, for instance by publicly confirming that he is the man the British are using to prolong their colonial hold. We have a complete dossier on General Amin's subversive activities and will make it available to you."

A little weasel of a man whom I had not noticed when I came in stood up and gave me an ironic bow. Even though I was used to the convolutions of African intrigues I felt stunned. I could not have imagined a more unlikely proposition.

The rivalary between Obote and Amin was notorious, and their fates had been linked from the start of their public careers. As a young man Obote had been Jomo Kenyatta's secretary when he led the Mau-Mau rebellion in 1952. Later, when the East African Federation broke up, he exploited the situation to create a political empire in his native country. He rose fast in Uganda, and was prime minister in 1963. But there was still the Kabaka of the federated kingdom of Buganda in his way, until Obote had his residence attacked by a battalion under a Lieutenant Colonel Amin, who was devoted to him in those days. The Kabaka fled to England, Obote made himself president of the Republic, and Idi Amin was appointed army chief of staff. Ever since then Obote had known that he was at the mercy of the man who had put him in power, while Amin himself, who was more artful and a lot more cautious than his forthright style suggested, was in no hurry to take over and preferred to dig himself in.

The minister was waiting for my answer, and I gave it to him straight: "What you are asking goes against my sense of honor. General Idi Amin has done a lot for the cause I have been defending, and I won't play your game."

The minister controlled his annoyance.

"All right. How much longer do you expect to remain in Kampala?"

"My plane leaves the day after tomorrow."

"Then you'll have time to reflect. I'll phone you before you leave. Perhaps you will have changed your mind."

That was all. I took my leave of the minister, and the other man walked me to the lift. On my way out a police officer came up to me.

"If you'll wait a few minutes, colonel, there's a car coming to pick you up."

How considerate, I thought, and sat down until a uniformed general arrived.

"Colonel Steiner, I have orders to escort you to police headquarters to settle matters with our immigration services. Also I am sorry to inform you that you must remain there till you leave. We are afraid that the British may be after you, and we want you in protective custody."

That was plausible enough. At police HQ in the city center I was given a comfortable room equipped with its own telephone and TV, and was asked not to leave it. At worst I thought that they might be trying to panic me into accepting the proposition, at the same time preventing me from warning Idi Amin. All I was really expecting was to be put aboard the plane without being allowed to contact anybody.

Next day I was visited by a second minister. He was on his own and putting on a friendly face.

"We quite understand that it is asking a lot to want you to testify against Idi Amin. You are both soldiers, and he has become your friend. But we want to know your price."

"Price? What price?"

"Come now, don't play the innocent. You're being offered money. How much?"

"You bastard, do you think I'm going to sell my friends out? A punch in the mouth would be too good for you. I said no yesterday and it's no today. I am not for sale. Get out."

He was incredibly thick-skinned and in spite of all my insults he kept returning to the charge using the same sugary voice, obviously convinced that my honor simply cost more than his other partners', and determined to stay in the auction. When he finally caught on he changed his tune.

"Be careful, Steiner. If you keep this up we have the option of sending you to Khartoum, and you know as well as I do that they'll hang you."

So angry that I could hardly speak, I managed to tell him once again to get out, and took a step toward him. He backed away, holding out a limp hand which I refused, and I slammed the door behind him. I didn't get the chance to slam it twice because there was the sound of a key turning in the lock.

Half an hour later the guards took me out of my comfortable room and into a cell in the basement.

The date was October 8, 1970. I was hoping for some intervention from Idi Amin, who had men of his own in the police and government and was bound to find out about my illegal arrest before long. In fact he got word to the West German ambassador, who asked to see me, and I was brought from my cell to the Parliament Building to meet him.

"Why are you being held?" he asked. "No one here can tell me."

I decided to put my foot in it.

"It's simple. I was being asked to compromise General Idi Amin, and I refused. They offered me money. Then they threatened that if I did not comply I would be sent to Khartoum, where I would surely be hanged. And to top it all they arrested me, which is where things stand now."

The silence dragged on, but the expressionless minister found nothing to say. It was the same with the ambassador, whose official position required him not to cause anyone to lose face over what might be only a regrettable incident that could be settled in a friendly way. As there was nothing he could do right then, he left, having first promised me (this time in German) that he would take legal advice about my case and do his best to get me freed.

A few days later he phoned to tell me: "There's no question of their being able to hand you over to the Sudanese. The lawyer I consulted is positive on that point. There is an extradition treaty between the Sudan and Uganda, signed in 1964, which specifically excludes political prisoners."

The game now seemed clearer. My arrest could only have been intended to implicate Idi Amin. This was a clever maneuver. By complaining that, for example, I had used material belonging to the Ugandan army in the service of a foreign cause, they were also disowning their commander in chief at the same time. Through me they were striking at Idi Amin.

I had been detained for over a month before the West German ambassador could get a promise to release me on condition that I swore never to return to any member country of the Organization of African Unity (OAU). I was asked to sign a document of the type signed by the mercenaries at Bukavu, in which I was supposed to plead guilty of subversive behavior against the peoples of Africa and to thank their rulers for their clemency.

"Gentlemen," I told them, "at this moment I cannot make any commitment concerning my future travels in Africa because I shall most likely be wanting to return."

And I refused to sign.

On November 29 there was a supposedly "mercenary" intrusion in Guinea and President Sekou Touré kicked up a row which had repercussions all over Africa. A meeting of the OAU foreign ministers in Lagos agreed on December 10 to extradite any mercenary taken prisoner in a member country to the country where he was accused of plying his trade. My own case was not unknown to the conference's host, General Gowon, and may have played its part in the decision. The only ambiguity had to do with the word "mercenary." Usually it covers people who can be proved to have taken money in return for fighting for a cause. Even my worst enemies could not put me in that category.

But that didn't make the situation any less bad for me or less advantageous for Khartoum. A minister now came back with a new proposition: "Do as you're told. You know what has happened in Conakry. Now it's easy for us to ship you to Khartoum."

They were starting to irritate me. This time, though, I didn't even need to take a step toward the man. I only had to look at him to send him scuttling.

In fact, as had to be expected, it did not take the Sudanese long to ask for my extradition. On January 8, 1971, Obote appointed a commission of six ministers to rule on my case. After an hour's deliberation it rejected Khartoum's request, arguing that the convention signed in 1964 was still valid. The West German ambassador and I were informed that I was not to be extradited to the Sudan but deported to a European country of my own choice.

On January 10, at eight o'clock in the evening, I phoned the ambassador for the last time on the guardroom telephone. I wanted him to send me a doctor for a malaria attack. He had still heard nothing, but expected to receive the papers next day.

At 11:30 I had a visit from a top civil servant who delivered the official deportation order, signed by Milton Apollo Obote. They told me that all my belongings had already been returned to the ambassador and that he was waiting for me at the airport.

All this seemed straightforward enough. We left for Entebbe airfield in a black Mercedes, escorted by two Land Rovers. It was dark when we arrived, and I was surprised to find that no aircraft was expected. Instead of stopping by the main entrance our convoy drove round to a service gate.

No ambassador. No plane. The cars drove along the strip toward the hangars, and now I could make out the silhouette of a plane in our headlights — first gray, then white, with green stripes. The colors of Islam. And Arabic characters on the fuselage.

So now I knew. The cars had pulled up and the plane's engines were idling. My escort stood silently by.

"But surely this isn't Lufthansa?" I asked ironically.

The man doing the dirty work simply said: "My orders were to convey you to this plane."

Without waiting to be told I left the Mercedes and walked the twenty meters to the plane, past the honor guard of escorting policemen. The door was open. No sound emerged, but there was light inside. The steps were in place, and I climbed on board.

To the left, the flight deck door was open. The light was coming from there, and I could see the outline of a man with his back to me. To the right, the cabin was pitch-black. It was when I set foot inside that the beating began.

I was thrown to the ground, kicked, trussed up with the kind of thick rough rope used in the country for tethering sheep, and hung by the wrists and ankles from the bars of the luggage racks, belly up. For good measure they then put a fifth rope under my kidneys and another round my neck, which half choked me with every move and jolt.

And there were plenty. Hanging a meter and a half above floor level I was conveniently placed for every boot, fist, and gun butt, which thudded in with clockwork regularity. I could barely make out the forms of my assailants but I could hear their hoarse breathing as they worked away silently and methodically, like demolition men.

Then the lights came on and I could see the expressions on their faces, twisted with hate. There were about twenty of them, Sudanese paras, armed with Kalashnikovs. Their blows became more accurate in the light, and they alternated with Arabic insults. I was kicked in the kidneys and between the legs, and when a gun butt struck the back of my head I made a sudden movement and my breathing was cut off. I started to choke, and my face must have turned blue, because I felt a hand untying the rope round my throat. The beating kept on and on, but I could no longer feel anything, and I just had time to hear the plane taking off before losing consciousness.

When I came to, the paras had cooled down and were sitting about in the cabin, smoking and joking among themselves. I was bleeding from the head and covered with saliva, but my hands and feet were totally numb and I felt as if I was floating in space. I was wet around the legs and stomach where the kicking had made me piss without knowing it. And for the first time in my life I said a prayer for myself and wished for the plane to crash in the south Sudan. I knew what the Arabs did to Anyanya prisoners.

After about an hour's flying the plane landed. Just before that the pilot dowsed the cabin lights, and the men kept strict silence all through the stopover. The plane was refueling, and their behavior told me that we must be at Juba, and that they were scared that the Anyanyas might have been warned and make some attempt to rescue me.

We took off again fast, and two or three hours later we landed once more, still in the dark. The lieutenant in charge of my para escort untied me and rubbed my ankles and wrists to restore the circulation. He even apologized for his men: "Sorry, sir, they were a bit jumpy." I would rather have had something to drink, but apparently it didn't enter his mind.

Another detachment now came on board and I was put on my feet with each wrist tied to a soldier's. You would have thought there wasn't a single pair of handcuffs in the Sudan. An officer offered a cigarette, which I refused. Through the open door came the cool, dry air of the desert at night. I asked whether we were in Khartoum and was told no.

At the bottom of the steps was the welcoming committee, a few civilians in capacious while djellabas, who appeared to inspire tremendous respect in my escorting soldiers. In the gloom I did not slow down to look at them — it would only have increased their satisfaction. I was taken to a Land Rover where I sank rather than sat down, the paras piled into trucks, and we took to the road. After about half an hour a kind of oasis came into view, a bunch of ghostly tamarisks around a low, colonial-style house with wooden arcades.

Our convoy halted and I was taken into a vast room which took up the entire ground floor. The only furniture was a big bed, a small table, and two armchairs standing in solitary state in the middle. Immediately after my arrival an officer entered and gave me a regimental salute. His look was frank, his mustache military, and his bearing upright.

"Major Zir, colonel. I have been instructed to look after you. If you need anything at all, tell your guards that you want to see me. What would you like to drink? Whiskey? Beer? Coffee? Tea?"

I asked for coffee and took advantage of his friendly attitude to ask where we were.

"At Kosti, colonel."

I rested for two or three hours. Toward midmorning Major Zir came in to announce visitors, and I was taken to the first floor, which had been fixed up as a conference room. Officers and officials drifted in in small groups. The entire government was queuing to see the wild animal which had just been captured. They introduced themselves: minister of this, minister of that. . . . They shook hands with me, deferential, polite, and absolutely ridiculous.

We talked about one thing and another. They seemed very

interested in the Israeli intervention and the army minister, General Hassan Abbas, tried his hardest to winkle impossibly precise details out of me. On the whole they behaved very correctly, with the exception of a little general who had introduced himself as a minister.

"Why do you wear general's insignia?"

"Because I belong to the Revolutionary Committee."

This man kept making sneering remarks about me which at first I pretended not to hear. Finally I had had enough.

"Could you repeat what you're saying in German or French? I can't make out your insinuations too well."

"Better in Arabic or Russian! I'm a communist, and I speak the language of free peoples. But since you only understand imperialist languages I will tell you in English that we know you are an agent of the Federal Republic, that Germany wants to make a colony of the south Sudan, that we shall not permit it, and that criminals like you will be hanged!"

I got up and took him by the throat. "Damned bastard! I'm ready to die, but you're not going to insult me!"

Other ministers intervened to separate us, then the guards with their Kalashnikovs hustled me back to my room.

Later that afternoon I woke up from a long-delayed sleep to find a man sitting in one of the armchairs watching me. He introduced himself as Colonel Babikir, the head of Sudanese intelligence, and said that he had dropped by just to make sure that I had everything I wanted and that his instructions about my treatment were being properly observed. Eventually he brought up his real reason for visiting: I was a mercenary, so would I turn my coat for money? In this case I was supposed to help the Arabs to crush the Anyanyas. I knew them well, and knew their hideouts; I would have no trouble running an antiguerrilla offensive. I refused, as usual, and he went away, convinced that he would be able to find an argument to win me over.

Three days after my arrival Major Zir woke me in the middle of the night to inform me that I was to be moved elsewhere.

"Right," I thought. "The intelligence fellow has thought it over: I said no to collaboration, and now I'm to be liquidated."

Once again I was tied by the wrists to two armed soldiers, and Zir made us get into the back of his car. He drove, and next to him sat a little captain I had not seen before. In the rear-view mirror I could see the headlights of a convoy following us — the execution squad, no doubt.

We drove for a hour. I already thought of myself as a dead man living on borrowed time. The desert flashed past us flat and bare, pebbles casting black shadows in the harsh light.

Suddenly the captain turned round and stared at me hard. He had a pistol in his hand. Our faces were almost touching. Still staring straight into my eyes he slowly and ostentatiously cocked his weapon and pointed it at my heart. My time had come. I was glad to be able to go this easily. And since I offered no reaction he started to play cat and mouse.

"I have to kill you," he said softly.

I was far away.

"I have to shoot you, right now!"

"Yes, I understand, no problem. Go ahead, do your job."

The answer did not please him. He wanted to frighten me and at the same time give himself pleasure by asserting his dominance over a white man. At other times I might have taken him seriously, but right then I didn't give a damn. The thoughts in my head had nothing to do with him or his gun — for me, it had been all over as soon as he was ready to shoot. It was at that point that Zir broke in.

"Game's over," he told the captain, tugging at his arm. Then, turning toward me: "Don't be afraid, colonel, he's bluffing. He has no orders to kill you now. And I am in command here."

Zir deposited me in an imposing three-story house, all in stone, with grounds sloping down toward a river. On the first floor there was a whole suite of rooms waiting for me, with thick carpets, air-conditioning, and a bathroom in marble. They gave me a cook and even an orderly who made my bed and cleaned my shoes. For the few days I stayed it was velvet glove treatment all the time.

Then early one afternoon Zir informed me that I was to meet the press.

"Don't expect a word out of me," I told him.

"There won't be any questions, you will simply be presented to the journalists."

It was January 18, 1970, the beginning of my blindfold period, because from then on the guards tied a black bandage over my eyes each time they took me out. The rest of the procedure remained the same, and I was tethered between two soldiers for the journey, which lasted only twenty minutes. The suspension of the Russian jeep was pretty rough, and a period of jolting on the way had told me that we were crossing a very long bridge which could only be on the Nile. So it had been a lie about us being at Kosti, and I knew when they removed the blindfold outside a great Victorian-style palace that we were in Khartoum and this was the Government Palace which had once been General Gordon's.

In a dusty office inside, a general and two colonels were waiting. A steward offered drinks, and I took a coffee. No one spoke to me, and the polite, frosty British silence dragged on for a quarter of an hour before the soldiers stood.

"Follow us, please."

We took a few paces toward the big doors at the end of the room, then they were flung open and I was dazzled by a fusillade of flashbulbs and television lights. It took nearly a minute for my eyes to adjust. I saw that the journalists were to my left, while to my right was a compact group whose age, formality, and racial diversity identified them as members of the diplomatic corps.

The exhibition only lasted long enough for the press to film and photograph me from all angles. I had nothing to say, not one diplomat or journalist made any attempt to enter into conversation, and all I had to do was listen to a speech from Dialo Tellé, the secretary-general of the OAU, making a special visit to express his pleasure that "the mercenary Steiner has been captured by the Ugandan army after being beaten and escaping to Kampala."

The worst of it was that all the ambassadors applauded. I could not understand why they should lend themselves to this charade.

I was left in peace for twenty-four hours, then in the morning it was back to the ropes and blindfold and we were on the road again. This time I landed in a barracks, surrounded by a lot of soldiers and a few civilians all talking long and hard to explain why it was in my interest to cooperate against the Anyanyas. Once more I said no.

The next day it was a different barracks and the same questions. This went on for four days, starting early and finishing late. I was being properly treated, but the daily battle of wills could only make matters worse for me. On the fifth day nobody came looking for me. It was like being given a day off after a hard week's work. Then in the afternoon I was visited by a group of officers bringing beer and cigarettes. They spent three or four hours trying with great patience to talk me into collaborating. I tried as politely as I could to make them see that they were wasting their time if they thought they could get me to betray people who trusted me.

Next day I visited another barracks — Khartoum was one

big garrison-town for me — but this time there was a change of tune. I remained there for two weeks, or perhaps three, I can't tell, and this is why.

They started with employing a specially nasty way to tie me against the wall, which dated back to some old Turkish customs of the eighteenth century. I was spread-eagled by ropes hanging from the ceiling beams, unable to sit down or turn round and facing a battery of powerful arc lamps of the kind used in film studios, which were kept pointing straight into my eyes and never switched off. The feeling became more and more terrible as time went by. Even by twisting my head as far as possible to left or right I could not avoid the fierce glare which burned my eyes and pierced my eyelids, no matter how tight I tried to screw them shut.

They left me like that all day and all night. There was no question of sleeping. The light, together with the wrenching in my wrists every time my legs gave way with fatigue, kept me awake and lucid.

At midday I was taken down, but the relief was short-lived. When they put a black bandage over my eyes I thought at first that they were going to continue alternating the rough with the smooth, and that I was to be taken back to my quarters now. But as soon as the blindfold was tied my eyes stung with an unbearable burning pain, and I realized that the material was covered in *piri-piri*, the powdered red pepper which the Arabs use in their food. Now I was led outside and made to climb aboard a canvas-covered truck where I was tied up again, still standing upright, with my arms spread out. The truck did not move. The sun, which in that season reaches a temperature of 60° to 70° Centigrade in Khartoum, made the inside of the truck an oven.

My guards had taken care to close all the outlets, and standing in the sun the truck quickly became a real sauna. After a few minutes I was drenched in sweat, which mingled with the *piri-piri* to fill my eyes with a blistering liquid which had me jerking uncontrollably, which chafed my wrists and ankles. The heat built up until I was literally stifling with thirst, and it was not till five o'clock, when the temperature dropped slightly, that they untied me, doled out a few drops of water, and took me back to the room with the arc lamps.

These tortures went on for two or three weeks, enough for me to lose all sense of time and of whether it was day or night. I wasn't fed for the first three days, and the water they allowed me was never more than a clinical minimum. My swollen tongue filled my mouth like a lump of leather. To put it simply, I was in hell.

My one thought was to hold out. I concentrated all my willpower on endurance, knowing that the pain would have an end. The time would inevitably come when they must call a halt, either to finish me off or to take me back to my quarters. In those moments, I didn't mind which way it went.

The cellar with the arc lamps was reserved for interrogations. Standing with my eyes dazzled, I could see nothing of my questioners, only hear their voices tirelessly asking questions, and always the same ones, in accented English: "Who sent you to Sudan? What were you doing there? Where did you get your orders?"

I would concentrate on answering, more and more mechanically: "That's no business of yours. I've said all I have to say."

From then onward, each time I opened my eyes I saw black circles. I still see them today. The faces of my torturers were never familiar, and the only person I remember, and whom I was to recognize at my trial, was one of the chiefs of the security services. He conducted the interrogations sitting a little ahead of the others, and I could make out his fat, swarthy face and thick black mustache on the rare occasions when the spotlights were dimmed.

I knew that I was in the hands of professional torturers because apart from their work there was never any unproductive brutality. Once, when I tripped on the step getting into the truck, they were even kind enough to help me get back up. All the same, I knew that those cold technicians were patiently waiting for their methods to take effect, and in spite of the pain and humiliation I would rather have died than give them that pleasure.

I was no longer counting the days. As a rule the arc lamp routine came at night and the truck in the daytime, and that rhythm provided me with a rough calendar.

In order to vary the routine, one day I tried to report sick and asked to see a doctor. Next morning I was taken down and the lights were switched off, then two doctors arrived to examine me — probably army men, and sworn to secrecy. Some soldiers also brought in a bed. I was mesmerized just by the sight of it, and once lying on it I had to make a superhuman effort to stay awake while the doctors were examining my eyes. I can't have been a pretty sight: there was no mirror, but I could feel with my fingers that the blend of sweat and *piri-piri*, brought to the boil by the lamps and the truck treatment, was producing spectacular effects. My eyelids were as bruised and swollen as a boxer's after fifteen rounds of continual hammering.

The doctors left after smearing ointment on my face, and another bunch appeared. These were talking too much to be interested in my health alone. I was too exhausted to make out what they were saying, but one name stuck in my mind because it kept recurring. I managed to force my eyes open enough to see a short, bustling man who expressed himself with the terse authority which characterizes leaders in Africa. He was holding a long tube in his hands and seemed to be explaining its use to an attentive audience.

"Keep still," he told me. "We are going to take a sample of your gastric fluid."

I had seen this done in military hospitals, and the man's convincing manner persuaded me to cooperate as he slid the tube down my throat. By now I was clearheaded again, and I watched as his assistants pumped the reddish contents of a big syringe into the tube. This did not surprise me too much, because I knew that specialists introduce a colorless liquid into the stomach so as to fix the juices for biochemical analysis. But the color was puzzling.

Right then I felt nothing. The supposed nurses jerked the tube out roughly, and everybody left. Only then did I begin to feel what at first was a smarting irritation deep in my throat but which kept growing with every second and soon became an intolerable burning sensation. Then, in a flash, I realized that the treatment had been the injection of liquid *piri-piri* into my stomach.

That was just the beginning. The pain I felt was only caused by the few drops of the stuff which had dripped into my mouth out of the tube while it was being removed. Soon the ordeal started: coughing, choking, cramps. The sensation was like having had pure alcohol poured into me. As if it had become independent of me my body went into all sorts of contortions as it fought against the pepper that was devouring it inside.

The effect of a stomachful of *piri-piri* is slow and progressive. It reaches its full intensity only after several hours. After a time the spasms got so violent that the guards decided to tie my arms and legs to the bedposts. When the *piri-piri* reaches the anus the pain becomes unimaginable. The body is on fire, flaming out of every orifice. . . .

Obviously now was the time for them to replace the bandage impregnated with *piri-piri* over my eyes. The means of torture didn't vary much, but you had to give credit for a certain genius in using them. Blind, and with my flesh on fire, I was a human lava flow, racked by irregular tremors, jaws clenched so as not to let out the moans which would confirm their triumph.

At that instant I admit that I was really afraid. Not of talking, which I could not have done had I wanted to, or even of crying with pain, but simply of going mad. Mad with pain, as people are stupidly liable to say without knowing what they mean, because the fire was burning my guts out. Yet the thought of suicide never occurred to me. I was fighting my last battle, which seemed to be a hopeless one, but suicide would have been a rout, a surrender, and I was ready to pay for the luxury of looking my executioners in the face.

The night hurt. At dawn an official looked in and authorized the guards to untie me and bring me something to drink. They gave me half a glass of water, then when I asked for more they gave me a bucketful, which I emptied in two hours, much to their amusement. They also took off the bandage. While I drank I decided to make this my last — from now on I would refuse all food and drink.

The day's work started, and again I was hauled up against the wall with the lights glaring. If I opened my eyes, they burned; if I closed them they burned more. Tears are the eye's natural defense mechanism, and they kept welling up to flush out the *piri-piri*, but it was far too strong for that.

I felt so drained that I was surviving in a trance, beyond sleeping or waking. Exhaustion anesthetized me.

That afternoon, in the truck, I tried to evacuate all the water I had drunk. As soon as I started pissing it burned as strongly as it had in the anus. It was red-hot iron, impossible to describe, but when I stopped by bladder swelled and scalded all the more.

In the evening, when they took me back to the wall, I couldn't stand it any longer.

"Please, I have to go to the lavatory."

They jeered at me, and brought me an empty jam jar, which I had to fill up publicly. It was too small, and I could not stop. They were doubled up with laughter.

During my stay in that barracks my jailers had kept me on survival rations — a bowl of clear bean soup a day, sometimes with a bit of bread. Obviously they still had hopes of making me talk. I also had noticed that they were not using knives or fire on me, so as not to leave traces, so I assumed that they were anxious to provide me no chance of giving evidence against them in the event of my release. I was fairly certain that they didn't want to finish me straight-away, although I was no less convinced that I was done for, and the relative consideration I received sometimes made me regret that they couldn't get it over with faster.

After the bucket incident I said: "I'm not playing any-more. From now on you can keep your water and your soup. I'd rather die."

And I started a hunger strike. That night I was hung up on the wall again like a coat on a rack, and I had two more days' roasting in the truck. Then when I persisted they left me alone — no more blindfold, no truck, no ropes. They took the arc lamps out of the cellar and let me lie down on the bed left behind by the army doctors.

They played their last card when a prison official in person brought in a tray loaded with hot food, fruit, and, in par-ticular, a carafe of iced water. He told me that it was mine if I agreed to help them. I turned my head away. The carafe stayed there, gleaming, and to test myself I did once lay a hand on the glass, but that was all.

Eventually they had me taken back to the villa with the marble bathroom. The contrast was unreal, as the orderly once again waited on me with his "What would you like, sir? Yes, sir. No, sir. . . ." I filled the bath with cold water and sank into it. It felt icy, and good.

I could hardly walk; all my joints felt rusted up. The

piri-piri produced caustic aftereffects. Even three months later I could feel it burn each time I went to the lavatory.

The worst remains to be told. I would rather avoid what follows, but I have no right to remain silent.

We have to go back to two days after the injection of the *piri-piri*, when I was taken to a cellar room near my own. In it a black man was hanging by the wrists, stark naked, with a bruised body and swollen face.

"Recognize him?" my guide asked, smiling.

"No."

"You don't recognize William Allau?"

I remembered the young Anyanya student who had unwittingly covered himself with glory at the time of the famous Kajo-Kaji raid. I stared hard into these bloated features, trying to recognize the fine intelligent face I had known. He was motionless and unconscious, in a semi-comatose state. They strapped me up alongside him and left us alone, after throwing a bucket of water over him in an effort to revive him. We remained side by side in the half-light for a long time, in a silence broken only by the sound of our own breathing.

Suddenly he turned painfully towards me and croaked: "Commander, most of all, say nothing. . . . Do not talk. . . . Better to die than talk to this scum. . . ."

Quietly as he had spoken, the listening guards had heard. The door opened and our torturers came in, one of them slamming his rifle butt into William Allau's stomach as he did so. Then the sergeant turned toward me and said: "Right, we're going to kill this son of a whore in front of you."

The body next to me stiffened. He let out a "No!" which was stopped by the soldiers as they began their rhythmic battering, their faces as matter-of-fact as if they were felling a tree. Allau gathered all his remaining life force and began to howl like an animal.

I was pushed in front of him. My hands were tied behind

my back, and joined to my ankles by a short rope which prevented me from standing up, as I wanted to do, to show my respect. All I could do was kneel. I turned my head away, not wanting to witness the death agony.

Time passed, the soldiers kept pounding, and Allau's howls diminished to cries, then to hoarse gasps. He had blacked out again. The executioners began slowly to sink their bayonets into his body, carefully probing. First his feet. Then his hands. Then his belly. I saw the muscles contract and heard the gasping resume. As the soldiers intended, none of these wounds was fatal. Blood trickled out of the wounds and dripped down to form a puddle at his feet.

Having done their job the soldiers left us, joking among themselves. It must have been dinnertime. I was left there with the dying man. His chest still rose and fell. I hardly dared to look.

An hour went by like that, maybe two, then the head stirred for the last time, the mouth opened as if to say a final word, but only a little reddish froth came out. The body jerked gently and subsided. Allau was dead.

A voice behind me said: "Now you know we are not joking."

23

Schmidt
und Schmidt

Two Europeans sat smiling at me from behind a desk, both of them blond and well fed. Their *"Guten Morgen"* told me that they were German, and they confirmed my assumption by dismissing the officer who accompanied me and producing drinking glasses and several bottles of Löwenbrau from a black leather briefcase. In the Sudan of 1970, whose pro-Communist sympathies were well known, they could only be East Germans.

It was my first German beer in a long time, and I took it slowly. My hosts put a packet of cigarettes on the desk, Bensons.

"It was Bensons you smoked in Biafra, wasn't it?"

I looked at beer, Bensons, and fellow Germans as if they had come down from the planet Mars. Whatever might happen later, I felt a deep satisfaction; it was like a few moments at home.

"We are not responsible for what the Sudanese have done to you," said the thinner of the two. "Just between ourselves, we think they've been stupid. You don't treat a soldier like that."

They introduced themselves, frankly admitting that they could not use their real names.

"Let's say we're called Karl and Hans. We are counsellors at the GDR embassy, and our job is to maintain friendly relations between the Sudanese government and the eighteen thousand technical helpers we are lending them. At the same time we have to deal with security questions, which is what brings us here."

The taller one had a strange resemblance to me. Slightly thinner, and with a bit more hair, he could have been my double when I was in good condition. The other was plump, balding, and as cheerful and talkative as his colleague was formal and dignified. They were both about my age. Since they weren't supposed to tell me their names, I made up my own for them. While I had been tied to the wall in the barracks I had noticed a tape recorder on a low table behind the battery of spotlights. A red and white flex ran from it into a next-door room, and deciding that my double must have been listening at the other end I called him Mr. Six-Volts. The second I baptized Bormann, which, as well as being the name of Hitler's lieutenant, means a man who digs or searches.

Our first meeting was not a working session but simply an introduction.

"We asked Numeiry to be allowed to talk to you alone to persuade you to relax your position. We know about your past record. We know that you were in Indochina, Korea, and Algeria. You were at Suez. We know all about your role in the Congo and Biafra. But we also know that you are not politically committed to the imperialists."

It was a cheerful mishmash of fact and fiction. They, too, must have been reading the papers. But they seemed well intentioned and it was the wrong moment to contradict them.

The second meeting lasted all day.

"Is it okay to call you Rolf?"

"If you want."

"Listen, Rolf, we are Germans too, and I think you'll believe us that we're trying to get you out of this."

"Maybe. But what do you want out of me?"

"First you'll have to call off your hunger strike. You're wearing yourself out for no reason. We guarantee that there'll be no more torture and that you will be properly tried. Also you'll hear nothing more from the Sudanese police. But we are asking you to collaborate with us. We're not asking you to betray your friends or ideas, just to provide us with some harmless facts we require for the investigation we are conducting."

"Our interest is in presenting a report to the government we are detached to," Bormann added. "The rest is up to you."

I was on my sixth day's hunger strike, apart from the beer the day before, which had done me a lot of good. I felt fine, and because their conditions seemed acceptable I answered their questions about my early years in Bavaria. We lunched in their office, and what with the pleasure of speaking my native language, their own good nature, and seeing an end to suffering without having to renege on my principles, I felt really at ease.

Next day Six-Volts and Bormann moved into my quarters, which were comfortable, but far too big, and I was glad to have some company. The next few weeks were like a vacation. Each morning there were two packets of Bensons by my bed. Six-Volts and Bormann would come in around eleven o'clock and stay till the evening. I was eating good European food, and on April 30 they even brought me a case of Munich beer to celebrate the anniversary of Camerone!

One day there was a hitch.

"It's no good," Bormann said. "We're going to have to start over again. You were not born in Munich, and your name is not Steiner."

"There must be a mistake somewhere," I told them when I

had recovered from the surprise. "It isn't on my side, because I don't tell lies. So it has to be yours. You'd better check your sources of information."

They told me that no trace of my name had been found in the records of my old school in Munich, the Plinganser Schule. I supposed that the upheavals of the war must be responsible, but there was an easy way for them to check up.

"My father's grave is in the Waldfriedhof cemetery in Munich. Send someone there. And he was a flier in the First World War: you'll find his name on the list of men decorated 'For Merit' [this is the highest German award]. If you want, we won't talk again till you've made sure."

A few days later they had details about my case which were so exact that some of them were unknown to me. For instance they told me that in 1923 my father had taken part in a flying competition at Frankfurt, and that during his display he had flown under the bridge on the River Main!

The test had reinforced our relationship, although I kept in mind that, though as Germans they might want to save me, as Communists they wanted me to talk. Still, during those conversations it became clear to me that my companions were not enthusiastic about their task with me. They were party officials, not militants, which explains the soft treatment I received, as well as the fact that they didn't give a hoot about the information they were supposed to be obtaining about the Anyanyas, and the subject never came up.

This situation went on for nearly three months. After a while they went back to Khartoum and our meetings became less frequent now that they had nothing much left to ask. Toward the end they were just dropping by for a drink.

It was during that period that I was confronted with Mohammed, the Arab tailor whose life I had saved in the south Sudan. The meeting took place in the presence of a top prison official in yet another barracks, and as soon as Mohammed saw me he ran up and embraced me. Obviously he did not know that I was a prisoner. I was allowed to talk to him for a few minutes, and he told me that on September 25, 1970, his village had been raided and he had escaped to Uganda. There he had been arrested and eventually handed back to the Sudanese, following in my footsteps. I was about to ask another question when the official gave a signal and the guards dragged him away. I think they started beating him as he was going out through the door.

Some days later this official produced another surprise. There had been an incident in the south Sudan when I had to intervene to save the life of a woman accused of poisoning another woman's child. I had spoken for her at her trial before the tribal chiefs, and they agreed to spare her, which also meant sparing her baby daughter, who would have died without her. The official said: "They say you saved a child's life in the south Sudan. We have another story — the mother's story. It is quite different."

And one June morning the guards brought in a young black woman, obviously straight from the bush.

I was sitting with Six-Volts, drinking coffee.

"Which is Steiner?" the interpreter asked her.

She pointed a finger at the innocent East German, and when the interpreter shouted at her she started to shake, changed her mind, and pointed at me, obviously wondering if she wasn't making another mistake.

She had learned her lesson badly, so to redeem herself she embarked on a ten-minute tirade, the interpreter limping along behind her. The climax involved me and a witch doctor called Baba. I was supposed to have ordered him to abort her in her seventh month of pregnancy, then to have personally thrown the newborn child to the crocodiles.

"Look," I said, "I'm sorry — this is all lies." And she left.

On July 10 Six-Volts asked me to meet the press again. I refused, but he insisted.

"You can speak freely. We know you now, and we know that you aren't a mercenary. They'll be journalists from East Germany. Tell them who you are."

Next day at ten o'clock an East German TV crew arrived, but I refused to appear. The prison official again paid me a visit the day after.

"Why won't you speak? We need your testimony against the Christians who used you and the imperialists who exploited you."

"I am no instrument of policy."

"Speak to the journalists. It is in your own interest and that of your friends. Remember how the traitor Allau died. We have other traitors. . . ."

I thought he was bluffing. I did not believe that they would start again. Things had calmed down; I was no longer being ill treated. But that afternoon, about four o'clock, I heard commotion on the stairs. The guards were bringing a man down, beating him as they went. I knew that two weeks before some black suspects had been transferred to the second floor, which I did not occupy. I was sure that they were not Anyanyas — they never reached jail; they were killed in the bush — but sometimes at night I could hear the cries jerked out of them by the dull thud of batons.

The noise had stopped. Suddenly, framed in the glass door of the veranda, I saw the bleeding head of an African. The naked man staggered, then collapsed. And the soldiers finished the job with their gun butts. The officer commanding them left the body outside my door.

The official returned to the charge.

"Talk. It would be stupid to let your friends be killed."

Two hours later another prisoner was brought to my door,

in very poor condition. On a shouted order from the officer some Arab paras armed with NATO rifles plunged their bayonets into his kidneys.

So I agreed to the German TV interview, and the date was set for July 17. Next time I saw Six-Volts and Bormann I protested against the shameful methods which had been used to make me give way. They had the grace to appear surprised, and honestly refused to believe me. Next day they informed me that the officer who had ordered those executions had acted on his own initiative and was to be severely punished.

On the morning of the seventeenth, twenty-two East Germans invaded my rooms with three cameras, and I was deluged with questions. It was the same on the eighteenth and nineteenth. They were supposed to come again on the twentieth, but they did not. That was the day of the coup d'etat.

I didn't know what was happening. Six-Volts and Bormann were nowhere to be seen, just armed Sudanese. Obviously there was something going on though, because all day long the soldiers' transistors were playing military music, like the radios in Algiers in May 1958.

The firing went on all night and the whole of the next day. That night it reached the villa. I had two armed guards posted outside my door, and one was removed and sent into action. On the afternoon of the twenty-first I was waiting for the end of the show, sitting in my room listening as the shooting came closer and then broke out all around the house. They were firing like Africans: shove in the magazine, then *brrrr*, loose off the lot, and in with the next magazine. Anywhere, anyhow. That showed me that it wasn't the Israelis: they look where they shoot.

That night the party continued. Looking out of the window I could see tracers flying in all directions. I didn't know who was fighting whom, but it has always seemed

crazy to me to sit around twiddling your thumbs when people are getting killed all around. I told the guards that if
they'd give me a weapon I would help.

At dawn the Communists took the house, and my guards
and the corporal disappeared. I expected trouble as the
victors' boots came pounding up the stairs, but they just
flung the door open, saw me, yelled something in Arabic,
and went off. Still I had no idea what was happening. It
was a private quarrel among Arabs, and there was no point
even in trying to take the opportunity to escape. There was
nowhere to go.

A few hours later the Numeirists counterattacked in
strength and the Communists fled. I was left in peace for
ten minutes before my guards came back as if nothing had
happened. I reassured the corporal when he asked about
my health, and he explained that the army had just prevented a CIA coup, which is all I knew for some time.

On July 30 the army minister came in person to inform
me that General Numeiry had given orders for my public
trial to begin in August 1, 1971.

Schmidt und Schmidt turned up the same day. They
brought sausages, cheese, beer, and cigarettes, and explained
that they had to leave, without saying exactly why.

"But what happened?" I asked.

"Never mind. We're going. But you are staying, and you'll
be needing a lawyer."

"Not at all, I have had time to prepare my own defense."

"No doubt, but it's like this: you admit we've helped you
a lot?"

"Certainly."

"Well, now we want you to do us a service. Ask for assistance from Salim Aïssa. He's a friend of ours, a Communist
educated in East Germany. He married a German girl and
speaks fluent German. At present he's in prison for political
reasons. That's all we can tell you. But if you insist on

having him and nobody else to defend you, Numeiry can't refuse."

I gave my promise.

A major, and bloody, political event had just happened, although I only heard the full story much later on, when I was sharing prison meals with some of the survivors of the uprising.

When they staged their coup, the Communists arrested Numeiry, but they made the mistake of leaving him alive. The tank corps had remained loyal, and they counter-attacked. The Communist officer who was holding Numeiry felt the wind change and escaped with him. That was on July 20. The revenge was terrible, and the massacre of the Communists went on for four or five days. There were also ten thousand arrests.

The bloodbath horrified the whole world, and to distract attention Numeiry decided to bring forward my trial and make it into a fantastic showpiece to retrieve his damaged prestige. He ordered all the hearings to be televised so as to give the Sudanese people a less disturbing entertainment than political repression.

24
The Trial

On Wednesday August 1, at eight in the morning, I was put on board a Russian amphibian tank equipped with a 105mm gun. Two similar monsters escorted me, mounted with heavy machine guns. With them in attendance I arrived at the scene of my trial, the Parliament Building. In order to create the kind of stir he wanted, Numeiry, who reckoned that my "crimes against Africa" deserved better than a mere courtroom, had booked the National Assembly for me. He even had it redecorated for the occasion.

I was deposited in the palace courtyard, watched by a noisy crowd outside the gates, where an armed infantry battalion stood guard. They took me to a quiet air-conditioned office and a steward asked me what I wanted for breakfast in the meaningless polite style which was still affected here, a hangover from the British Empire. A quarter of an hour later he returned with a luxurious breakfast, luxuriously served, complete with a vase of imported flowers.

I was thinking about a lawyer over my breakfast coffee. In my ignorance about both charges and procedure I was in no hurry to ask for one, especially as I had no illusions about the likely outcome, which seemed to me to be a foregone conclusion. But I had kept Salim Alïssa's name in reserve to return the favor to the two East Germans.

Sitting waiting in a comfortable armchair, it took no effort to be relaxed. I even felt some pleasure about the prospect of going into action. All I had to do was to collect myself in anticipation of the coming attack.

I have often been asked why I appeared at the trial with my head shaved. The reason is simple. During the period when I was spending my time between wall and sweat-truck, I was standing under the arc lamps one day when I collapsed with fatigue. All my weight came onto the ropes suspending me by the wrists from the roof beam, and the left one must have been frayed by my earlier struggles because it suddenly snapped. My dead weight pulled on the other rope, and I swung around and down to crack my head open on the floor. To treat this wound my torturers shaved my skull, and subsequently they went on shaving it. Probably they thought it made my face a bit more Arab-looking. After that, partly out of derision and partly because in the heat of the Sudan it was practical, I kept it that way.

The guards sprang to attention and a brigadier general made his appearance, wearing red epaulets and the caduceus of the medical corps. He was supposed to examine me, he said, to make sure that I was fit for trial. More play-acting.

"I'm not ill," I told hm.

"It is the law," he answered.

The examination showed that my condition was weak but adequate. I then informed the general that I had no lawyer.

"I was told that you did not want one."

"It's just that I haven't had the opportunity to ask."

"Who do you want?"

"Salim Aïssa. Can you inform the presiding judge of my request?"

The next general had three stars and no caduceus.

"I am the presiding judge. I am delighted with your

decision to take defense counsel. It will look better for international opinion. All the press is here, and we want the journalists to be convinced that we are impartial. The Sudan has had such a bad press, you know."

He was almost apologetic, a fat timid man, visibly crushed by the weight of the mission given him by Numeiry. Ignoring his possible embarrassment, I told him that there might be some difficulty getting hold of Salim Aïssa, at having to extricate my lawyer from one of their own jails.

"You shall have him, you shall have him," he assured me.

An hour later a colonel walked me down a long corridor toward another man, also with an escorting officer, coming the other way. When we met our guardian angels halted.

"Colonel Steiner."

"Doctor Aïssa."

"Some friends of yours suggested I should ask for you."

"Yes, I thought it must be that. But I'll have trouble defending you, you know. I'm sorry to say that apart from your being Steiner, 'the big mercenary chief,' I know nothing about you. I have only just been told and" — he spoke with a smile — "where I have been I haven't had much chance to inform myself."

Salim Aïssa seemed lively and sympathetic. He spoke perfect German. His broad gestures, stout figure, and dark skin identified him as a southern Sudanese, and I guessed his age to be around forty. His short, curly hair was black and he had a black mustache and wore a black tie knotted over a crumpled white shirt which he must have picked up in a hurry.

Anyway, come on!" he sighed. "We'll soon see."

The double doors swung open, spotlights glared, and guards stood solemnly to attention. We made our entrance in utter silence, preceded by the colonel, stiff as a tailor's dummy. At once the flashbulbs popped and blazed into my sore eyes and forced me to screw them up until I could see nothing except the colonel's back as he led me to a table bristling with microphones. I sat down and the fusillade continued, with photographers standing and kneeling at pointblank range, swarming around like flies. I had a strong urge to give one of them a punch in the eye, to show him what my head felt like, but at long last the assault subsided.

I found myself in the middle of a huge hall, half church, half clinic, with walls of a restful sea-green, and equipped with tiered rows of seats filled by a silent crowd. To my right, on the rostrum, were the judges, five tanned officers doing their best to look appropriately dignified. I recognized the presiding judge by his red-trimmed cap. His concentration was so heavy that it removed all expression from his face. Behind him sat a dark-suited civilian holding a dossier, obviously the legal adviser.

The place was stuffed with microphones, cables, spotlights, and cameras; they sprouted out of the floor, dangled from the ceiling, and crowded into every corner. Against this background stood paras armed with machine pistols. All eyes were turned on me: those of the advocate general standing at his desk; of the two hundred journalists crammed into the press gallery; of the public themselves, where the white shirts of civil servants mingled with the pale djellabas of those inhabitants of Khartoum who had been picked to see justice done.

Salim Aïssa sat next to me and asked me to put on the headphones. Behind us the simultaneous interpreters were shuffling papers. The cameras hummed and the presiding judge opened the hearing, speaking in a halting voice fortified by the translator's: "Rolf Steiner, there are four charges against you. First . . ." A pause as he reached for the right dossier. "First, you are accused of illegal entry and residence in the Republic of the Sudan. Do you plead guilty or not guilty?"

"Guilty."

"Second, you are accused of secretly importing material and medicines, and of illegally practicing medicine. Guilty or not guilty?"

"Guilty."

"Third, you are accused of having fomented subversive activities aimed at overthrowing the legitimate government of the Sudan on behalf of foreign powers. Guilty or not guilty?"

"Not guilty."

"Fourth, you are accused of having headed an armed rebellion and so of having endangered the unity and security of the Republic. Guilty or not guilty?"

"Not guilty."

I had replied automatically, without thinking. At that moment my lawyer rose to ask for a recess, explaining that since he had met me only five minutes before the opening of the trial he had not had time to prepare my defense. The request was granted, and the court adjourned for three days.

I was taken back to the house in the middle of the armored convoy, without the customary ropes and blindfold. There were too many photographers around. My lawyer followed the convoy and I told him what he needed to know about me and my activities in the Sudan. In his opinion, in view of Article 4 of the extradition treaty with Uganda, I ought not to have been arraigned for entering the country without a proper visa.

"You had ceased your supposedly subversive activities in the south Sudan by the time you were arrested in Kampala. Now, you may not know that Numeiry altered his policy some time ago and now wants a negotiated settlement with the Anyanyas. During the course of your stay in Khartoum a decree has been issued proclaiming an amnesty for those involved in the rebels' operations. You should have benefited from it. If they refuse that because you are a white man, it is racism, and illegal."

"Illegal" was a word that passed his lips several times as he pored over the indictment. He was a pugnacious man, clearly not in agreement with his country's system of justice. Not that it mattered whether he was right or wrong: I was going to be tried by a special made-to-measure court whose officers knew nothing about the law. They were there to play out their assigned roles, and the outcome was up to the court's creator, General Jaffar Mohammed al-Numeiry.

For the start of the second hearing I arrived before the judges. There was the same reception, but this time I was ready for it, and under control.

The first witness that day was a major in the Sudanese army, who was sworn in on the Koran and went on to tell a story which seemed to have nothing to do with me. On September 29, 1970, he said, he had commanded a helicopter raid on Morto, a big village which was General Taffeng's HQ at one time. It was possible. I had not been there. I wondered why this witness had been called, and had concluded that it was some kind of propaganda exercise for the benefit of all these pressmen when the translation on the headphones produced: "I occupied Morto on October 1. Steiner was commanding the enemy defenses in person, and he was wounded while escaping."

I stood up to reply to this ridiculous claim. In fact I had heard about the major's operation, which had happened like this: in late September a northern Sudanese para company had landed by helicopter thirty kilometers north of Morto and had run true to form by burning down a small village in the area. The inhabitants had hit back by destroying one of their helicopters and had come to warn me. I was then about four days' march from Morto which, now that it was no longer General Taffeng's HQ, was of no strategic importance whatever, and I radioed the commander of the place not to defend it but to disperse into the bush, burning what he could not evacuate. So it was an empty base that the Arabs had captured.

I was about to speak when my lawyer stood up to question the major.

"No, not you," I said; "you don't know about this business."

"But you are not allowed to speak," Salim Aïssa answered.

I was furious.

"In that case I'd rather handle my own defense."

There was a stir in the courtroom, and the presiding judge intervened to call a half-hour recess for us to settle our disagreement. Aïssa and I went to the office where I had been taken on the first day, and were joined by the presiding judge and the prosecutor. They put their heads together and agreed that I should speak whenever I thought it necessary.

Back in the courtroom I asked the witness: "How can you state that I was wounded while defending Morto, and that I ran away? Did you see me yourself?"

"No."

"What did you find when you reached Morto?"

"The place was empty and the houses burned."

"Did you meet any resistance?"

"None."

"In that case, how can you talk about an attack on a village that I had ordered evacuated three days previously?"

No answer. I had nothing else to ask him. It was just that I could not tolerate his claim that he had defeated me in a regular battle.

Next day the star witness for the prosecution was a top prison official. He undertook to read out the Arabic translation of my conversations with Six-Volts and Bormann, which came back over the headphones retranslated into German. It was no surprise to me: I had made no objection to their taking notes. But we had spent a lot of time in conversation, and it took three or four sittings to read everything into the court record. When the reading ground to an end, Salim Aïssa stood up.

"Sir, was it you who took down everything you have been reading for the past few days?"

"Yes."

"It was you who interrogated the accused?"

"Yes."

"So it was to you personally that he made the statements we have heard?"

"Yes."

At that point I flared up again and took over. The secret police boss had to eat his own report because I made him admit that the document in question had originally been written in German then translated into Arabic, since he, the prison official, did not speak a word of German; that consequently he could not have collected the information himself; that, after his own methods had proved ineffective, all the work he was claiming for himself had in fact been done by the special services of the GDR.

He had to admit that he had not been present at the time of these conversations, which constituted a public admission that he had violated his oath. There was no immediate reaction, but after that day he made no more appearances in court. After its anti-Communist crusade the government of the Sudan preferred not to be reminded about East German aid.

Mohammed was next. When I had first seen his name on the list of witnesses I had thought it was a mistake, but there was no list of defense witnesses, so I awaited his intervention with curiosity. Even in the middle of the hall he gave the impression of hugging the walls, and he darted an agonized look at me as he stood there between his guards. He had to be prodded before he would take the oath.

Then he turned the tap on. I was a jackal, a wild animal

who had killed hundreds of Arabs. With every new denunciation he would bow and scrape toward the platform, studding his sentences with Allah this and Allah that, while at the same time his mournful eyes denied the words he had been taught.

It was a sad performance. All his "evidence" contradicted what he had said when we were brought face to face in the barracks, and I told Salim Aïssa about it. The prison official was still there, and my counsel asked him: "What did the witness do on the day he saw Colonel Steiner again?"

"He said: 'Colonel Steiner saved my life.'"

"Was he answering a question or did he speak out of his own accord?"

"Of his own accord."

"And how did he behave?"

"He embraced the accused," the official admitted sulkily.

Witness number four was the crocodile girl, still bubbling with confidence, ready to take her oath on the Koran and peddle her crazy accusations. I had nothing to say, but my lawyer did not leave things there.

"You say that Colonel Steiner ordered this man Baba to give you medicine to abort your child. What language was he speaking?"

"English."

"Do you speak English?"

"No."

"In that case, how could you understand what he said?"

"But what is there to understand? It was English, that's all!"

Salim Aïssa continued: "After your abortion, which you say happened an hour after taking this medicine — which is medically impossible — you have stated that Colonel Steiner took your baby by the foot and threw it to the crocodiles. Did you see him?"

"No."

"Then how did you know?"

"What is there to know? The white man killed my baby, that's all there is to it!"

My lawyer sat down, the prosecution had no questions to ask, and she was starting another tirade when the judge interrupted to thank her for her evidence. She walked out, darting me a hate-filled look.

Two other prosecution witnesses were listed. They were supposed to prove that I had been in touch with the Israelis and to testify that they had seen me conferring with them and Colonel Lagu at Owing-Kibul. The job must have been beyond them because they never showed up.

There were no witnesses for the defense. It would have been hard to find any in three days in a country where I knew nobody.

The next day's program was a closed session. Even the guards were excluded. I was alone in front of the judges. During this sitting the prosecution tried to compromise the Catholic Church and the "imperialist nations" and produced a letter from Julia concerning the publication of photos of atrocities committed by the soldiers of Khartoum in the south Sudan, photos which I had provided. This letter had been addressed to General Taffeng and stated that it was impossible to publish these documents because they were too horrible. Even the German magazines had refused them.

He also read out extracts from a correspondence between Taffeng and General Idi Amin. This had nothing to do with me either, but since in the meantime Amin had seized power in Kampala I realized that Numeiry was looking for clues from me about the possible intentions of Uganda's new leader. I asked the presiding judge how the Sudanese had obtained this material and he made no difficulty about telling me that in late January the Khartoum army had attacked Lagu's HQ at Owing-Kibul and had retrieved stacks of records, among them papers confirming my appointment as commander of the Anyedi armed forces.

After the closed session I took the floor. Since we were on stage, I might as well speak my piece. I had prepared a twenty-page speech defending all my actions. In the course of it I said:

"I have never been a mercenary, either in Biafra or the Sudan. I have never been in the service of any power, religious or political. My choices have always been guided by a concern for justice and my sense of honor. And the only reason for my presence in the Sudan is the genocide that your army was committing there."

That brought the prosecutor to his feet, of course, but I did not intend to be interrupted.

"I wanted to help that nation, and that meant helping the insurgents who were fighting for their freedom. They respected me because I was the only white man prepared to live with them in the jungle, and because I treated them as equals."

"What, does an agent of the imperialist powers dare to speak about the equality of men?" the prosecutor grated.

Till then the trial had run smoothly, but I was starting to feel hostile.

"Don't get your sides mixed up, Mister Prosecutor. Your government has recently noticed that imperialism comes in all colors. And the type that you yourselves are practicing over the wretched black peoples of your country is one of the worst there is, because it is the most hypocritical. The Universal Declaration of Human Rights was not made only for colonized peoples, but for oppressed peoples, whatever power is oppressing them."

The prosecutor was choking with rage. "I have no lesson to learn from a mercenary!" he shouted. "From a stateless man who has served a foreign power for money since adolescence! A mercenary — that's what you are. Like the ones in the Congo, who fouled the soil of Africa, or those who sold their services two hundred years ago to fight against American independence."

"The prosecutor has been misinformed. On the English side there were no mercenaries in the modern sense. At that time the related kings of Europe customarily lent each other their regiments. It is true that there were regiments from Hesse and Brunswick who were sent overseas in the services of the king of England, but there were also foreigners fighting with the Americans. Take Lafayette. . . ."

"Mercenary! Mercenary!" the prosecutor chanted, trying to din the word into the journalists' skulls.

The judge called for order, and a few moments later a guard whispered a message and the prosecutor left the courtroom. He came back pale but collected. That evening I heard from my lawyer, who had it from the judge himself, that General Numeiry in person had called him to the phone to instruct him to let me speak. He had been following the trial on TV and felt that it looked bad to interrupt me.

"I'm fighting my last battle as a soldier," I concluded. "Fighting for my honor, not my life. And I will be proud to sacrifice my life in order for the Africans of the south Sudan to be free. Whatever happens I shall go on fighting. I will never give up my ideals."

At the next hearing it was the prosecutor's turn to present his indictment, but it wasn't the same prosecutor! The previous day's had been dismissed, obviously for excessive zeal. Not that his replacement, a major, had no fight in him. He painted me as an enemy of humanity, and especially of blacks. Coming from a Khartoum Arab that was a pretty daring paradox. I did not listen, having removed my headphones, but I could read his flights of fancy on the prepared text, which he followed slavishly. He too was plugging the tried and tested theme of the paid killer.

"A man of war," he concluded, "cannot be a humanist. Clemency for Steiner would do damage. His condemnation must be a lesson to other mercenaries and so convince the world that Africa is quite determined to get rid of his kind. In the name of all free African peoples I demand the death penalty for the accused."

Then came the speech for the defense. My lawyer had not had time to prepare his speech and he improvised a good deal, but on the whole he followed my recommendations. He did not ask for pity, and wound up his remarks like this:

"This man is not guilty of the crimes he is accused of. He has always acted nobly, in accordance with the dictates of his conscience. He ought to be set free."

The end of the pleading also maked the end of the trial. In the Sudan the accused does not know the verdict straightaway. If he is condemned to death he is notified later, and hanged shortly after that.

So I left through a noisy, struggling crowd fighting to get closer to me, and again I had to run the flashbulb gauntlet. I had to admit that, apart from the phony witnesses, the trial had been properly conducted. Numeiry had made a big effort to put on a performance worthy of a great civilized nation; the judges had never departed from extreme politeness.

They took me back to the villa in my Russian tank, and I did not hear the verdict until November 9 — fifty-eight days after the end of the trial. For me it was borrowed time. Every morning except Friday (the Arab Sunday) I told myself it might be today they came to fetch me. I had never before taken such an interest in the calendar.

From the material viewpoint I was still being properly treated, as the East Germans had decided. The food and service were good, and the only change was no longer having anything to read. Six-Volts and Bormann were gone and

I already knew the books they had left for me: even a condemned man does not read Marx, Engels, and Lenin twice in six months.

I slept well enough, having said definitive good-byes to everything, convinced that they would hang me. In fact this way my only worry, and before leaving Salim Aïssa I had asked him not to make any appeal, but to ask for a firing squad instead of a gallows when the execution date was announced, so that I might die like a soldier.

Then on Tuesday, November 9, 1971, with some ceremony, they came to inform me of the sentence. It was another performance. Numeiry's emissaries were preceded by an invasion of journalists and cameramen. At least in Biafra the vultures used to wait outside. . . .

For the occasion, the guards had pushed the bed away from the middle of the room and replaced it with two chairs and a table. At 12:30 a resplendent colonel sat down at one end, and I at the other, and he took a dossier from under his arm. Cameras started whirring, and since this particular production was mainly intended for export the colonel addressed me in English.

"Colonel Steiner, you have been found guilty on the first charge, not guilty on the second, guilty on the third and guilty on the fourth. For the latter two, you have been condemned to death."

This was no news to me. I simply thought: "Right, that's it," and I think I might have heaved a sigh of relief if I had not felt all those eyes and cameras zooming in on the slightest change of expression.

The colonel waited a few beats, as a master of suspense, either to let the press do their job or because he thought that what he had to say deserved a frame of silence.

"But by the grace of our generous president, the death sentence is commuted to twenty years' criminal detention."

25
Kober Jail

So began what was, for me, a very long period of detention. It would take another book to describe it day by day, so I shall stick to writing about the place and the main characters and events.

Twenty-four hours after the notification of the verdict some officers arrived to take me to jail — no blindfold or ropes, and no tank, just a plain civilian vehicle. The prison governor, a colonel, of course — the Sudan is a military democracy — received me with honors all the same. A job like that in a country like that can only make its holder more cautious: you never know if the minister who visits today will be your prisoner tomorrow, or vice versa.

A captain showed me to my new quarters, while a common-law prisoner carried my gear. After leaving the main building which housed the administration and the governor's office, we advanced into the interior of the camp along alleyways between the brick-colored buildings which made up the various sections.

This central prison, Kober Jail, in the north of Khartoum, was built by the British in 1907. Since independence a booming business had kept it expanding until it overflowed into the surrounding area. Like all prisons it had its own smell, but here it was not a blend of cold ashes and cabbage soup but the strong odor of nutmeg and pungent urine common to all the fortified villages of the North African desert.

The fierce heat intensified the smell. The beaten sand pathways were wet with slops and waste, and swarmed with flies. Most of the building were just one-story concrete shacks, cooled only by their eighty-centimeter-thick walls. Some quarters had their own surrounding walls, and every time we reached one of these the warder had to let us through a heavy iron gate.

My status as a European won me one of the places kept for special guests: a rectangle of about two hundred and fifty square meters, surrounded by a wall four meters high, with what I came to call my "cage" standing in the middle. It was a shack measuring around seven meters by five, with bare brick walls pierced by holes which let in all the winds that blew. There were no door and no bars, because one side was left open, overlooking the big courtyard. In the season, my cage was swept by the simoon.

Thank God there is no lack of space in Arab prisons! The ground was desert sand. The roof, the only technical innovation since the days of the British, was a concrete slab six centimeters thick. The furniture was simple — an iron bedstead, a mattress, and two blankets. Later I found out that I was the only prisoner in the whole country who had that privilege. Even the former prime minister who occupied the cage next to mine slept on a mat on the ground. A sanitary pail in one corner marked the position of the washroom. It was made of rusty iron, without a lid, and had obviously seen plenty of service. Its one advantage was that is sidetracked the flies. But I did have running water, out of a tap fed by ground-level pipes constantly exposed to the sun, so that I could shower in the morning while the temperature was still bearable. Even in winter it was never cold. Sleep was difficult, and there was no way to cool off, which was even harder to bear than the perpetual mosquitoes that bred in the Nile a hundred meters away.

In the Sudan a prisoner never stays shut in his cell. He spends his time squatting in the doorway, sleeping, smoking, or drinking tea with the warders. I was by myself. There was nobody in charge of me, and unlike the common-law prisoners I had no watchman. In my open-air prison I was like a zoo bear on its rock, except that nobody could see me from behind the surrounding wall, and I could see nobody. There was no kind of timetable, and my only links with the outside world were the prayers of the muezzin five times a day, amplified by loudspeakers, and the dull mutter of response from inside the jail.

I had no cause for complaint about the warders, whom I never saw except at mealtimes and when they emptied my bucket, once a day, into an unlined hole dug in the ground beside my cage. I persuaded them to send common-law prisoners morning and night to water the area round my shack, which had a slight cooling effect. But I never managed to get quicklime poured into the latrines, and they drew flies by the thousand.

My consul had guaranteed that I would be given suitable food. In fact I calculate that I was getting about five hundred calories a day in the form of bean soup, more or less thick according to whether my turn came at the beginning or the end of the pot. There was never any meat and no fresh vegetables, so no vitamins. Later on, when diplomatic relations were resumed between the Sudan and the Federal German Republic, things improved and I received sporadic supplements. But it was not till January 1974, when a new Munich-trained doctor arrived at the prison hospital, that I was able to get proper food — meat, eggs, and fish — on prescription.

All the same I had not had to wait for his arrival before finding a few extras on the menu from time to time. There were hundreds of south Sudanese in Kober Jail, and to them I was a VIP whether I liked it or not, as the white man who had sacrificed himself on behalf of their people. Since they were not political prisoners, these blacks could receive visitors, and they had been able to organize a comprehensive communication system with the outside, including a supply service. The prisoners who cleaned my shack were the carriers and the warders took a cut for looking the other way.

The prison rules allowed me to write one letter a month, which I could not do because I was refused pencil and paper. They also allowed me a monthly visit, which came from the ambassador, not the consul, of the Federal German Republic, because a month after my imprisonment Khartoum had further changed its spots by resuming relations with Bonn. He was a courteous, dynamic man, and made every effort to improve my conditions all through my detention.

To begin with his role was confined to bringing me oranges, books, and cigarettes, but he was also keeping an eye on developments between the Anyanya rebels and the Numeiry government. On my hundred and eleventh day in jail, when open negotiations between the two in Addis Ababa produced a sort of armistice followed by a general amnesty, he was quick to notice that I was the only one not to profit by it.

"Your position is starting to become illegal," he told me with a smile.

Inside my two hundred and fifty square meters I was at liberty, but there were very few people to meet. First there was my next-door neighbor, the ex–prime minister, who arrived in mid-1972. His name was Doctor Mustapha, and he was the head of the government that preceded the Communist coup d'etat, and a specialist in tropical diseases. His place was just like mine, minus the bed. We could visit each other whenever we liked. The warders made no difficulties about opening the gates between our two estates.

After Mustapha's arrival we played chess or cards all day long. We also talked politics. He had managed to get hold of a transistor radio, through one of his many friends, and we were able to keep in touch, if not with world affairs, then at least with the Arab scene.

It was sometime later that my lawyer returned, this time on his own account, with thirty-one colleagues who had signed a petition stating that it was illegal to keep amnestied prisoners under lock and key. They were all thrown into jail.

There was also a Palestinian. This one had fallen out with his comrades, who occupied a barracks in town, and he had had to be separated. His name was Kassem, and he had been one of the participants in the massacre of the Israeli team members at the Munich Olympics. Freed thanks to compatriots who had hijacked a Lufthansa aircraft, he surfaced in Khartoum on March 1, 1973, when he liquidated three hostages and made a clumsy attempt to grab two Arab ambassadors considered to be too lukewarm.

As an Arab among Arabs, Kassem naturally came in for princely treatment. He was a tall man of around twenty-five, spoke fairly good English, and always looked confident and well dressed. I suppose he was drawn to me by the very different means through which we had gained our notoriety; at any rate he arranged to meet me, and after that he used to stop by for coffee in the morning. In spite of our ideological differences I saw no harm in this, especially when he was providing the coffee.

Those conversations between the "Palestinian terrorist" and the "Biafra mercenary" would have come as a surprise to the people who never look behind a label. He used to tell me how Black September operated, and about the techniques of the *fedayin* commandos. I need not stress how much I disapproved of these methods, and it was obvious to Kassem also. We were in opposite camps, and he knew it. We hardly ever got ourselves into arguing our irreconcilable viewpoints, and when I asked him why he and his friends did not attack the Israelis on the battlefield his answer was: "Because they are too strong. But that is no reason to submit."

When I arrived there, Kober Jail contained about six thousand prisoners, and about five thousand of these were Communists. The prison had been intended to hold four hundred people.

The quarter near my cage held only the serious cases: those with long sentences, those accused of murder, and those who had been condemned to death. The executions took place next door to me. I saw quite a few.

If an execution was arranged for next day at dawn, the condemned man was informed at noon. He was then removed from the communal room he occupied with a number of others and put into an isolation cell measuring one meter by two. Clearly the warders now saw him as no longer belonging to this world, because they didn't even bother to beat him any more, but contented themselves with lashing his hands and feet to the door bars, which made it impossible to sit down. No cigarettes, no food, and the man stood, knowing that he had only a few hours to live. Still, humanity did permit him a family visit in the afternoon, even though the farewells were rather inhibited by his being tied to the door.

The execution usually took place at four in the morning. At two the prisoner was taken out of his box. There was an empty room nearby, with a heavy iron ring fixed to the ceiling, like one of those rings that ships are moored by. The hanging itself was preceded by a macabre ritual. The guards produced a short chain, passed it through the man's bound ankles and wrists, and pulled. Bent like a bow, he was then hung by the chain on a hook in the wall, some-times for as much as two or three hours.

Fatalism is deep-rooted in Africa, and it was rare for men to cry out or even to complain about this treatment. During my stay it did happen two or three times. I could hear young men gently whimpering — the first time I thought it was a dog. But generally the victim suffered in silence, as if he wasn't there. Black or Arab, the "hard" men had that much in common: when they win they are often cruel, and when they lose they do not expect pity.

Beneath the iron ring a wooden podium was placed, a box with sides a meter square. On top of it was a painted circle half green, half white, divided by a black line. The con-demned man was unfettered and had to stand with one foot on either side of the circle, with his head muffled in a black bag. A warder, always the same one — he was paid two pounds a head — performed the various operations, starting with putting the platform in place. Then he tied the rope to the ring. The noose had an iron spur which stuck out so as to snap the vertebrae at once with the impetus of the drop. The executioner pulled a lever, the circle collapsed, and down the man came. His feet dangled about a foot off the ground.

After three and a half years in Kober Jail, I cannot think about that period without hearing the ritual prayers that marked each execution, the clack of the trapdoor opening under the falling body, and the snap of the neck as it cracked like a bundle of twigs. I can still recollect the jerky rhythm of the body thumping against the wall; it might take as long as ten minutes for the thudding to quiet and stop.

In May 1972 I fell ill and the German ambassador was authorized to have me taken to a civilian hospital where I was installed in one of their best rooms, at the expense of the Federal German Republic. When the doctors took samples they found practically the entire range of tropical microbes and viruses: typhoid, dysentery, malaria, and I don't know what else. I stayed there for two weeks, with my temperature in the low hundreds and no sign of improvement. Then the *piri-piri* expert happend to visit the hospital in his capacity as a health official and noticed two guards standing outside my door with their Kalashnikovs. He asked who was in there, and two hours later I found myself back in prison.

At the jail there was nobody competent to look after me. My neighbor, Dr. Mustapha, was qualified, but had no medicines. This situation went on until June 1973, when the West German ambassador again managed to have me transferred to a hospital. The Sudan happened to be looking to West Germany for financial backing at that time, and the ambassador had to be buttered up. . . . I spent another three weeks in the doctors' hands. But the decision had been taken while Numeiry was away on an official visit. When he returned he ruled that I was being mollycoddled and again the soldiers took me back to prison.

This time I really saw red and made up my mind to resort again to my favorite weapon, the hunger strike. Apart from the monthly visit I had no contact with the ambassador, so I was advised by my partner in trouble, Dr. Mustapha. As a medical man he was concerned about my health, but as a former prime minister he doubted whether I would get quick results unless I could find some way to force the hand of the authorities. I was getting weaker all the time, and needed urgent treatment.

Two days later, with his support, I decided to make a fake suicide attempt by opening my wrist, a delicate operation for which he pointed out the right vein, found me a new blade, and even brought me a white shirt. "Put this on," he said. "It will look more impressive."

I pressed the blade deep into my left wrist and a spurt of blood stained the immaculate shirt. It didn't hurt at all. I called out to Mustapha, who was waiting a bit nervously by the gate of my cage: "Done it."

"Good. Now you lie down."

He led me toward the bed, letting the blood trickle over my shirt and the blanket. It looked very good. Then he fixed a tourniquet.

"Everything's going fine," he said, as if to reassure himself. "Now lie still while I call a warder."

There was a half-hour wait before a stretcher could be found, then I was driven to the hospital. I had time to glimpse a crowd of veiled Arab women waiting to take food in to sick relatives. Then I blacked out.

When I woke up I was on a trolley being pushed along a corridor. A nurse called Zuleika, whom I remembered from my previous visits, took me to my room and helped the orderly to lift me onto the bed.

"You've just come out of the operating theater," she told me while she attached a saline drip feed. "We've given you a transfusion and sewn you up again. Is there anything I can do?"

I asked her to phone the German ambassador and my lawyer. The ambassador was away, but half an hour later the first consul and Salim Aïssa, who was still free at that time, ran up the stairs. When he heard how callously I was being treated the consul exploded.

"This can't be tolerated. They're going too far!"

He introduced himself. "I'm Manfred Holden. I shall report this whole thing to the ambassador, and I promise you that Mister Aïssa and I will make a vigorous appeal to the president."

They must have done so, because I managed to stay a

whole day and night in the hospital, nurses and doctors alternating at my bedside, before the soldiers came to collect me again.

The whole jail knew about my suicide attempt. Next day I was summoned by the governor. He had lost his initial courtesy and informed me icily that I was to receive a three-year addition to my sentence for trying to kill myself in his establishment. As a supplementary punishment I was to be put into a disciplinary cell.

Two Sudanese policemen took me there. Having heard the governor's angry tone they saw their chance to rub the lesson in. I was in too weak a condition to react as they pushed and pulled and kept me running along with them when I barely had the strength to walk. I just had to let myself go limp in their hands. When I asked them to take it easy and told them that I was ill they thought I was feeling sorry for myself, and that made them even more brutal. They laid into me with boots and gun butts, and I felt one very painful blow crunch into the small of my back. It was a genuine relief to be thrown into a sort of stone coffin with a door grille, which I recognized as the condemned men's cell.

They took my clothes and left me there naked, without food or water. There was no mattress, no blanket, no sanitary pail — nothing. I was aching all over, and covered with bruises, and I started to pass blood. Later on, when the embassy kicked up enough fuss to get me returned to the hospital, the doctors found that my right kidney was out of action.

I remained in the cell for two days, dead to the world, before the new prison doctor came to see me. He had only just heard that I was there, and was astonished that I had not sent for him. When I told him that I had in fact asked the warders to see him, he went straight to the governor to inform him that I was not malingering and that in my

condition I could not take much more ill treatment. I was
returned to my cage. For the next three weeks, torn between
Numeiry's orders and the doctor's warning, the luckless
governor resolved his problem by ruling that I was to be
taken to the hospital in the morning and brought back to
jail at night.

26
Free

A white Volkswagen. Day was just breaking. I must be dreaming . . . that's it, I'm dreaming that I have just woken up and taken my usual stroll around my territory to watch the dawn.

"Pick up your belongings, colonel, they're waiting."

I opened an eye and saw the chief warder. It was an odd time for a visit.

"Shut up, I'm trying to sleep."

"Wake up, colonel, you are to be released."

They had tried this before. It must be a joke.

"Get out. I'm ill; I will only get up to go to the hospital."

"Come on, Rolf, get up. You're free."

This time it was real. I recognized the voice as Manfred Holden's. He was bending over me, and outside the gate of my cage there really was a white Volkswagen parked.

"You'll get a hospital all right," he growled, with a wide smile. "A German one! We've been fighting to get you out of here for three years, and you aren't going to stay by pleading illness. Come on!"

I was dazed and flabbergasted. The whole thing was so unexpected that I didn't know what to think and walked like a robot. I felt cold, the effect of fever. On the way out we looked in on the prison governor, who congratulated me and offered to shake hands. I refused, and he gave me an awkward smile.

"Come now, colonel, don't take it so badly. Everybody has been to jail some time or other. Good luck, and come back to see us!"

That woke me up. "If I do," I promised him, "it will be with an atomic bomb!"

The sentries saluted when we drove out through the gates, and Manfred took me to his house in the residential quarter on the bank of the Blue Nile, not far from the villa where I had been kept at the start of my detention. It was certainly a fine, comfortable place, but to me it seemed like a palace. And the Nile seemed to me to be the same color as Strauss's Danube — and with as little reason. Pool, green lawns, clumps of multicolored flowers, the contrast was overwhelming.

I was overcome with emotion, hardly able to believe that I was only a few kilometers away from the dung-heap where I had been rotting just half an hour before. A short time ago the morning beans were still due, a stinking wind had been scouring my cage in the world where the muezzin called, the dawn came with the sound of snapping vertebrae, and Dr. Mustapha waited to start our game of dominos. . . .

It was over, all over, and it was beer they were bringing, in a glass covered with condensation, and as cool to the touch as the surrounding air was fresh. A German beer, of course. I had my first beer since September 12, 1971, at eight o'clock on the morning of March 30, 1974.

Sitting in the garden in a white wicker chair with flowered cushions, I was fascinated by the water sprinkler making its thirty revolutions per minute on the Victorian lawn, like all the others which were making their metronomic progress around the English lawns bequeathed to fine houses in fine suburbs in all the former colonies of the British Empire. It stood for a bygone order, as if nothing had happened since Steiner had been arrested, Montgomery had conquered at Alamein, Lawrence had recaptured Aqaba, and Kipling had created Mowgli . . . I was rambling. And here was this pretty young woman, Manfred's wife, smiling as she brought me another beer. It was so unreal that I rubbed my sore eyes.

I washed in Manfred's bathroom, dressed in some of his borrowed clothes, all far too big, and was taken to a room occupied by a bed with a mattress, bolster, two pillows, and real clean sheets. Frau Holden switched on the air-conditioning, drew the curtains, and tiptoed out. I was flat out before the door closed.

When I woke up it was six o'clock and night was falling. Manfred called me into his office. I had a midnight plane to catch, and he was arranging my passport. I could provide my date of birth, but no identity photo, and all the photographers had shut up shop for the night. So after a moment's thought he put the Chancery stamp in its place.

Some people arrived from the embassy. A vice-consul brought a shirt and trousers nearer my size than Manfred's. The ambassador arrived, and we drank an aperitif together. The dream was continuing. Sitting in the garden, its romantic atmosphere created by discreet lighting hidden by foliage, we were no longer even in Africa. When Frau Holden appeared to ask me what I felt like eating, the question struck me dumb, but I managed eventually to ask for sausages and sauerkraut, and felt high just with the sight of the steaming plate when it came.

At the airport there was an hour's wait. My friends did not leave me for a second. My baggage caused no trouble for the customs, but my presence made more than one problem for the police. I had no exit visa, and since I had also no entrance visa the passport controller took on a baffled expression. Flipping through my passport, he then came across the embassy stamp where my photograph should have been, and he started thinking that there was something fishy going on. He frowned when he learned that I had just left prison, but everything was all right when he heard my name. He had certainly been notified in advance, but probably could not read.

I arrived in Cologne, via London, at ten in the morning, after a sleepless trip. The seats had been comfortable enough, but I was not, with so many conflicting feelings in my head. Of course I was happy and relieved to have left behind one of the most painful episodes of my life, but I also felt totally disoriented by the suddenness of the unexpected shift. While I racked my brains about what came next, I was also afraid that I might finally have become accustomed, as old lags sometimes do, to the idea of spending the rest of my life inside. At the same time I was not afraid of the future, but kept thinking: Hell, what am I going to do for a start?

For the time being, my story stops there. Today I live on my own, in Germany. One of my kidneys no longer works, and I lost thirty percent of my vision under the arc lamps in Khartoum, but I get up at five o'clock and train to keep fit. This is a different Germany, with its tidy fields, brand-new villages, gigantic towns, ultramodern factories, and docile crowds. It is hard for me to adapt, and I haven't yet got my bearings.

Of the causes I have defended, not one has triumphed. There is no point in resurrecting Indochina. *Algérie française* is a badly healed scar which aches now and then. I don't feel bitter about that. I had no personal responsibility in any of these setbacks. I was a small cog in the machinery, trying to do my job.

It is not like that with the other two causes I have been devoted to. First Biafra. For me, Biafra is not a lost cause. In any case, it is my own. Biafra's territory is at present occupied by Nigerian troops, but sooner or later the Ibos will win. No matter how hard you shake the bottle, the oil always comes back to the top. It is a simple question of density.

In January 1970, when the news of the surrender reached me in the bush, I at once wrote to Ojukwu reminding him of de Gaulle's words: *You have lost a battle; you have not lost the war.* I still consider myself a Biafran.

The Sudan? I was satisfied to hear that an accord had been signed between Numeiry and the people he had once called "rebels." They gained some major advantages. In the south there are no more Arabs, and the blacks practically have a status of internal self-rule. Their priests are back, the refugees have come home, and the peasants have emerged from the bush. The south Sudan is finding its feet again. Khartoum needs the support of the south.

In the face of this example, I cannot help thinking that if the south Sudan did not surrender it is because it got something more than milk powder from its allies. By sending arms, Israel made peace possible. If France had stood up to Britain and Russia by deliberately restoring the balance in arms and munitions instead of venturing into some kind of hesitation waltz, Biafra would never have lost the war. And even if it had not won, it would have had the means to preserve its identity.

And that is enough about regrets.

So what has become of the men? I hear regularly from Ojukwu, who is living in Abidjan. The tensions caused by the French secret services and their clumsy pressures are finally forgotten. Emeka is looking after my son Felix and often writes to me. And I am also in touch with the zones of resistance which still exist in Biafra, although it is too soon to mention them here.

General Gowon lost power to my partner General Mohammed, whom I often encountered on the northern front. Unfortunately for him he did not keep it long. He was assassinated on February 13, 1976. My other direct adversary, the "Black Scorpion," Adekunle, had his political ambitions smashed by a drugs scandal.

In the Sudan I have not lost sight of General Taffeng. The old chief has withdrawn into the mountains with five thousand Anyanyas. He respects the agreement signed, because it is in his people's interest, but he is suspicious and holds himself in reserve. Once the Israelis had been turned out of the south Sudan Joseph Lagu changed his tune: he became one of Numeiry's ministers.

Everybody knows about General Idi Amin's career in Uganda. He clearly has no need of me or anyone else to handle his public relations. Milton Obote took refuge in Tanzania after his deposition, which I indirectly caused.

All the others are dead, or looking for the next venture.

At the time of writing, one thing still vexes me. I still suffer from the label of mercenary, which sticks like glue. I am not a mercenary. I did not fight for money either in Biafra or the Sudan. Before then I never wanted to profit by my military experience, although there was no lack of opportunity. I never showed up in Yemen or the Congo. As for the Legion, nobody in his right mind can believe that a young man would join it to make his fortune: in 1950 our weekly pay would buy one packet of Gauloises.

The other account I have to settle is with those who have accused me of racism. I can solemnly swear that if I had been born black in the suburbs of Durban I would have fought with the African National Congress, and that had I been born an Indian in the slums of Bogotá I would have become a guerrilla. They are my brothers. Twice I have fought alongside Africans in their struggle for freedom. Why reject me because I am white? Who is the racist then?

Who am I? A man of war? Certainly. I have never liked it, but it fascinates me. Each battle is a race to your own limits. When you get there your reward is the joy of surviving. What is to replace such a school of courage and self-control, which ruthlessly shows its pupils to themselves as they are, knaves or knights?

The square is the symbol of life, my personal emblem. I am for order when it is in the service of justice, and for discipline when it makes for effectiveness. A square is a frame, a solid structure for my own certitudes. The military framework is one that I at first endured then re-created because, although I was critical of some of its aspects, I recognized its merits. I have always been involved with that kind of setting, from school and the *Jungvolk* to the Legion, the OAS, the Santé, Biafra, the Sudan, and even Kober Jail. Yet no one has ever exerted a decisive influence over me. The chiefs I modeled myself on were already like me. Although I was destined for communal life, I have always been the odd man out in the team. Even when the fame machine went to work on me later on, I remained a solitary man.

Corporal, sergeant, colonel, general, the names mean nothing. What counts with me is the obsession to do things *well*. You have to be up to the job, and the greater the responsibility the more worthy you have to prove. To me, it is indispensable to set an example. Once people have put their trust in me, I cannot disappoint them. In Biafra I held some very important posts, rising higher by the month. My greatest satisfaction was being able to say to myself as I left that I had not failed in the missions entrusted to me.

I always respect my adversary. The battlefield is a square of red which encloses the opponents like boxers in a ring, or footballers on the playing field. No ball here, but bullets. And strict rules which I must not break even if the other side cheats. I am my own referee. For or against me, the officers and volunteers are those who have had the nerve to take risks, and have agreed to put up their lives as the price of their education. The others, conscripts, rankers, those who do not fight of their own free will, are only tools of policy. But once they have come in, they are committed. All they had to do was refuse. I admire pacifists, especially militant ones. I have the greatest respect for conscientious objectors. But when war has been declared it cannot be brought to a conclusion by means of nonviolent philosophies; otherwise you lose. All the rest is hypocrisy.

I am not the inhuman brute that some people imagine. I am fond of animals, and I have preserved a little of my childhood in my heart. When I am in combat, firing or giving orders to fire on people, I am aware that they, too, may have good motives and believe in their cause. Yet if I kill a man in battle I feel no moral qualms. Left-wing intellectuals will blame me for that, I suppose. I don't think: My God, this fellow facing me has a wife and children — maybe even a couple of kittens, like me. I know he is my brother, and he is there to die. Those who have accepted the struggle have to play out the game. A man who walks onto the field of red knows what is waiting for him. He can't complain when someone does to him what he was ready to do to them.

I found the law of warfare in the Legion. The rule of Camerone is quasi-monastic. If the motto "Honor and Fidelity" has fascinated me so much, it is because without doubt it was not a discovery for me but a meeting. My own natural tendency was already taking me in that direction, and there was nothing meritorious about arriving.

I am not ashamed to say it: for me the word "honor" still has a strict meaning. I hate compromises and I am not easygoing; in fact, I am irritatingly righteous sometimes. I may violate laws — they are the letter, not the spirit — but I have never stretched my principles. I despise and condemn aerial bombing, the taking of hostages, and reprisals against civilians. During the Algerian war, if some officer had said: "Sergeant Steiner, you are to torture that man!" I would have answered, "No!" These are the disfigurements of war, as theft, crime, and prostitution are blots on peace. In battle it is part of my job to keep my men clear of them.

When a man is so involved in his craft, he neglects his personal life. I haven't had much room for love and for women, although I am a man and constituted like other men. But there have been affairs. I have loved, yes, but with a cool head.

I realized too late that marriage was not for me. I was not cut out for wife, kids, office, retirement, and a house on the hill. In 1967 I was up against two alternatives. Either I stuck to the kind of insidious family life that wears down the soul day after day, and gnaws into both of you until life together threatens to disintegrate into mediocrity and routine; or else I got out and went back to the search for noble feelings, comrades, a cause to be devoted to, soldiers to love and be loved by, and loyal right-hand men like Emeka . . . something else again.

I had to choose, and I chose. I have always preferred the warmth of the team to the lukewarmness of the hearth.

Field of red, green beret, black legion, that is my life. Red, green, and black — the colors of Biafra. The counterpoint of my past has been furnished by all the dead men who have escorted my existence. I have seen a lot of people die — friends, enemies, unknowns, all of them as dead as they would have been in old age, having simply accelerated the natural course of things. I do not know whether I have a need for violence, but I believe that I have ennobled it by putting it in the service of just causes.

"Honor and Fidelity" was a challenge against my own solitude when I was seventeen. Since all life leads to death, best to look it straight in the eye on your way toward it.

Letting Go

by Linda Richards

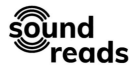

Set 2: Book 10

Letting Go
Sound Reads Set 2: Book 10

Written by Linda Richards
Illustrations by Laura Eckersley
Edited by Catherine White

First published and distributed in 2021 by Gatehouse Media Limited

ISBN: 978-1-84231-230-8

British Library Cataloguing-in-Publication Data:
A catalogue record for this book is available from the British Library

Cover Image: Stock photo. Posed by model.